Osteology Guidelines for Oral and Maxillofacial Regeneration
Preclinical Models for Translational Research

W. V. Giannobile, M. Nevins
(editors)

Osteology Guidelines for Oral and Maxillofacial Regeneration
Preclinical Models for Translational Research

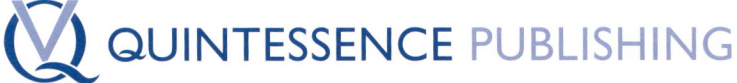
QUINTESSENCE PUBLISHING

London, Berlin, Chicago, Tokyo, Barcelona, Beijing, Istanbul, Milan, Moscow, New Delhi, Paris, Prague, São Paulo, Seoul and Warsaw

Imprint

Cover
Histologic section illustrating the tooth attachment apparatus. The collagen fibers of the periodontal ligament span between bone and the root surface and insert as Sharpey's fibers into the cementum and into the bundle bone. Undecalcified ground section, unstained and viewed under polarized light. (Courtesy of PD Dr. sc. nat. Dieter D. Bosshardt, Head of the Robert K. Schenk Laboratory for Oral Histology, School of Dental Medicine, University of Bern, Switzerland)

British Library Cataloguing in Publication Data
Osteology guidelines for oral and maxillofacial regeneration : preclinical models for translational research.

1. Dentistry, Operative--Research--Methodology.
2. Maxilla--Surgery--Research--Methodology.
3. Face--Surgery--Research--Methodology.
4. Animal models in research.
I. Giannobile, William V. II. Nevins, Myron.
617.6'00721-dc22

ISBN-13: 9781850972112

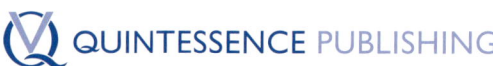

Quintessence Publishing Co., Ltd,
Grafton Road, New Malden,
Surrey KT3 3AB,
Great Britain
www.quintpub.co.uk

Copyright © 2011
by Quintessence Publishing Co, Inc
All rights reserved. This book or any part thereof may not be reproduced, stored in a retrieval system, or transmitted in any form or by any means, electronic, mechanical, photocopying, or otherwise, without prior written permission of the publisher.
Editing: Quintessence Publishing Co, Ltd, London, UK
Layout and Production: Quintessenz Verlags-GmbH, Berlin, Germany
Printed and bound in Germany by Bosch-Druck, Landshut/Ergolding

Preface

The Osteology Foundation was created to support progress in the field of oral and craniofacial regenerative medicine for the benefit of patients. The foundation supports research, education, and collaboration among scientists and clinicians. The objective is to make new techniques and products available in clinical practice more quickly and with greater determination toward the desirable goals.

It has been established that the best results in clinical medicine are achieved by performing treatments based on sound scientific and clinical evidence. This evidence is created through well-performed research including laboratory-based, preclinical, translational, as well as clinical research. People conducting research in any of these areas need to be well qualified in order to perform state-of-the-art research leading to meaningful results. The process of acquiring the necessary knowledge and skills to qualify as a competent researcher is cumbersome and strenuous.

The aim of the present book is to provide young researchers beginning their career with high-quality guidelines to conduct preclinical animal research. At the same time, the book is intended to serve as a valuable reference for scientists who wish to build on the experience of people with a track record in preclinical and translational research.

The editors, Dr William Giannobile and Dr Myron Nevins, recruited a team of experienced researchers to write the various chapters on different aspects of preclinical animal research. The first part of the book covers basic aspects of animal research including phylogenetics and physiology, and aspects of ethical and regulatory issues, and deals with study design and methods of statistical analysis. The remaining contents reflect the many topics of research in the field of tissue regeneration in the oral and maxillofacial area. Experimental designs to study bone regeneration in different clinical situations are dealt with in various chapters. Guidelines are provided on how to proceed in designing experiments in the rather novel area of oral soft tissue regeneration as well as in the thoroughly studied field of periodontal regeneration. Methods are described for exploring integration and disintegration of implants in the oral and maxillofacial tissue environment. Recommendations are provided in Chapter 5 with respect to screening models for questions regarding materials and mechanisms of tissue engineering. In all these topics various experimental designs are described and qualified assessments are provided regarding advantages and disadvantages of specific design possibilities.

This book will be an important building block in improving knowledge and skills of researchers conducting animal research in oral tissue regeneration. By doing so, the quality of experimental results will be increased and lead to more meaningful answers. As a next step, this knowledge will be translated into new and improved clinical procedures and novel biomaterials. A resulting task of the Osteology Foundation will then be to use its educational channels to bring this new state-of-the-art information on best clinical practice to the dental profession in clinical practice.

Christoph Hämmerle
President, Osteology Foundation

Acknowledgements

The editors first of all acknowledge the authors for their excellent reviews of the preclinical models enclosed in this book. We believe this text is unique to the disciplines of oral, dental, and maxillofacial regeneration as the first of its kind devoted to preclinical investigation in the field.

We also greatly appreciate the creative vision of the Osteology Foundation, our generous founder Dr Peter Geistlich and our dedicated president Prof Christoph Hämmerle. The excellent support of the authors and editors in the preparation of this book is greatly appreciated. This book underscores the Osteology Foundation's mission of promoting regenerative medicine initiatives in the oral and maxillofacial complex.

We would also like to thank Mr Johannes Wolters and Mr Daniel Jenk from Quintessence who have been supportive of the timetables and layout of the book. We also appreciate Ms Karen Gardner for her efforts in handling the manuscript revisions for the editors. At the Osteology Foundation we appreciate the capable leadership of Dr Kay Horsch, Executive Director, in moving forward this concept as the inaugural textbook endeavor for the Foundation. Lastly, and very importantly, we speak not only for the editors but also the authors in expressing our gratitude for the excellent support of Dr Kristian Tersar, Scientific Project Manager of the Foundation. Kristian was fundamental at all stages in the organization, execution, and completion of this book. His high degree of enthusiasm and attention to detail at each and every stage were of critical importance in the creative vision of this textbook.

William V. Giannobile
Myron Nevins

Dedications

I would like to dedicate this book to my mentor Dr Samuel Lynch who guided me during my development in preclinical research; the creativity and inspiration of my students; and to the devoted support of my wife, Angela.

William V. Giannobile

I would like to recognize the inspiration provided by Ulf Lekholm to concentrate on translational research and continuing investigations, and to thank my wife Marcy for enthusiastically supporting my activities and being the wind beneath my wings.

Myron Nevins

List of contributors

Editors

William V. Giannobile, DDS, MS, D.Med.Sc.
Najjar Professor of Dentistry and Biomedical Engineering
Director, Michigan Center for Oral Health Research, University of Michigan School of Dentistry College of Engineering
Ann Arbor, MI USA
william.giannobile@umich.edu

Myron Nevins, DDS
Associate Clinical Professor of Periodontology
Harvard School of Dental Medicine
Clinical Professor of Periodontics
University of Pennsylvania School of Dental Medicine
Swampscott, MA USA
nevinsperimp@aol.com

Authors

Khalid A. Al-Hezaimi, BDS, MSc
Assistant Professor
Director, Eng.A.B. Research Chair for Growth Factors and Bone Regeneration
King Saud University School of Dentistry, Riyadh, Saudi Arabia
kalhezaime@ksu.edu.sa

Maurício G. Araújo, DDS, MSc, PhD
Department of Dentistry
State University of Maringa
Maringa, Parana Brazil
odomar@hotmail.com

Andreas Bachmann, Dr. phil.
CEO Ethik im Diskurs
Ethik im Diskurs GmbH
Zurich, Switzerland
bachmann@ethikdiskurs.ch

Jürgen Becker, Prof. Dr. med. dent.
Department of Oral Surgery
Heinrich Heine University
Düsseldorf, Germany
jbecker@uni-duesseldorf.de

Michael M. Bornstein, PD Dr. med. dent.
Assistant Professor and Head
Department of Oral Surgery and Stomatology
University of Bern School of Dental Medicine
Bern, Switzerland
michael.bornstein@zmk.unibe.ch

Dieter D. Bosshardt, PhD
Senior Scientist and Head
Robert K. Schenk Laboratory of Oral Histology
University of Bern School of Dental Medicine, Bern, Switzerland
dieter.bosshardt@zmk.unibe.ch

Thomas M. Braun, PhD
Associate Professor
Department of Biostatistics
University of Michigan School of Public Health, Ann Arbor, MI USA
tombraun@umich.edu

Daniel Buser, Prof. Dr. med. dent.
Professor and Chairman
Department of Oral Surgery and Stomatology
University of Bern School of Dental Medicine, Bern, Switzerland
daniel.buser@zmk.unibe.ch

Christer Dahlin, DDS, PhD, Dr. Odont.
Assistant Professor Department of Biomaterial Science
Institute for Surgical Sciences & Department of Oral Maxillofacial Surgery
The Sahlgrenska Academy, University of Gothenburg
NÄL Medical Centre Hospital
Trollhättan, Sweden
dahlinchrister@hotmail.com

Reinhard Gruber, PhD
Medical University of Vienna
Bernhard Gottlieb School of Dentistry, Department of Oral Surgery, Vienna, Austria
reinhard.gruber@meduniwien.ac.at

Christoph H.F. Hämmerle, Prof. Dr. med. dent.
Chairman
Clinic for Fixed and Removable Prosthodontics and Dental Material Science, Vice-Dean Medical Faculty for the University of Zurich Center of Dental Medicine
Zurich, Switzerland
christoph.hammerle@zzm.uzh.ch

Carina B. Johansson, PhD, Dr. Odont.
Professor, Örebro University School of Health and Medical Sciences
Department of Clinical Medicine & Department of Biomaterial Science, Institute for Surgical Sciences
The Sahlgrenska Academy
University of Gothenburg
carina.johansson@oru.se

List of contributors

Ronald E. Jung, PD Dr. med. dent.
Associate Professor and Vice Chairman
Clinic for Fixed and Removable Prosthodontics and Dental Material Science, University of Zurich Center for Dental and Oral Medicine and Cranio-Maxillofacial Surgery, Zurich, Switzerland
ronald.jung@zzm.uzh.ch

Darnell Kaigler, Jr., DDS, MS, PhD
Division of Periodontics
Department of Periodontics and Oral Medicine,
University of Michigan School of Dentistry, Ann Arbor, MI USA
dkaigler@umich.edu

David M. Kim, DDS, DMSc
Assistant Professor
Department of Oral Medicine, Infection and Immunity
Harvard School of Dental Medicine, Boston, MA USA
dkim@hsdm.harvard.edu

Ulrike Kuchler, MD, DDS
Medical University of Vienna Bernhard Gottlieb School of Dentistry, Department of Oral Surgery, Vienna, Austria
ulrike.kuchler@meduniwien.ac.at

Rainer Lutz, DDS
University of Erlangen-Nuremberg, Erlangen, Germany
Rainer.Lutz@uk-erlangen.de

Juliana C. Mesti, DDS
Department of Dentistry
State University of Maringa
Maringa, Parana Brazil
julianamesti@hotmail.com

Marc L. Nevins, DMD, M.M.Sc
Assistant Clinical Professor of Oral Medicine, Infection and Immunity
Harvard School of Dental Medicine
Boston, MA USA
marc_nevins@hms.harvard.edu

Hector F. Rios, DDS, PhD
Assistant Professor
Department of Periodontics and Oral Medicine
University of Michigan School of Dentistry, Ann Arbor, MI USA
hrios@umich.edu

Isabella Rocchietta, DDS
Foundation IRCCS Cà Granda Maggiore Policlinico Hospital
Department of Reconstructive Surgery Science and Diagnostics
University of Milan, School of Dentistry, Institute for Dental Research and Education
Milan, Italy
isabella.rocchietta@gmail.com

Martin Sager, Priv. Doz. Dr. med. vet.
Animal Research Institute
Heinrich Heine University
Düsseldorf, Germany
Martin.sager@med.uni-duesseldorf.de

Karl Andreas Schlegel, DDS, MD
Professor of Oral and Maxillofacial Surgery, University of Erlangen-Nuremberg, Erlangen, Germany
Andreas.Schlegel@uk-erlangen.de

Beat P. Schmid, PhD
Swissmedic, Swiss Agency for Therapeutic Products
Head, Preclinical Review & GLP-Monitoring Compliance
Berne, Switzerland
beat.schmid@swissmedic.ch

Frank Schwarz, Prof. Dr. med. dent.
Department of Oral Surgery
Heinrich Heine University
Düsseldorf, Germany
Frank.Schwarz@med.uni-duesseldorf.de

Cléverson O. Silva, DDS, MSc, PhD
Department of Dentistry
State University of Maringa
Maringa, Parana Brazil
prof.cleversonsilva@yahoo.com.br

Massimo Simion, MD, DDS
Associate Professor, Department of Periodontics
Foundation IRCCS Cà Granda Maggiore Policlinico Hospital
Department of Reconstructive Surgery Science and Diagnostics
University of Milan School of Dentistry, Institute for Dental Research and Education, Milan, Italy
m.simion@studiosimion.it

Myron Spector, PhD
Professor of Orthopaedic Surgery (Biomaterials)
Brigham and Women's Hospital
Harvard Medical School
Director, Tissue Engineering
VA Boston Healthcare System
Boston, MA USA
mspector@rics.bwh.harvard.edu

Stefan Tangl, MS
Medical University of Vienna
Bernhard Gottlieb School of Dentistry, Department of Oral Surgery, Vienna, Austria
stefan.tangl@meduniwien.ac.at

Daniel S. Thoma, Dr. med. dent.
Assistant Professor
Clinic for Fixed and Removable Prosthodontics and Dental Material Science, University of Zurich Center for Dental and Oral Medicine and Cranio-Maxillofacial Surgery, Zurich, Switzerland
e-mail: daniel.thoma@zzm.uzh.ch

Thomas von Arx, Prof. Dr. med. dent.
Associate Professor and Vice Chairman
Department of Oral Surgery and Stomatology, University of Bern School of Dental Medicine
Bern, Switzerland
thomas.vonarx@zmk.unibe.ch

Falk Wehrhan, DDS, MD,
University of Erlangen-Nuremberg, Erlangen, Germany
Falk.Wehrhan@uk-erlangen.de

Contents

Preface   V

List of contributors   VII

Chapter 1   Preclinical Model Development for the Reconstruction of Oral, Periodontal, and Craniofacial Defects   1
William V. Giannobile, Darnell Kaigler, and Myron Nevins

Chapter 2   Ethical Considerations for Performing Research in Animals   9
Andreas Bachmann

Chapter 3   Good Laboratory Practice (GLP) in Nonclinical Investigations   23
Beat Schmid

Chapter 4   Research Design and Biostatistical Considerations in Preclinical Research   31
Thomas M. Braun

Chapter 5   Screening Models for Tissue Engineering   45
Myron Spector, Khalid Al-Hezaimi, and Marc L. Nevins

Chapter 6   Soft Tissue Regeneration   57
Daniel S. Thoma, Ronald E. Jung, and Christoph H.F. Hämmerle

Contents

Chapter 7   Preclinical Protocols for Periodontal Regeneration   77

Hector F. Rios and William V. Giannobile

Chapter 8   Osseointegration of Implants   103

Christer Dahlin and Carina B. Johansson

Chapter 9   Ridge Preservation   123

Maurício G. Araújo, Cléverson O. Silva, and Juliana C. Mesti

Chapter 10   Horizontal Ridge Augmentation   141

Michael M. Bornstein, Dieter D. Bosshardt, Thomas von Arx, and Daniel Buser

Chapter 11   Vertical Ridge Augmentation   159

Isabella Rocchietta, David M. Kim, Khalid Al-Hezaimi, and Massimo Simion

Chapter 12   Sinus Floor Augmentation   175

K. Andreas Schlegel, Rainer Lutz, and Falk Wehrhan

Chapter 13   Peri-implantitis Defect Model   197

Frank Schwarz, Martin Sager, and Jürgen Becker

Chapter 14   Compromised Bone Healing: Implantation Model   225

Reinhard Gruber, Stefan Tangl, and Ulrike Kuchler

Index   245

CHAPTER 1

Preclinical Model Development for the Reconstruction of Oral, Periodontal, and Craniofacial Defects

William V. Giannobile, Darnell Kaigler, and Myron Nevins

1.1 Introduction

The treatment of oral and craniofacial diseases and anomalies accounts for a significant proportion of the healthcare burden, with the manifestations of these conditions being functionally and psychologically debilitating. New medical formulations (NMFs) are critical to the development, maturation, maintenance, and repair of craniofacial tissues by establishing an environment conducive to cell and tissue growth (Fig 1-1). Tissue engineering principles aim to exploit these properties in the development of biomimetic materials that can provide an appropriate microenvironment for tissue formation. These materials have been assembled into devices that are used as vehicles for delivery of cells, bioactive factors, and DNA, for eventual clinical use. In this chapter, an overview of the rationale and targeted preclinical development for NMF evaluation will be described with an eventual goal to deliver these devices, drugs, or biologics to the clinical arena for the treatment of patients (Fig 1-2).

The development of NMFs is based on the understanding of the etiology of the disease, its progression, and the general principles of tissue repair. However, knowledge in these areas does not necessarily allow conclusions about the safety and efficacy of NMFs to treat oral and craniofacial defects. This situation is reflected by the regulatory approval agencies such as the European Medicines Agency (EMEA), the US Food and Drug Administration (FDA), and other international bodies that demand a sequence of preclinical evaluations before clinical studies can be conducted. Based on these demands, preclinical studies pave the way for clinical studies that lead to the approvals for NMF products for the promotion of craniofacial bone regeneration (Pellegrini et al., 2009). Planning of a preclinical study must be adapted for the purpose. It does not necessarily mean that an NMF which successfully improves long bone regeneration is also

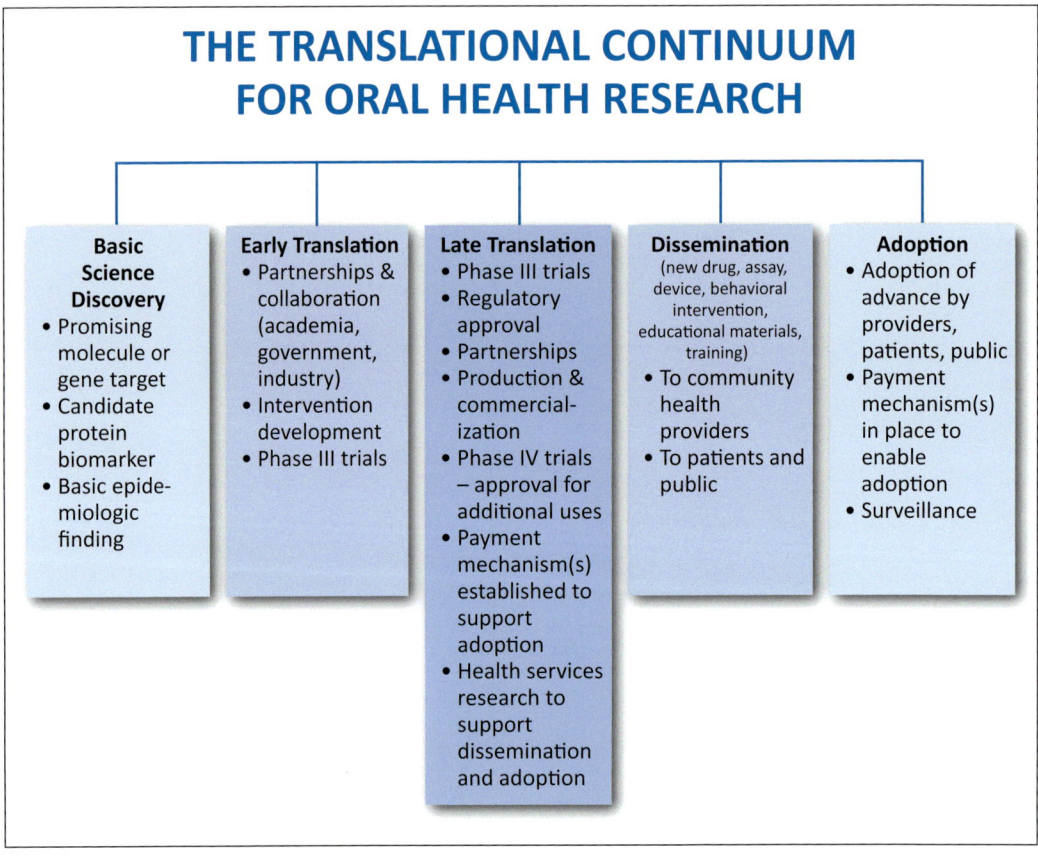

Fig 1-1 The translational continuum from basic science discovery to preclinical translational research to eventual adoption into dental practice. Adapted from National Cancer Institute (2009).

appropriate for the treatment of craniofacial bone defects and vice versa. Moreover, the objectives of a preclinical study must relate to the efficient and effective design of a reconstructive therapy. The choice of the endpoints is therefore a critical issue in the study design. Overall, planning a preclinical study to test an NMF requires decisions about animal species, the defect type, study endpoint, and study duration (Fig 1-3) (Dannan and Alkattan, 2008). Moreover, endpoints have to be defined to estimate the sample size necessary to achieve the desired power (see Chapter 4). Considerations about the size of the defects as well as morphologic changes related to the anatomic defect that can occur over time can help to estimate the appropriate study duration.

The selection of preclinical models usually takes the phylogenetic tree into consideration; however, this can be hampered by the differences in anatomy and healing characteristics between rodents and larger animals. It is the aim of this chapter to provide a summary of commonly used preclinical modes to evaluate

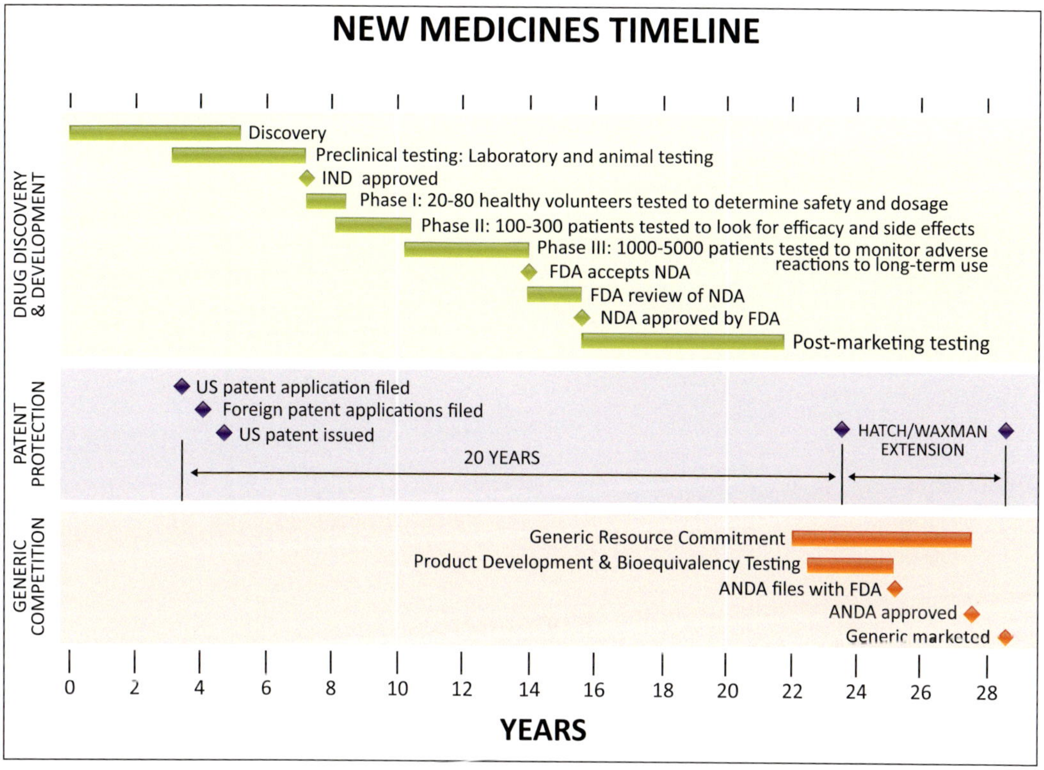

1.1 Introduction

Fig 1-2 New medicines timeline: This trajectory demonstrates the steps required for the development of a medical device for application to an oral/craniofacial defect. FDA, Food and Drug Administration; NDA, new drug application; IND, investigational new drug; ANDA, abbreviated new drug application. Adapted from Pharmaceutical Research and Manufacturers of America (PhRMA; www.phrma.org).

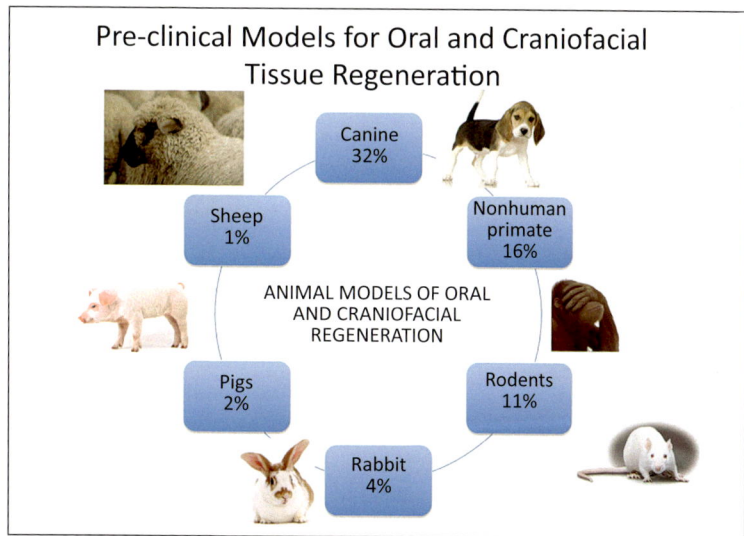

Fig 1-3 Animal models used in preclinical research and the proportion used in oral tissue regeneration studies.

Table 1-1 Materials for oral and craniofacial bone repair

Biomaterial	Trade name
Allografts	
Calcified freeze dried bone, decalcified freeze dried bone	Grafton®, Lifenet®, Musculoskeletal transplant Foundation®
Xenografts	
Bovine mineral matrix, bovine-derived HA	Bio-Oss®, OsteoGraf®, Pep-Gen P-15®
Alloplasts	
HA, dense HA, porous HA, resorbable HA	
Tricalcium phosphate (TCP), calcium phosphate cement	Synthograft®, α-BSM®
Hard tissue replacement polymers	Bioplant®
Bioactive glass (SiO_2, CaO, Na_2O, P_2O_5)	PerioGlas®, BioGran®
Coral-derived calcium carbonate	Biocoral®
Polymers and collagens	
Collagen	Helistat®, Collacote®, Colla-Tec®, Gelfoam®
Poly(lactic-co-glycolic acid) (PLGA)	
Methylcellulose	
Hyaluronic acid ester	Hy®
Chitosan	
Growth factor	
Platelet-derived growth factor (PDGF)	
Enamel matrix derivative (EMD)	Emdogain®
Bone morphogenetic protein (BMP)	
Fibroblast growth factor-2	
Insulin-like growth factor	
Growth factor + scaffolding material	
Collagen + BMP-2	Infuse®
β-TCP + PDGF-BB	GEM21S®

HA, hydroxyapatite.

periodontal and oral reconstructive therapies, highlighting those related to devices and biologics (Table 1-1). We briefly describe surgical protocols and study duration of each approach. This book considers commonly used endpoints and morphological characteristics of bone and soft tissue healing for a variety of tooth and oral implant-associated defects. This information should serve as a guide to choosing the appropriate preclinical models to help the translation of NMFs into the clinical arena.

1.2 Purpose of Preclinical Research: Bringing New Therapies to Treat Patients in Need

1.2.1 Drugs

On average, it takes about 12 years and over US$350 million to bring a new drug from the development stage in the laboratory to the market stage on the pharmacy shelf (Kaigler *et al.*, 2010). Testing in the laboratory and animal (preclinical) phase can take 3–4 years prior to applying to the FDA, EMEA, or other national–international regulatory authorities for initiating clinical trials. Only one out of every 1,000 compounds that undergoes this initial phase of testing will ever reach the next phase of testing in humans (Center for Drug Evaluation and Research [CDER], 2011). Assuming regulatory approval for human testing following submission of an investigational new drug application, three phases of clinical trials typically follow:

- *Phase I* – designed for establishing safety of the drug
- *Phase II* – designed to gain preliminary data relative to the efficacy of the drug
- *Phase III* – often designed to be multi-centered, randomized, and controlled in order to definitively determine efficacy of the drug.

1.2.2 Medical Devices for Reconstruction of Craniofacial Defects

The initial step in the approval process for a device is to determine whether the product is actually a device. While this may seem rather intuitive, the FDA and EMEA have very specific definitions regarding what constitutes or is considered a medical device (Center for Devices and Radiological Health [CDRH], 2011b). The FDA has established descriptions of roughly 1,700 different "generic" types of devices, and organized them into 16 medical specialties, referred to as panels. Each of these "generic" types of devices, described in depth within the appropriate panel, is assigned to one of three regulatory classes (CDRH, 2011a). The "class" of a device is determined by the level of regulatory oversight necessary to assure safety and efficacy of the device. In general, the higher levels of classification (II and III) demand more documentation from the manufacturer prior to distribution. Thus, once it has been determined that the construct is a device, it must then be determined how a regulatory agency may classify the device into one of three possible classes. The three classes are described below in the list of definitions:

- *Class I* – General controls (with or without exemptions)
- *Class II* – Special controls (with or without exemptions)
- *Class III* – Premarket approval (i.e., dental implants and bone graft-related products).

It is the preclinical development of Class III devices which is the overall focus of this book.

Unless the product is deemed exempt, the classification of the device will determine the process by which the manufacturer has to proceed in order to obtain approval for marketing. Once it is determined which pathway for approval is required, it is necessary to prepare a marketing application including all relevant data and pertinent information regarding the device. For some submissions, an essential component of this application is the product's clinical performance data. In the end, the regulatory agencies of the respective country make the final determination of the device classification.

1.2.3 Biologics

In recent years, a significant increase in therapeutic demands for more "biologic" approaches for treatment of a number of different diseases and conditions has resulted in substantial rises in "biologic" product sales, with global sales expecting to reach US$105 billion in 2010 (Belsey *et al.*, 2006). Individuals or companies that manufacture biologics are required to hold a license for introduction into interstate commerce. Following initial laboratory testing and the appropriate preclinical studies, safety and effectiveness of a biologic are evaluated in human clinical trials (beginning with Phase I) under the governance of an investigative new drug application. If the findings of the clinical studies demonstrate that the product is safe and effective for its intended use, the data are submitted to the Center for Biologics Evaluation and Research (CBER) as part of a biologics license application for review and approval for marketing. Following approval, the biologic is subject to lot release, which means that the manufacturer is required to perform certain tests on each lot of the products before it is released for distribution. In addition to quality control tests performed by the manufacturer, the CBER may perform its own tests to help ensure the safety, purity, potency, and effectiveness of products, prior to their release for distribution (Kaigler et al., 2010).

1.2.4 Combination Products

Due to the rapid increase in cutting-edge technologies that have the potential to incorporate biologics with devices, devices with drugs, and drugs with biologics, the FDA has recently developed the Office of Combination Products (OCP, 2011). Though this branch of the FDA has broad responsibilities covering the regulatory process for combination products, the primary oversight of these products remains with one of three product regulatory centers: CDER, CBER, or the CDRH (Beltran-Aguilar and Manz, 2010). The OCP's responsibilities include: assignment of a combination product for review and jurisdiction to one of the three centers; insurance of timeliness and consistency of premarket review; assessing appropriateness of post-market regulation; serving as a liaison between the three centers regarding overlap of jurisdiction of a product if necessary; update and review regulations regarding combination products. Thus, the OCP is not directly involved in the initial review of the product, but plays an integral role in determining where and how timely it will be reviewed.

1.3 Methodologies in the Evaluation of New Biomaterials in the Preclinical Research Setting

1.3.1 Common Animal Models Used in Periodontal Research

A variety of different animal models have been used in periodontal regenerative studies such as rats, dogs, and nonhuman primates (Pellegrini et al., 2009) (Fig 1-3). The rat periodontal model has been frequently used for bone regeneration studies (King et al., 1997; Jin et al., 2004; Huang et al., 2005). It is quite valuable as a screening model for regenerative molecule assessment due to cost-effectiveness, ease of handling, etc.; however, the typical defect size is relatively small making visualization challenging, thus requiring the use of surgical microscopes for defect creation (see Chapter 5). Large animal models, such as the canine or nonhuman primate, make a logical next step. The canine wound healing kinetics and tooth anatomy have many similarities to the human situation (Wikesjö et al., 1991, 1995). Nonhuman primates are highly desirable to evaluate the safety and efficacy of new molecules because their anatomic and biologic features are very close to humans (Giannobile et al., 1994). However, their economic burden and handling difficulties prevent them from being more highly utilized. One should select the preferred animal model according to the study requirements. This text reviews the variety of animal models used for preclinical research in periodontal areas, oral implants, sinus floor augmentation, and localized alveolar ridge reconstruction, among others.

1.3.2 Animal Welfare Guidelines

A study should not be proposed if a clear endpoint goal has not been established which will eventually have an impact on human health or disease. Animal-based research has led to significant improvements in the quality of life for every human being (Voigt and Borysiewicz, 2010). However, these advances must be the result of humane use and care of animals used for research and instruction (see Chapter 2). Every investigator should adhere to the Public Health Service Policies on Humane Care and Use of Laboratory Animals, incorporating principles from the Guide for the Care and Use of Laboratory Animals while executing any work with vertebrate animals (specific guidelines vary from country to country). Individual institutions have specific guidelines utilizing policies put in place by the national or regional governing agencies, and it is necessary to review these guidelines before initiating any efforts in animal research. Proper maintenance of documentation and medical and surgical records is also an essential component of compliance with federal and institutional guidelines.

1.4 Surgical Models for Reconstructive Therapies for the Craniofacial Complex

Before performing any *in vivo* regenerative experiment, the specific animal model should be selected based on outcome. Critical-size defects can be made in some animal models, while others heal spontaneously and are considered as kinetic defects. Thus, it is very important to choose the appropriate model to effectively analyze the effects of bioactive molecules in a specific study (Pellegrini *et al.*, 2009; Seol *et al.*, 2010). Rodent, canine, and nonhuman primate models are most often used for these experiments. The following chapters will outline critical aspects in the proper research design, surgical methods, biopsy assessments, tissue preparation protocols, and imaging assessments to determine the appropriate endpoints of assessment prior to human clinical assessment. This book provides specific details pertaining to the most common oral and periodontal regeneration models that have been successfully used for specific endpoint goals.

1.4.1 Directions for Preclinical Research for Regeneration of Craniofacial Bone Defects

The use of preclinical animal models remains a critical component in the development of NMFs for human clinical investigation. It is clear that *in vivo* models compared with *in vitro* studies provide distinct advantages in the understanding of the complex molecular, cellular, and tissue reactions that occur in response to delivered scaffolds, proteins, cells, or genes to oral and craniofacial defects. Despite the limitations of preclinical models for human disease, *in vitro* investigations for the simulation of human disease continue to remain inappropriate prior to testing for national regulatory agencies. The increasing development of biologics and devices for oral regenerative medicine application requires a thorough examination of when and how the appropriate endpoints can be evaluated prior to entry into human clinical trial testing. With continued innovations in noninvasive biomedical imaging and *ex vivo* model systems, the needs for extensive preclinical testing will probably decrease.

Advancements are still needed for the better exploitation of preclinical animal models for the evaluation of NMFs prior to human testing. These include obvious differences in host immunology and defect and disease development in animals and humans (Graves *et al.*, 2008). Furthermore, the size of osseous defects found in humans makes assessment of tissue neogenesis, oxygen and nutrient diffusion through prototype scaffold matrices, especially in large defects, challenging (Cancedda *et al.*, 2007). Continued development of disease of systemic factors (e.g., simulating common disease conditions that alter wound repair such as diabetes mellitus, cigarette smoking, obesity, etc.) may aid in the continued refinement of preclinical animal models to allow for more targeted and refined human clinical trial testing.

As the clinical practice arena enters the realm of pharmacogenomics and individualized patient medicine, host susceptibility and identification of those patients who best respond to NMF may aid in the improvement of safety and effectiveness (Pellegrini et al., 2009). The ultimate result of enhanced preclinical testing will greatly advance patient care for the public.

Acknowledgments

The authors appreciate the collaboration of preclinical researchers Drs Hector Rios, Gaia Pellegrini, Po-Chun Chang, Yang-jo Seol, Qiming Jin, and Reinhard Gruber, who have contributed to the research team's expertise in this chapter. The authors appreciate the assistance of Dr Hector Rios for the preparation of Figure 1-3. This work was supported in part by NIH/NIDCR DE 13397 and NIH/NCRR UL1RR-024986.

References

1. Belsey MJ, Harris LM, Das RR, Chertkow J (2006). Biosimilars: initial excitement gives way to reality. *Nat Rev Drug Discov* 5:535–536.
2. Beltran-Aguilar ED, Manz MC (2010). Post-marketing surveillance. In: *Clinical research in oral health.* Giannobile WV, Burt BA, Genco RJ, editors. New York: Wiley-Blackwell, pp. 247–264.
3. Cancedda R, Giannoni P, Mastrogiacomo M (2007). A tissue engineering approach to bone repair in large animal models and in clinical practice. *Biomaterials* 28:4240–4250.
4. Center for Drug Evaluation and Research (2011). New drug approval process. Available at: http://drugs.com/fda-approval-process.html (accessed Jan 12, 2011).
5. Center for Devices and Radiological Health (2011a). Classify your medical device. Food and Drug Administration. Available at: http://www.fda.gov/cdrh/devadvice/312.html (accessed Jan 12, 2011).
6. Center for Devices and Radiological Health (2011b). Is the product a medical device? Medical device definition. Available at: http://www.fda.gov/cdrh/devadvice/313.html (accessed Jan 12, 2011).
7. Dannan A, Alkattan F (2008). Animal models in periodontal research: a mini-review of the literature. Available at: http://www.ispub.com/journal/the_internet_journal_of_veterinary_medicine/volume_5_number_1_2/article/animal_models_in_periodontal_research_a_mini_review_of_the_literature.html (accessed Jan 12, 2011).
8. Giannobile WV, Finkelman RD, Lynch SE (1994). Comparison of canine and non-human primate animal models for periodontal regenerative therapy: results following a single administration of PDGF/IGF-I. *J Periodontol* 65:1158–1168.
9. Graves DT, Fine D, Teng YT, Van Dyke TE, Hajishengallis G (2008). The use of rodent models to investigate host-bacteria interactions related to periodontal diseases. *J Clin Periodontol* 35:89–105.
10. Huang KK, Shen C, Chiang CY, Hsieh YD, Fu E (2005). Effects of bone morphogenetic protein-6 on periodontal wound healing in a fenestration defect of rats. *J Periodont Res* 40:1–10.
11. Jin Q, Anusaksathien O, Webb SA, Printz MA, Giannobile WV (2004). Engineering of tooth-supporting structures by delivery of PDGF gene therapy vectors. *Mol Ther* 9:519–526.
12. Kaigler D, Fuller K, Giannobile WV (2010). Regulatory process for the evaluation of dental drugs, devices, and biologics. In: *Clinical research in oral health.* Giannobile WV, Burt BA, Genco RJ, editors. New York: Wiley-Blackwell, pp. 55–78.
13. King GN, King N, Cruchley AT, Wozney JM, Hughes FJ (1997). Recombinant human bone morphogenetic protein-2 promotes wound healing in rat periodontal fenestration defects. *J Dent Res* 76:1460–1470.
14. Office of Combination Products (2011). Overview of the Office of Combination Products. Available at: http://www.fda.gov/oc/combination/overview.html (accessed on Jan 12, 2011).
15. Pellegrini G, Seol YJ, Gruber R, Giannobile WV (2009). Pre-clinical models for oral and periodontal reconstructive therapies. *J Dent Res* 88:1065–1076.
16. Seol YJ, Pellegrini G, Franco LM, Chang PC, Park CH, Giannobile WV (2010). Preclinical methods for the evaluation of periodontal regeneration in vivo. *Methods Mol Biol* 666:285–307.
17. Voigt J, Borysiewicz L (2010). Uniting research into human and animal health. *Vet Rec* 166:406–407.
18. Wikesjö UM, Selvig KA, Zimmerman G, Nilveus R (1991). Periodontal repair in dogs: healing in experimentally created chronic periodontal defects. *J Periodontol* 62:258–263.
19. Wikesjö UM, Sigurdsson TJ, Lee MB, Tatakis DN, Selvig KA (1995). Dynamics of wound healing in periodontal regenerative therapy. *J Calif Dent Assoc* 23:30–35.

CHAPTER 2

Ethical Considerations for Performing Research in Animals

Andreas Bachmann

2.1 Introduction

In many industrialized countries it is a legal requirement that before an animal experiment can be approved, the human interests in the advancement of knowledge and the development of new drugs or therapies must be weighed up against the animal interests in freedom from pain and a species-appropriate life. This weighing of interests aims at a rational choice between the available options for the performance of the planned experiment. Deliberations of this kind are always *ex ante*: not only do the extent of harm and benefits have to be taken into account but also the probability of their occurrence. This is tantamount to comparing risks and benefits with the aim of choosing, on the basis of the comparison, a morally acceptable option.

Asking researchers to weigh up human interests against animal interests makes sense only on the basis of the assumption that animals have some kind of moral status. If animals had no moral status there would be no need for taking them into account at all. Weighing the harms and benefits would simply be superfluous since animals would have no moral weight. What then is the moral status of nonhuman animals, especially in comparison with human beings? This will be the first question to be dealt with in this chapter (Section 2.2). It will be seen that the answer the majority of the population in Western countries would subscribe to is unsatisfactory. For this reason it is necessary to take a closer look at the answers given by the most prominent ethical theories. As will become apparent, there is no agreement among these theories regarding the moral status of animals. As a consequence, they also disagree with regard to the way animal testing should be ethically evaluated. Provided such testing is permitted how should it be performed? This is the next question we will turn to (Section 2.3). By means of three examples it will be discussed how animal interests can be weighed up against human interests and why the three-R principle is not the exclusive criterion for the ethical assessment of animal experiments.

2.2 The Moral Status of Animals

2.2.1 (Modern) Common Sense

According to our everyday beliefs (most) animals do have some moral value. However, between the human and animal there is a considerable, ultimately unbridgeable, moral gap: Humans have higher moral value than animals. Thus, assigning too much moral importance to animals is ethically questionable. Two examples may suffice to illustrate this point: (1) sacrificing animals and sacrificing humans are judged to be two completely different things; and (2) most people agree that animals, unlike human beings, may be caught, kept in captivity, and sold.

Regarding animal experimentation this implies that the suffering of humans carries more weight than the suffering of animals. This is why it is morally and legally required to test new therapies or drugs on animals before testing them on humans. If humans and animals had the same moral value this could not be justified. In that case testing drugs or therapies on animals or humans would have to be forbidden or it would be admissible to test them directly on humans.

The question then is whether human beings really have a higher moral standing than animals. Is this common sense belief justified? Given that our common sense beliefs, i.e., our pre-theoretical moral intuitions are the product of history, culture, and upbringing, and not a reflection of objective moral values, we can better assess their validity if we take a look at their origins. In Western culture they have two historical roots:
- *The Bible*. According to the Bible, man is made in the image of God. So to equate human beings to any other animal degrades humankind. God placed animals on earth for the benefit of humankind; therefore humans have the right and obligation to use animals as needed. The main problem of this argument is that in secularized societies, religious beliefs cannot claim validity for all. They are ultimately nothing more than private creeds.
- *Natural right theory*. According to this theory which traces back to stoicism, a school of Greek philosophy founded in the third century BC, the ability to reason constitutes the fundamental moral difference between human beings and nonhuman animals. Unlike animals, humans are able to think and to reason. Therefore animals exist only for the benefit of humankind. The main problem of this argument is that it does not show why cognitive capacities – language-based reasoning and accountability – have a special ethical value, even if it was true that only human beings have them.

2.2.2 Speciesism

Neither the biblical nor the stoic justification of the special moral status of human beings is convincing. Therefore, many people opt for another approach called speciesism. According to this approach human beings have a special moral status, i.e., they are more valuable than members of nonhuman species, because they belong to the species *Homo sapiens*. Hence human and nonhuman beings may be treated differently because they are members of different species. However, speciesism cannot be warranted since there is no reason why a bare biologic divide – marked by reproductive isolation – should be morally relevant (Rachels, 2006a).

Thus far we have found no plausible justification for a morally relevant difference between human beings and nonhuman animals. Regarding animal experiments this means: The dominant ethical (and legal) position according to which animal testing is admissible in order to achieve scientific and medical goals provided that animal suffering and use is minimized is harder to warrant than its supporters believe. This position is usually based on some of the arguments sketched above, which are deeply ingrained in our culture. However, if these arguments cannot withstand critical scrutiny they must be abandoned. This does not necessarily entail that the dominant ethical position cannot be warranted. Doing that requires more plausible arguments, though.

Such arguments may be found if we ask which features of individual beings are morally relevant irrespective of species (or race or sex). There are mainly three features that must be mentioned: Pain and suffering/pleasure (fulfillment of desires), autonomy, and dignity.

The basic idea of this approach is that individual beings who have some or all of these features count morally, regardless whether they are human beings or nonhuman animals (Rachels, 2006b). How much they count, however, is an open question (Gruen, 2003). Do they all deserve the same respect and the same degree of protection? Or are there justifiable differences? The four single most important systematic ethical theories answer this question differently. These theories are Kantianism (deontology), strong egalitarianism, utilitarianism (consequentialism), and contractualism (interest-based moral theory).

2.2.3 Kantianism (Deontology)

Kantianism is the most prominent case of a moral view called deontology. From a deontological point of view certain acts, such as the intentional killing of an innocent person, are morally wrong in themselves, i.e., irrespective of their consequences. Such acts are prohibited even if they would increase or maximize net benefit (Timmons, 2002).

On a Kantian approach the ethically decisive feature is autonomy: the ability to reason or, more accurately, the ability to set oneself goals based on reasons and, in doing so, to be guided by what is morally right (in Kantian parlance the categorical imperative). Only individual beings with this ability morally count for their own sake. And all beings with this feature count alike.

According to Kant autonomous beings have an absolute value. This is what he calls dignity. In this sense autonomy is coupled to dignity. Having dignity implies that autonomous beings must never be used as mere means to an end. With regard to experiments in general this means: No autonomous being may ever be used in any experiment without prior consent, not even if thousands of lives could be saved. This is the deontological aspect of Kantianism: There must be no trade-offs between autonomous beings – irrespective of the consequences. The main problems of this ethical theory are the following:

1. It must be able to show by means of rational argument, that is, without recourse to religious or metaphysical assumptions that autonomy has an absolute value. Whether this is possible appears highly doubtful.
2. According to Kantian hierarchism most animals are not autonomous because they do not have the ability to reason. This is why we have no direct moral duty to animals, we owe nothing to them (Gruen, 2003). Yet Kant himself clearly opposed wanton cruelty to animals, but mainly because "he who is cruel to animals becomes hard also in his dealings with men". This, however, does not change the fact that animals – insofar as they lack autonomy – are "there merely as a means to an end. That end is man" (Kant, 1997).

Kantians thus claim that we have an indirect duty to animals. However, whether such a duty can be justified is questionable. Kant does not deny that animals can suffer. Nor does he deny that the suffering of animals may engender feelings of compassion. Nonetheless, cruelty to animals is not morally prohibited per se but only insofar as it may affect autonomy since autonomy is the only morally relevant feature. However, if we are aware of this there is no reason why we should not be able to differentiate clearly between cruelty to nonautonomous animals and cruelty to autonomous human beings. And if we have this ability there is no reason why cruelty to animals should necessarily tend to turn into cruelty to human beings. If this is correct Kant's argument collapses. This would entail that animals may be used for any kind of experiment and that any kind of cruelty may be inflicted on them.

Attitude Towards Animal Experimentation
Because humans are the end and animals mere means, animal experiments that help or are likely to help maintain and foster autonomy or prerequisites of autonomy (like health) are morally justified. In other words: the interests of autonomous human beings – as far as they affect their autonomy – always outweigh the interests of nonautonomous animals.

2.2.4 Strong Egalitarianism (Animal Rights Movement)

According to strong egalitarianism – mainly represented by the American philosopher Tom Regan (1983) – the decisive moral feature of an individual being is its inherent value. Beings with inherent value have moral rights or dignity.[1] They must therefore be respected. This means that we must never use them as mere means to some end. In this sense strong egalitarianism is a version of Kantianism: Dignity can only be assigned to autonomous beings. What lies at the basis of dignity is the value of autonomy. Strong egalitarianism radically differs from Kant, however, with regard to the interpretation of dignity (inherent value) and autonomy. It claims that animals have dignity just like human beings. This implies according to its understanding of dignity that animals are just as autonomous as human beings.

If dignity is explained in terms of autonomy, autonomy usually refers to the ability to reason and to take decisions on the basis of reasons. Obviously most animals do not have this kind of autonomy. This is why strong egalitarians suggest interpreting autonomy in a different way. To them autonomy does not mean the ability to reason but the ability to have one's desires fulfilled, which implies the ability to form desires and beliefs as well as the ability to remember things and have a sense for things to come. Thus understood, at least most mammals are autonomous – or so strong egalitarians claim.

In the present context, this conception is problematic mainly for the following reason: Even if we accept the extension of dignity to animals it remains hard to see why we should accept that dignity is an incomparable or infinite value.[2] It may even be argued that the abil-

---

[1] According to Regan dignity means the same as inherent value.

[2] To do justice to Regan's account it must be added that this value is not absolute in the sense that trade-offs are absolutely prohibited. It is always wrong to treat an autonomous being merely as a means to the ends of others. This implies that it is invariably morally reprehensible to harm others in order to generate benefits for oneself or other autonomous beings, whatever these benefits may consist of. To give an example: We must not, ever, hurt any autonomous animal in an experiment even if this were the only way to develop a life-saving therapy for other autonomous beings. However, there are situations where, whatever we do, we violate the rights of others. In such situations trade-offs between autonomous beings become inevitable. We should then follow the "miniride principle" and override the rights of as few autonomous beings as possible, given each affected individual would be equally harmed. When the individuals involved would not be equally harmed, the "worse-off principle" should be applied. This principle says that in situations where the right of several individuals not to be harmed will unavoidably be violated we should override the right of those individuals who would suffer less harm than the others. What this implies can be illustrated using lifeboat cases. Imagine a lifeboat with four humans and one dog vying for space. One being must go overboard as there is only room for four. Regan claims that the dog ought to go overboard. The reason for this is that death would cause a greater harm to each of the (normal healthy) humans than to the dog. Why? Because there are more possible sources of satisfaction in a normal human life than in the life of a dog. Note that this argument is based on a contentious view of the disvalue of death: the so-called deprivation view on which death is bad for the dead because it deprives them of the positive goods they would have experienced had they not died. This also makes clear that Regan does not fall back on a speciesist position: The dog should not be sacrificed because it is a non-human animal.

ity supposedly underlying this kind of dignity, i.e., the ability to be the subject of a life and to have one's desires fulfilled, has no particular moral value at all.

Attitude Towards Animal Experimentation
According to Kant the dignity of a person is only respected if his/her autonomy is treated as an incomparable value. This means that there must be no trade-offs with other values of any kind. Furthermore, since autonomy is an infinite value and this value is equal to dignity one cannot say that 10 persons have more dignity than one person. Strong egalitarianism claims that the same applies to animals as far as they are autonomous: Their value is infinite. Hence, one cannot say that one ape has less dignity than 1,000 apes or 1,000 human beings. In terms of weighing interests this means: No human interest can ever outweigh the interest of just one mammal not to be harmed. For this reason harming or sacrificing autonomous animals can never be justified. As a consequence, strong egalitarians are opposed to any kind of animal experimentation, provided that autonomous animals are affected.

2.2.5 Utilitarianism (Consequentialism)

Utilitarianism is the paradigm case of an ethical view named consequentialism. According to this view the rightness of an act solely depends on its (expected) consequences. Consequentialism requires choosing among those acts available, the act having the best consequences. From a utilitarian point of view this means that in each case the action must be chosen that presumably results in most happiness for all those being affected. Hence, there is just one moral duty: the duty to maximize happiness (Timmons, 2002). Happiness refers to the ability to feel pleasure and pain or, alternatively, to desire fulfillment. Only individual beings with this ability morally count. And all beings, with this ability, i.e., all sentient beings count alike (Singer, 1975).

Note that utilitarianism does not only differ from Kantianism with regard to the morally relevant feature. Rather, the structure of the theory is different. In utilitarianism there are no inherent values that allot dignity or moral rights to individual beings. Hence there are no rights that serve as constraints on utility considerations. Sentient beings – including human beings – are just receptacles of pleasure and pain. As such all of them have the same value: They all count as one and nobody for more than one (Bentham, 1781/1982). However, what actually matters is not their individuality or personhood but the pleasure or pain they are able to experience: They are mere units of utility. Morality requires maximizing this utility, i.e., the aggregate happiness of all beings affected by an action. The technical term for this is total utility or net benefit. Net benefit is defined as the total amount of pleasure (pleasant feelings) minus the total amount of pain (unpleasant feelings).

Utilitarianism is faced with a whole array of problems. In our context two need to be mentioned:
1. It is hard to see how the principle of maximization can be rationally justified. Why should everybody have a moral duty always to maximize the net benefit?
2. Weighing pleasures and pains and summing them up presupposes a common scale, a common currency, as it were, that allows adding and subtracting them. But what does this currency consist of?

Attitude Towards Animal Experimentation
Animal experiments are justified if they help to increase the expected net benefit (the well-being of all affected beings). Of course, this does not require predicting the results with certainty. Experiments are necessary exactly because we do not know the outcome for sure. Yet in many cases the accumulated scientific knowledge allows estimating the probability with which the hypothesis to be tested in the experiment may be corroborated and the hoped for goal(s) thus achieved.

The expected net benefit if the experiment were performed would consist of the following aspects: the probability of reaching the goal(s) of the experiment; the overall decrease of human pain (or increase of pleasure) to be expected if the goal(s) can be achieved; and the foreseeable (probable) pain or suffering inflicted on the animals used in the experiment. It is crucial to bear in mind that if the suffering of two individuals is alike it must be given the same weight irrespective of species, i.e., irrespective of whether it is a human being or a nonhuman animal (Singer, 1975). This explains why for utilitarians it is just as important to determine the severity of pain inflicted on the animals in an experiment as to determine the quantity of human pain that may be reduced due to the experiment.

2.2.6 Contractualism (Interest-based Moral Theory)

According to contractualism, morality is based on the self-interest of rational beings. It is better for each person that everyone should follow certain restrictions than that nobody (or few people) should follow these restrictions. To abide by moral rules is thus a question of prudence: Rational people, interested in their long-term well-being, voluntarily bind themselves to certain moral norms and are willing to enforce morality as a public good by sanctioning those who do not stick to these norms. They do so because the institution of morality – publicly accepted by all – fosters and safeguards their long-term individual welfare.

In the standard version of this theory it is prudent for every rational person to take all beings into consideration that are able to punish their noncompliance. It is also prudent to care for other human beings in need since each person may one day find him or herself in a situation where they need other people's help. From this it follows that certain moral rights such as the right to physical integrity or the right to assistance and the corresponding duties should be accepted. According to this understanding of contractualism animals do not have moral standing because they cannot help or sanction us. They only matter indirectly, i.e., insofar as rational persons care for their well-being and strive to avoid their suffering. There is thus no duty to respect them for their own sake (Carruthers, 1992).

There is, however, an alternative version of contractualism according to which animals do have moral rights, justifying a duty to respect them for their own sake. Suppose, as all contractualists agree, that we have an interest not to be harmed as well as an interest to be protected when we lack power of judgment or when we are unable to act and need other people's help. This applies to old people just as much as to young children. If we base this approach on the hedonistic idea that it is in no one's interest to suffer, it would even apply to all sentient beings. This would entail that animals (at least vertebrates) also have moral rights, such as the right to physical integrity (Rippe, 2008).

From a rational point of view the main strengths of contractualism are that it is not based on ontologically queer entities such as objective values and that it does not implicitly presuppose any moral norms. Nevertheless, some aspects of contractualism are problematic. Why, for instance, should strong persons have any interest in accepting moral constraints if they do not have to fear sanctions? Furthermore, would it not be better for every rational person if all other persons abided by the rules except themselves? And if so why should they not act accordingly? Finally it may be objected that contractualism does not unequivocally answer the question about the moral status of animals: On the standard version animals have no moral rights, on the alternative version at least vertebrates have moral rights.

Attitude Towards Animal Experimentation

Depending on the version, the attitude towards animal experimentation varies. The standard version takes a positive attitude as there are no direct duties to animals but direct duties to other actual and potential persons, especially a duty to help them if they cannot help themselves. The alternative version takes a critical attitude. If vertebrates have a moral right to physical integrity this entails that animal experimentation can only be justified if the right of human beings to get help in specific emergency situations is so important as to outweigh this right.

Table 2-1 summarizes the four widely known ethical approaches to animal welfare.

2.3 Weighing Up Interests in Animal Experiments

The basic idea of weighing up human interests against animal interests is that an animal experiment is morally admissible if the expected net benefit for humans is greater than the suffering and distress the affected animals have to expect. This basic idea can also be formulated in deontological terms, namely as a conflict between the duty to help human beings and the duty not to inflict pain and suffering on animals. An animal experiment would be morally justified if the former outweighs the latter. Whether or not this is the case can only be decided on a case-by-case basis.

This idea is not the idea underlying the three-R principle – replacement, reduction, refinement – a concept introduced by Russell and Burch at the end of the 1950s – since this principle assumes a basic precedence of scientific knowledge and the duty to help human beings over animal protection interests (Russell and Burch, 1959). Accordingly there is no need to perform the weighing procedure. There is only a moral duty to reduce the suffering of the affected animals as much as possible. However, from the perspective of the three-R principle a scientifically relevant experiment may never be prohibited on the ground that it inflicts too much pain on the affected animals.

Regarding the ethical evaluation of specific animal experiments the normative moral theories outlined above may yield different results. Ultimately there is no way of rationally comparing human and animal interests, no method or procedure that is independent of these theories. At this point we have to be more specific, though. At least one of the theories, namely strong egalitarianism, always prohibits trade-offs between human and animal interests. This theory completely rejects any kind of weighing of interests since at least mammals are just as autonomous as (most) human beings and thus have dignity (absolute value). At the other end of the theoretical spectrum is utilitarianism. Utilitarianism demands allocating a weighing to the respective human and animal interests every time someone intends to conduct an animal experiment. Kantianism allows comparing human and animal interests as long as autonomy is not affected. If, however, an animal experiment helps to protect or promote autonomy it must be conducted, provided only non-autonomous animals are used, irrespective of the amount of pain that has to be inflicted on these animals. The standard version of contractualism takes a similar stance even though it does not focus exclusively on autonomy and its prerequisites. The alternative version of contractualism is closer to strong egalitarianism. In this theory, insofar as they are sentient beings, animals have moral rights such as a right to physical integrity. These rights may only be weighed up against human interests if the interests are important enough, i.e., if they are linked to claim rights such as the right to assistance. Otherwise trade-offs between animal and human interests are not admissible.

2.3.1 How to Do the Weighing

What could the weighing of interests in animal experiments concretely look like? One option is to understand it as a deliberative process consisting of three steps. The first step aims at formulating arguments for the experiment. The

Table 2-1 Overview of the most prominent normative ethical theories and their attitude towards animal experimentation

Ethical theory	Type	Morally relevant feature	Moral status of animals	Attitude towards animal testing
Kantianism	*Deontology* Certain kinds of actions are wrong as such, i.e., regardless of their consequences	*Autonomy*, understood as the ability to reason and to do what is morally required	(Most) animals do not have autonomy and therefore lack dignity. Hence, there is no direct moral duty to animals. However, there is an indirect duty to refrain from cruelty to animals	If animal experiments contribute to preserving or fostering autonomy or its prerequisites they are morally obligatory. Otherwise they may only be performed if the attitude underlying the experiment is free from cruelty towards animals and if the experiment is not suited to promote an attitude of brutalization
Strong egalitarianism	*Deontology*	*Autonomy*, understood as the ability to have desires (to be the "subject of a life")	All animals (at least mammals) are autonomous. Hence, they have dignity and must be respected like any other individuals with dignity	Animal experiments cannot be justified. They must be completely banned
Utilitarianism	*Consequentialism* The rightness of acts of any kind solely depends on their consequences	Ability to feel pleasure/pain or ability to have desires	All beings – including all animals – who can feel pain basically count alike	Animal experiments are justified and must be performed if they help to increase the expected net benefit. If they are not likely to increase the expected net benefit they must not be performed
Contractualism (standard version)	*Deontology*	Self-interest (interest not to be harmed and to be helped in situations of need)	Animals have no direct moral standing. Hence, they have no moral rights. Therefore, there is no duty to respect these rights. However, they matter indirectly insofar as rational persons are interested in their well-being.	If animal experiments contribute to the protection or promotion of the moral rights of rational persons they are morally obligatory. Otherwise they should not be performed – at least not on animals whose well-being matters to rational persons.
Contractualism (alternative version)	*Deontology*	Self-interest (interest not to be harmed and to be helped in situations of need)	All sentient beings – including animals – count alike: They have moral rights that must be respected	Animal experiments can only be justified if the right of human beings to get help in concrete emergency situations outweighs the animals' right to physical integrity

aspects to be taken into consideration include in particular: the expected gain in knowledge and its significance; and, if it is applied research, the expected applications and their significance for the health or life quality of the affected human beings. Also part of the first step is the promotion of the three Rs. The second step aims at identifying arguments against the experiment. The aspects to be taken into consideration include in particular: the number and kind of animals being used, and the expected pain and suffering inflicted on them (severity levels). In addition, the researcher is asked to reflect on his knowledge of animal husbandry and animal behavior: Is he really acquainted with the symptoms of suffering in the animal species being used in the experiment? Do the conditions in which the animals are kept meet the standards required to avoid unnecessary pain and stress? The third step consists of weighing the pros and cons against each other. It seeks to determine whether the pros outweigh the cons or vice versa, i.e., whether or not the planned animal experiment is morally justified.

The main problem of this reading of the deliberative process is that it does not seem possible to quantify the individual steps. To justify the outcome of the third step with mathematical precision is therefore out of reach. Nonetheless, from this it does not necessarily follow that the results of the deliberation are arbitrary. Qualitative comparisons, especially of degrees of suffering, are possible. Note, however, that this way of conceptualizing the weighing of interests looks very much just like a utilitarian interpretation: We compare the expected benefits and harms, i.e., perform a benefit-risk analysis. If the conclusion is that the benefits for the affected human beings are greater than the risks the affected animals are exposed to, more precisely that the probability that the humans will gain more than the animals lose is greater than the probability that the animals lose more than the humans gain, the experiment is considered to be morally sound.

From a deontological point of view things look rather different – provided weighing up human against animal interests is deemed to be admissible at all. The main question here would be what rights and duties are affected by an animal experiment and in what way. This question cannot be answered by simply summing up the amount of benefit to be expected for human beings and the amount of harm to be expected for the animals involved in the experiment. Rather, what we would have to know is on the one hand whether the pain inflicted on the animals in case the experiment takes place is of a sort that violates their right to physical integrity and if so how severe this violation is; and on the other hand whether the hoped for benefits for human beings are firmly linked to the right to assistance (and therefore a corresponding duty to help) and how bad it would be to disregard this right in this situation.

2.3.2 Three Examples

Some examples may help to clarify further how the different ethical theories evaluate animal experiments.

- *Example 1: Experiments on rabbits in order to test new cosmetic ingredients*

Described in terms of interests, rabbits have an interest not to suffer, the consumers of cosmetic products have an interest to increase their well-being by using new products of this kind. How would the theories outlined above evaluate animal testing for this purpose? The answer is clear: They would unanimously reject it regardless of whether there are alternatives to animal testing. This, however, for different reasons. Strong egalitarians are vehemently opposed to any kind of animal experiments. Supporters of the alternative version of contractualism would argue that weighing up animal interests against human interests is inadmissible in this case since there is no conflict between different duties or moral rights. There is just one moral right affected: the right of rabbits as sentient beings to bodily integrity – and thus just one duty: The duty to respect this right. Whereas there is no moral right on the side of consumers, i.e., no legitimate moral claim to new cosmetics. It would be morally wrong therefore to violate the right of rabbits to bodily integrity in order to enhance the well-being of some humans.

From the standpoint of standard contractualism and Kantianism comparing the human and animal interests involved would be the adequate way to decide whether cosmetic experiments on rabbits may be admitted. Both theories would deny that rabbits have a right to bodily integrity. Nevertheless, rabbits have an interest not to suffer which should be taken seriously. We should not inflict pain on animals without good reason because if we do this, it might lead to a similar behavior in our relations with other persons. A good, even compelling reason would be experiments that were necessary to protect human autonomy. This is not the case here: New cosmetics have no repercussions on autonomy. They may improve the well-being of some consumers, but that does not justify inflicting pain on rabbits, even more so as there are already a lot of cosmetics.

Utilitarians would subscribe to this conclusion. However, they would adduce other reasons to substantiate it. They would urge to weigh the animal and human interests involved by comparing the pains inflicted on the rabbits when testing cosmetic ingredients on the one hand, and the pleasure consumers may experience when using new cosmetics on the other hand. From their point of view moral rights are just as irrelevant as autonomy. The only thing that matters is the net amount of happiness, i.e., the total amount of pleasure minus the total amount of pain. The crucial argument would be that performing these experiments would presumably produce more pain and less pleasure overall than not performing them. Note that this claim might be false. In this case utilitarians would have to revise their verdict and approve of experiments on rabbits to test cosmetic ingredients.

- *Example 2: Experiments on mice in order to develop a therapy for treating childhood leukemia*

Expressed in terms of interest, mice have an interest not to suffer and die, and the affected children have an interest not to suffer and die prematurely from a severe disease. There is no unanimity among the various moral theories on how to appraise this example. Provided mice are "subjects of a life" and in this sense autonomous, strong egalitarianism would oppose these experiments even if they were indispensable for the development of a therapy for treating childhood leukemia. The alternative version of contractualism would take the same view since mice are sentient beings and therefore have a right to physical integrity that must not be disregarded in order to help others.

Kantianism and the standard version of contractualism would agree that in this case weighing up animal interests against human interests is morally prohibited (given that this procedure is performed because it is an open question whether more weight should be given to human or to animal interests). They would argue that these experiments must be performed if there is the slightest chance that they may help to reach the goal of developing a therapy for leukemia. Kantians would emphasize that the mice must be sacrificed since we have a duty to do everything in our power to avoid that autonomy is harmed and since leukemia is a serious threat to autonomy and therefore to dignity: it is a disease which, if left untreated, has fatal consequences, thereby making the development and preservation of autonomy impossible.

Supporters of standard contractualism would point out that children have a right to get help, especially if the consequences of not helping are as grave as in the case at hand.

Since they have this moral right there is a corresponding duty to help them as much as possible. Mice on the other hand have no such right. They have no rights whatsoever. This does not mean that we are free to harm them as we please. They are sentient beings, able to feel pain and pleasure. We should not make them suffer without any reason. Yet mice have no right to physical integrity; therefore there is no moral duty to respect this right. For this reason there is no conflict between our duty to help affected children by developing a therapy for leukemia on the one hand and the suffering inflicted on the mice that are used as means to reach this goal on the other hand.

The only ethical theory in favor of weighing up animal against human interests in this case study is utilitarianism. Utilitarians would argue that the experiment is morally justified if the expected amount of pain reduction is greater than the amount of pain produced. They would then ask the researchers to figure out the net amount of pain inflicted on the mice used in the experiment as well as the net amount of pain reduction that would result if the experiment were successful. However, they would formulate a proviso: Since what is required is a risk-benefit analysis the experiment would only be warranted if there is a reasonable probability that using mice would indeed contribute to developing a therapy for childhood leukemia. Given this probability there is a moral obligation to conduct this kind of experiment. Otherwise performing it would be inadmissible.

- *Example 3: Experiment on Beagle dogs in order to perform an immunohistochemical evaluation of guided bone regeneration using different types of barrier membranes (Schwarz et al., 2008)*

The main aim of this experiment is to compare different barrier membranes with regard to their ability to support bone regeneration. It is designed as an *in vivo* experiment since *in vitro* comparison is not possible. For this purpose 12 Beagle dogs, aged 20–24 months, with fully erupted permanent dentition would be used. These dogs would be subjected to two surgeries. In the first surgery the second premolar and first and second molars are planned to be extracted bilaterally in both jaws. In the second surgery after 4 months of healing, dehiscence-type defects will be created followed by the insertion of titanium implants. Subsequently, all defects will be filled with a bone-grafting material and covered by different types of barrier membranes. After a healing period of 1 to 12 weeks the dogs will be sacrificed, their jaws dissected and blocks containing the experimental specimens will be obtained.[3]

In terms of interest the Beagle dogs have an interest not to suffer and die prematurely, the scientists have an interest to compare the functionality of barrier membranes *in vivo*. However, the experiment can also be seen as part of a more comprehensive effort to help human patients whose bone structure makes the use of certain conventional dental implants impossible. After all, the reason for using Beagle dogs is not just that they are pleasant animals, but mainly that the morphology of their jaw bones and their chewing behavior is similar to that of humans.

From the perspective of strong egalitarianism, this experiment is unjustifiable like any animal experiment and should therefore not be performed. Kantian moral theory would reject the experiment if it is viewed in isolation, arguing that there is no connection between the expected gain in knowledge and the protection of autonomy. Furthermore, the pain inflicted on the dogs appears to be disproportionate in

---

[3]The main result of the study was that "all membranes investigated supported bone regeneration on an equivalent level" (Schwarz et al., 2008, p. 413). Note, however, that the experiment must be evaluated *ex ante*, i.e. before performing it and hence without knowing the result. So even though it was actually approved and then performed the issue here is whether it was morally right to approve it.

relation to new insights that might result. This verdict may be modified if the experiment is seen in a larger context, i.e. if the ultimate aim is the development of a new or improved technique for specific dental implants. This is only the case, however, if the experiment is a necessary intermediary step on the way towards this aim and if the aim itself is indeed directly linked to the protection or promotion of autonomy or its prerequisites.

The standard version of contractualism would put forward a similar argument. From the point of view of this theory inflicting considerable pain on dogs just for the sake of comparing the functionality of certain barrier membranes can hardly be morally warranted, especially since rational persons are usually more interested in the well-being of dogs than, say, in the well-being of rats. If, however, the experiment is a necessary means to the end of helping human beings with a specific health problem this assessment changes because that would mean that it contributes to the protection of a moral right of rational persons – the right to get adequate medical treatment. In this case performing the experiment would be morally mandatory.

The alternative version of contractualism would also oppose the experiment as such since dogs have a moral right to physical integrity that must not be violated in order to find out more about the functionality of barrier membranes. The reason for this is that moral rights may only be weighed up against other moral rights, not against interests (such as the interest in more knowledge) that are not protected by moral rights. The situation might change if comparing barrier membranes for guided bone regeneration using dogs is a precondition for an application of this surgical procedure on human patients. Then the question would arise whether these patients have a moral right to receive assistance and if so, whether this right (and the corresponding duty to help) outweighs the dogs' right to physical integrity. If the answer is yes, the experiment is morally justified and should be performed; if the answer is no, the experiment is not justified and ought not to be performed.

According to utilitarianism it is essential for the assessment of any kind of animal testing that animal interests are weighed up against human interests. In this regard utilitarianism differs from the other relevant moral theories. In view of the experiment to be evaluated this means that the pain inflicted on the dogs must be weighed up against the expected gain in knowledge. If the net amount of pain is greater than the expected net amount of pleasure associated with the gain in knowledge the experiment is not justified; if it is the other way round it is justified.[4] Given that considerable pain would be inflicted on the dogs, utilitarians would question whether this pain can be outweighed by the knowledge which may be obtained. This evaluation may change, however, if the experiment can be regarded as an essential step in the development or improvement of a surgical procedure for a certain group of human patients. If the amount of human pain that presumably could be alleviated by this procedure is greater than the amount of pain inflicted on the dogs the experiment would be morally justified. There would be a moral duty therefore to perform it.

---

[4]Some utilitarians are value pluralists. They would argue that scientific knowledge is not only instrumentally, but also intrinsically valuable, i.e. valuable for its own sake regardless of whether it is needed for developing new technological or medical applications and regardless of whether it is associated with any kind of pleasant feelings. This view is problematic for two reasons. First, it is unclear why knowledge should be regarded as an intrinsic value. Second, if knowledge is deemed to be intrinsically valuable, comparing and weighing interests becomes even more difficult. For now not only pleasant and unpleasant feelings must be taken into consideration when summing up the pros and cons in order to calculate the net benefit, but also, as an independent aspect, the gain in knowledge. It is hard to see, however, what the "common currency" would be that allows comparing and aggregating these different values.

2.4 Conclusion

Ethics as a science aims at a rational justification of moral norms and actions. From an ethical point of view all animal experiments need a justification of this kind. This is a more challenging task than one might think at first sight – at least if it is correct that human beings do not have a special moral status just by virtue of being human. The relevant normative ethical theories agree that this is the case. From their perspective it cannot simply be taken for granted that basic or applied scientific research is morally warranted by the aim of benefiting humankind. We cannot just assume that animal experiments are justified if they are necessary for scientific progress and if the pain inflicted on the animals is minimized. Whether such experiments are admissible can only be decided on the basis of a case-by-case analysis. The main challenge here is that there is no agreed on set of criteria regarding the ethical evaluation of specific experiments as each normative ethical theory has its own criteria. This difficulty can be overcome if it is possible to determine which of these theories is the most plausible one. There is no reason to think that this is not possible. To show, however, which theory should be favored is beyond the scope of this chapter. Suffice it to say that despite their differences there is one issue about which all theories agree: When thinking about the ethical assessment of animal experiments the three-R principle is one criterion to be taken into account. It is not sufficient, however, to justify these experiments. From a justificatory perspective it is not enough to minimize the numbers of animals being used and the pain inflicted on them. Rather, this negative aspect must be weighed against the positive aspects of an experiment, i.e., the scientific objectives one strives to achieve. This is an open-ended process. The objectives may be important enough to justify the infliction of pain and suffering on the animals. If they are not important enough, however, it is a moral duty to refrain from performing the experiment.

References

1. Bentham J (1781/1982). An introduction to the principles of morals and legislation. London: Methuen.
2. Carruthers P (1992). The animals issue. Moral theory and practice. Cambridge: Cambridge University Press.
3. Gruen L (2003). The moral status of animals. Available at: http://plato.stanford.edu/entries/moral-animal/ (accessed April 3, 2010).
4. Kant I (1997). Lectures on ethics. In: Heath P, Schneewind JB, editors and translators. Unpublished lectures originally held in the 1780s. Cambridge: Cambridge University Press.
5. Rachels J (2006a). Darwin, species, and morality. In: Rachels J, editor. The legacy of Socrates. Essays in moral philosophy. New York: Columbia University Press, pp. 15–31.
6. Rachels J (2006b). Drawing lines. In: Rachels J, editor. The legacy of Socrates. Essays in moral philosophy. New York: Columbia University Press, pp. 32–46.
7. Regan T (1983). The case for animal rights. Berkley: University of California Press.
8. Rippe KP (2008). Ethik im ausserhumanen Bereich. Paderborn: Mentis.
9. Russell WMS, Burch RR (1959). The principle of humane experimental technique. London: Methuen & Co Ltd.
10. Schwarz F, Rothamel D, Herten M, Wüstefeld M, Sager M, Ferrari D et al. (2008). Immunohistochemical characterization of guided bone regeneration at a dehiscence-type defect using different barrier membranes: an experimental study in dogs. *Clin Oral Implants Res* 19:402–415.
11. Singer P (1975). Animal liberation. A new ethics for our treatment of animals. New York: New York Review of Books.
12. Timmons M (2002). Moral theory. An Introduction. Lanham: Rowman & Littlefield Publishers, Inc.

Good Laboratory Practice (GLP) in Nonclinical Investigations

Beat Schmid

3.1 Introduction

Good laboratory practice (GLP) is a quality system covering the organizational process and the conditions under which nonclinical health and environmental safety studies are planned, performed, monitored, recorded, archived, and reported. The present chapter aims to provide a general overview of the principles of the quality system of GLP and its organizational processes, as well as the framework in which it is embedded. The discussion has been purposely presented in general terms and does not endorse a particular item or product.

Government and industry are concerned about the quality of nonclinical health and environmental safety studies on which hazard assessments are based. To avoid different schemes of implementation that could impede international trade in chemicals, the Organisation for Economic Co-operation and Development (OECD) has developed a quality system and has established criteria for the performance of these studies, which interested OECD Member Countries have pursued over the past three decades with international harmonization of test methods and GLP. Through this, multiple testing can be prevented, avoiding unnecessary use of animals and their suffering. Also, common principles for GLP facilitate the exchange of information and prevent the emergence of nontariff barriers to trade, while contributing to the protection of human health and the environment. In a recent note by OECD on "Cutting Costs in Chemicals Management: How OECD Helps Governments and Industry", an analyses of the GLP system for assessing and managing chemicals estimated it to cost around €150 million each year (Sigman, 2010).

3.2 History of GLP

The OECD principles of GLP were first developed by an expert group on GLP established in 1978, under the Special Programme on the Control of Chemicals, and the principles of GLP were formally recommended for use in member countries by the OECD Council in 1981. They were set as an integral part of the Council Decision on Mutual Acceptance of Data in the Assessment of Chemicals, which states that "data generated in the testing of chemicals in an OECD Member country in accordance with OECD Test Guidelines, and that OECD Principles of Good Laboratory Practice shall be accepted in other Member countries for purposes of assessment and other uses relating to the protection of man and the environment" (OECD, n.d.,a). At a meeting in 1983 concerning the mutual recognition of compliance with GLP, the OECD recommended that implementation of GLP compliance should be verified by laboratory inspections and study audits.

In 1997 the OECD council extended the concept of GLP by adapting it to the scientific and technical progress made, and also expanded the principles of mutual acceptance of data to nonmember countries wishing to cooperate with OECD. Today, a series of publications on the OECD principles of GLP, guidance documents for compliance monitoring authorities, consensus documents, and position papers have been published and are publicly available on the OECD website under the chapter "OECD Series on Principles of Good Laboratory Practice and Compliance Monitoring" (OECD, 1998).

The European Community (EC) adopted the OECD principles and a number of directives stipulate that tests must be carried out in accordance with the principles of GLP and also that EC member states should incorporate into their laws the requirements for all the nonclinical safety studies that are listed in the sectoral directives, to be conducted to GLP, and that premises conducting such studies must be inspected by a national authority. The revised principles of GLP and compliance monitoring were adopted by the EC in October 1998 and issued as Directives 99/11/EEC and 99/12/EEC.

In Switzerland, the first GLP guidance on GLP was published in 1981 for pharmaceuticals and extended in 1986 to chemicals, and subsequently in 2000 the GLP Ordinance was laid down, with revisions in 2005 (OECD, 2005). Information on GLP and the ordinance relevant to Switzerland are available on the GLP website of the Federal Office of Public Health (2006).

3.3 Scope of GLP

The scope of the GLP principles covers the nonclinical safety testing of test items contained in pharmaceutical products, pesticide products, cosmetic products, and veterinary drugs, as well as food additives, feed additives, and industrial chemicals. These test items are frequently synthetic chemicals; however, they also include those of natural or biologic origin. The tests are also applicable to domains where nonclinical safety studies are being conducted for registration/notification dossiers to be submitted to authorities.

3.4 GLP Framework

The regulations not only set out the rules for good practice, but also help scientists and laboratory personnel to perform their work in compliance with their own pre-established plan and the standardized procedures worldwide. Lastly, the receiving authorities can build on a well-established quality system (Fig 3-1).

It is important to state that the GLP regulations are not concerned with the scientific or technical content of the research or development program, and do not aim to evaluate the scientific content or value of such studies. To be able to work within the GLP framework a number

3.4 GLP Framework

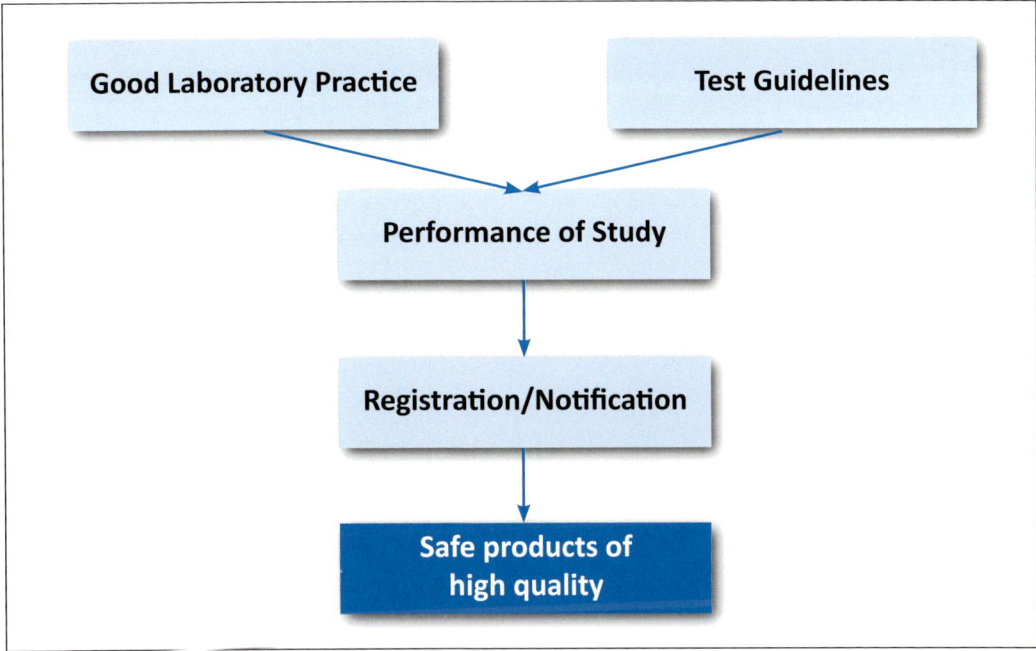

Fig 3-1 The test and good laboratory practice (GLP) guidelines represent a sound basis for the performance of a study with regard to content and quality, which, through the registration or notification process, will ultimately lead to safe products of high quality.

of basic requirements need to be fulfilled in order to adequately conduct GLP studies.

While the necessity of monitoring the compliance of test facilities with the principles of GLP is obvious, the OECD has not provided a general directive for the formation and establishment of the national authorities with regard to other governmental structures. As a consequence, countries have taken different approaches for their GLP compliance monitoring authorities. The spectrum stretches from governmental offices dealing with monitoring GLP compliance to inspectorates charged with the supervision of all quality systems – from International Organization of Standardization (ISO) standards and accreditation to entire good practice surveillance systems. As indicated above, what the compliance monitoring authories share in common is their relationship to the receiving registration or notification authority.

At this point, the GLP compliance monitoring program has therefore to be mentioned, as the implementation of GLP principles established within a test facility will sooner or later be controlled and certified by the GLP monitoring authorities. The latter will thoroughly investigate on the following sections during the inspection of the test facility:

- Organization and personnel
- Quality assurance program
- Facilities
- Apparatus, material, reagents
- Test systems
- Test and reference items
- Standard operating procedure
- Performance of the study
- Reporting of study results
- Storage and retention of records and materials.

Further, specific audits of a particular study can be initiated *ad hoc* when there is a request to verify data, records, reports, etc. as they may not comply with GLP standards. Such study audits can be triggered on the initiative of the GLP compliance monitoring program unit itself, or at the request of another competent authority in another country or region.

GLP certified test facilities are ultimately being added to the GLP-OECD list; removal and also noncompliance is generally communicated to GLP countries, and, in general, also to receiving authorities. Inspection intervals for the maintenance of the test facility in the GLP program vary from country to country, but generally are around 2–3 years.

Further, monitoring authorities have the duty of participating in the OECD mutual joint visit program in order to continuously improve and harmonize inspections, and they participate in OECD working group sessions, and contribute to the interpretation of GLP principles on a national and international level. They also maintain regular contact with the receiving authorities to discuss relevant topics which are of common interest to both parties (e.g., cross-contamination issues in control animals), and integration of training courses for new GLP inspectors into the process of GLP monitoring.

3.5 Test Facility Structures

Firstly, visible structures within the test facility conducting the test under GLP conditions need to be established as fundament for the implementation and daily surveillance of the quality principles, which are represented by management, quality assurance, and the study directors.

Adequate organization of the activities being carried out within a company/test facility regarding nonclinical laboratory safety investigations is essential, and a representative scheme is given in Figure 3-2.

3.5.1 Test Facility Management

Test facility management is responsible for ensuring compliance with the GLP principles throughout the facility as a whole, as well for the setting up of initial and continuous training of all personnel involved in GLP activities. In order to ascertain its responsibility, a number of measures have to be implemented, such as hiring an adequate number of appropriately qualified and experienced staff throughout the facility, including those specifically required to perform quality assurance functions.

Although sponsors had been defined in the original OECD principles, their role within a GLP study, if not acting as a test facility management, remained not clearly defined. There are, for example, no indications as to which responsibilities are to be taken over by the sponsor, a situation which has led to a number of difficulties. Since the connections between sponsor and study will be mainly through the test facility management and the study director, and/or the principal investigator, the sponsor should be particularly aware of their responsibilities towards the study, and especially of the fact that the full responsibility for the entire study remains with the study director. With regard to the submission of the study to health authorities for market application, the company should either monitor the selected Contract Research Organization (CRO) prior to the initiation of the study, or the respective national compliance monitoring authority may be contacted to determine the current compliance status of the test facility.

3.5.2 Quality Assurance

Quality assurance is the internal system for ensuring that the GLP principles are applied in an optimal manner, and that the studies that are conducted at the test facility comply with the principles to the necessary extent. The rules governing this will have to be laid down in a quality assurance program as defined for the test facility. The program on GLP standards has

3.5 Test Facility Structures

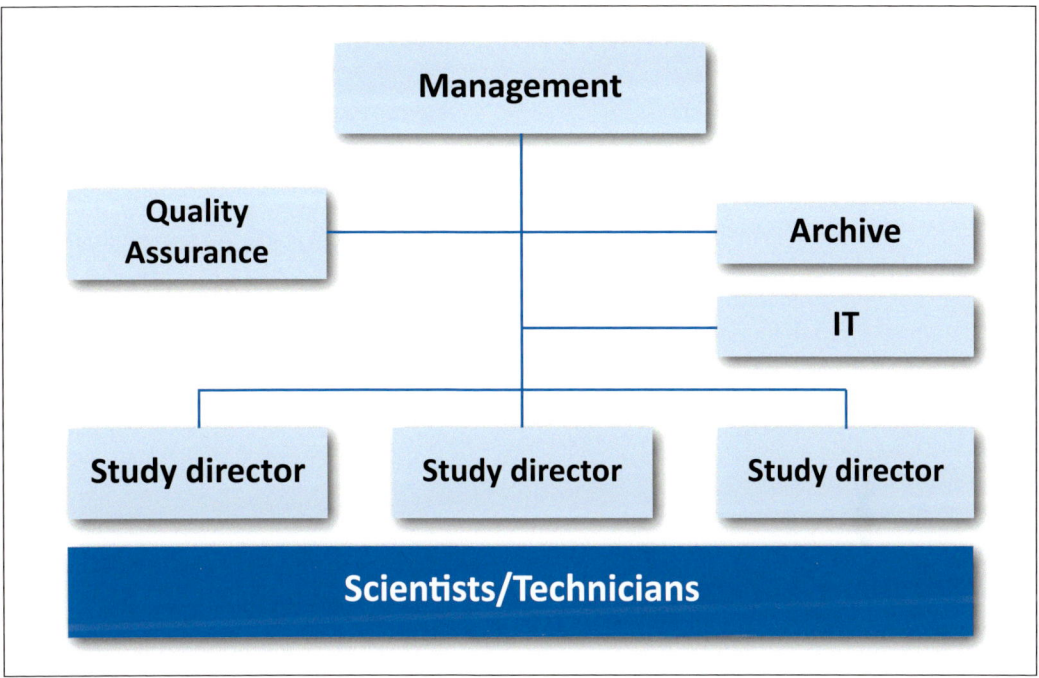

Fig 3-2 Scheme for the necessary structures at a company/test facility for the carrying out of good laboratory practice (GLP) studies.

to be implemented in the everyday work of a test facility, and it has to be considered in this context that the program can only be as good as the involvement of the quality assurance manager in daily activities and issues of individual persons or departments from receipt of the original complaint to its final resolution. It is also important that the quality assurance function is independent from the actual study conduct. Any activities conducted by quality assurance should not compromise the independence of the quality assurance operation and should not incorporate quality assurance personnel in the conduct of the study other than a monitoring responsibility. In addition, it should be guaranteed that the appointed person for this position has direct access to the different levels of management, particularly the top-level management of the test facility; quality assurance has to be able to inspect the test facility and running GLP activities at any time and bring any deviations to management's immediate attention, in order to define and put into place corrective action.

To clarify responsibility sharing between management and quality assurance, the scheme depicted in Figure 3-3 can be followed.

3.5.3 The Study Director

The study director is the single point of study control, and the responsibilities for the content and the GLP conduct of the study from the signing of the study plan to his signature on the study reports are centralized in this role. This can only be accomplished through coordination of the inputs from management, scientific/technical staff, and quality assurance. Although some of the duties of the study director may be

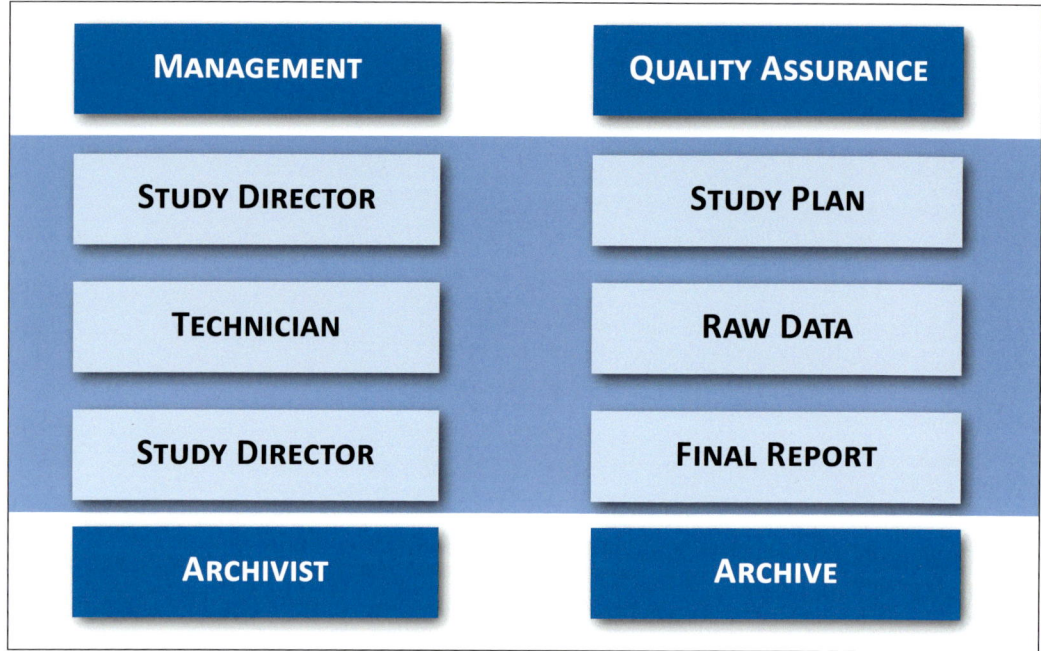

Fig 3-3 Scheme illustrating the division of responsibilities between management and quality assurance.

delegated to a principle investigator, as is the case for subcontracted phases of studies, or a specialized responsible scientist (as may be the case for analytical or histopathological work as part of an animal safety study), it is only the study director who has the overall responsibility for a given study: he or she finally acknowledges this by signing the GLP statement in the final report of the study they have directed.

3.5.4 The Archivist

The archive serves to store the complete materials, records, and other documentation specifically related to individual studies, and for the test facility in general. An archivist has to be specifically nominated by the test facility management as the only person authorized by management to have access to the archives. It should be mentioned, however, that at the delivery point of the materials (documents, raw data, tissue, histopathological slides, etc.) for archiving, the study director is responsible for the completeness of the study-related materials, and has to trigger the transfer to the archivist. There has also to be a well-designed system for keeping track of any material that is leaving or returning to the archives, and movement of material in and out of the archives has to be properly recorded. It is self-explanatory that the necessary security and fire protection measures should be in place to protect the materials in the archive to guarantee reconstruction of a study. In this context GLP defines the general conditions under which archives should be operated in order to ensure the availability and to guarantee traceability of such materials at any time. GLP does not provide specific definitions of storage period, as different countries have different legal requirements, but simply refer to the national rules and laws.

3.5.5 IT Personnel

Computerized systems have taken over an increasing number of tasks in the conduct of safety-related nonclinical GLP studies within test facilities, and are not only applied during the planning, conduct, and reporting of studies, but are also used to make internal standard operating procedures (SOPs) immediately accessible globally, as well as for data transfer from automated instruments, and the recording, processing, reporting, general management, and storage of data. It is important to note, however, that whatever the scale of computer applications is, the GLP principles have to be followed, and that such systems require detailed GLP validation before being used in the daily activities. In this context, the basic principles in the use of computerized systems within regulatory safety studies indicate that all such systems used for the generation, measurement, or assessment of data intended for regular submission should be developed, validated, operated, and maintained in ways that are compliant with the GLP principles. Controls for security and system integrity should also be adequately addressed during the entire lifecycle of computerized systems. IT responsible personnel are being more and more involved in GLP studies, particularly in context with validation of GLP studies. This should be considered early by test facility management, and IT personnel included in the GLP program at an early stage.

3.6 GLP Documentation

With regard to all GLP documents, whatever their origin or the industry targeted, the following topics have to be covered:
- Resources: organization, personnel, facilities, and equipment
- Rules: protocols and written procedure SOPs
- Characterization: test items and test systems
- Documentation: raw data, final report, and archive.

Of the indicated topics, written SOPs relating to the important aspects of test facility operations are considered one of the most key management techniques for controlling facility operations. Indeed, the availability of a complete set of SOPs for the steering of the everyday activities and procedures in a test facility is a prerequisite for GLP compliance, and is defined as: documented procedures which describe how to perform tests or activities normally not specified in study plans or test guidelines. The compilation of SOPs cover the whole GLP process, and will include organizational and managerial issues on one hand, and technical issues, such as the conduct of studies, use of equipment and apparatuses, on the other hand. Computerized systems will certainly occupy an important position in the resources with regard to the establishment and the implementation of SOPs in GLP, with extensive guidance on the validation of computerized systems. SOPs on the use of SOPs will also have to be established, in which the responsibilities of GLP personnel are described and the approval process, distribution process, maintenance, review and revision, and finally archiving processes – including the timing intervals for review and revisions – are established.

Last but not least, the traceability of the test item needs to be stressed, which means that there has to be a continuous line of evidence that the test item – which is finally submitted for marketing authorization or notification – can be followed and documented throughout the entire GLP process.

3.7 The Study, and Multisite Studies

The safety study represents the basis of all the assessments on which ultimate decisions about the safe use of the tested items, and the products derived from there, will be made by the respective authorities. In this context, GLP defines the quality frame for an experiment or set of experiments in which a test item is examined under laboratory condition, or in the environment, to obtain data on its properties and/or its safety, intended for submission to appropriate regulatory authorities.

Complexities have increased with globalization in general, and the globalization of companies has also impacted on the way nonclinical studies are conducted. The splitting of the GLP process occurred partly as a consequence of outsourcing of certain phases of nonclinical safety studies, and also through specialization in certain areas (e.g., analytical work, histopathology) which are confined to different competence centers all over the world. The responsibilities of a study director to control all the aspects of a study led to the establishment of the OECD consensus document on multisite studies, and was ultimately described in the OECD series (no. 13) on principles of good laboratory practice and compliance monitoring (OECD, 2002). According to this document, certain responsibilities of the study director have to be transferred to another role, the principle investigator, who would then be fully responsible for the GLP compliant conduct of the particular defined task within a study. The principle investigator is "an individual who, for a multi-site study, acts on behalf of the study director and has defined responsibility for delegated phases of the study" (OECD, 2002). The ultimate responsibility for study conduct, however, still remains with the study director as it is given in the principles that the "study director's responsibility for the overall conduct of the study cannot be delegated to the PI; this includes approval of the study plan and its amendments, approval of the final report, and ensuring that all applicable Principles of GLP are followed" (OECD, 2002).

3.8 Summing Up

Overall, the nonclinical GLP system provides a sound quality system which can be used for data assessment and reporting in nonclinical safety studies, in order to ensure that data are reproducible and traceable. Although regulated through individual countries, congruence and harmonization have been achieved by including and maintaining the GLP principles and compliance monitoring in the international framework of the OECD, governed by its guidelines, concept papers, and documents for consideration on the one hand (OECD, n.d., b), and national legal and administrative practices on the other hand, hence providing international acceptance of the data and the quality system, and avoiding duplicative testing.

References

1. Federal Office of Public Health, Federal Office for the Environment, Swissmedic. (2006). Good laboratory practice. Available at: www.bag.admin.ch/themen/chemikalien/00253/00539/index.html?lang=en (accessed 22 November 2010).
2. OECD (1998). Principles on good laboratory practice. ENV/MC/CHEM(98)17. Paris: OECD Environment Directorate.
3. OECD (n.d.,a). Decision of the OECD Council concerning the mutual acceptance of data in the assessment of chemicals. C(81)30 (final).
4. OECD (2005). Ordinance on good laboratory practice 2002. DOK 813.112.1.
5. OECD (2002). OECD series on principles of good laboratory practice and compliance monitoring. No. 13. Consensus Document of the Working Group on Good Laboratory Practice: The Application of the OECD Principles of GLP to the Organisation and Management of Multi-Site Studies (2002/9). DOK JT00128856.
6. OECD (n.d.,b). OECD series on principles of good laboratory practice and compliance monitoring. Available at: www.oecd.org/document/63/0,3343,en_2649_343 81_2346175_1_1_1_1,00&&en-USS_01DBC.html (accessed 22 November 2010).
7. Sigman R (2010). OECD: Cutting costs in "chemicals management". How OECD helps governments and industry. Issued under the responsibility of OECD's Joint Meeting of the Chemicals Committee and Working Party on Chemicals, Pesticides and Biotechnology. Available at: www.oecd.org/dataoecd/17/59/44982952.pdf (accessed 22 November, 2010).

Research Design and Biostatistical Considerations in Preclinical Research

Thomas M. Braun

4.1 Introduction

Biostatistics is the study of biologic phenomena, referred to as the signal, in the presence of variation, referred to as the noise. From a set of data, biostatistics attempts to determine if the magnitude of the observed signal relative to the magnitude of the observed noise is simply due to chance or is evidence of a true signal. As such, biostatistics plays two important roles in preclinical research. First, biostatistics is necessary *before* any research study commences so that hypotheses, outcomes, study design, and sample size are all clarified and justified so that the study is able to detect a true signal in the presence of the expected level of noise. Second, biostatistics is necessary *after* any research study is completed to help analyze the data so that the level of noise in the data is appropriately accounted for, thereby increasing the ability to detect any true signal present in the data.

Many investigators mistakenly assume that there is very little need for biostatistics in preclinical research, as they believe that biostatistics plays a role primarily in human research where the amount of variability is enormous and fairly impossible to control. However, preclinical experiments often involve highly precise technology that is sensitive to many sources of variation, including general measurement error, the use of multiple lab technicians, and between-batch variation of assays. Unless they are tightly controlled, all these and other sources of variation will serve to weaken the strength of any experiment. Biostatistics is the set of tools to help account for sources of variation so that the signal, when present, has an increased likelihood of being detected.

It is also emphasized that the role of biostatistics goes far beyond sample size calculations and generating *P* values.

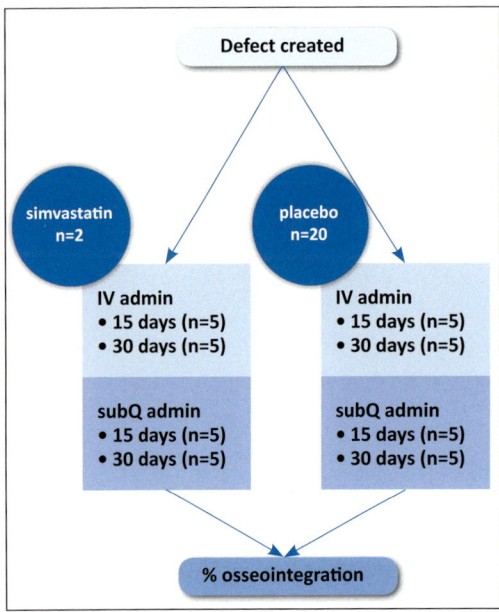

Fig 4-1 Schematic of study design used in Example 4.2.1.

4.2 Illustrative Examples

4.2.1 Example 4.2.1

Anabinder and colleagues describe an experiment studying the effects of simvastatin on bone regeneration (Anabinder et al., 2006). Figure 4-1 shows the design of the experiment. Forty mice were first divided into two groups. One group contained 20 mice of which 10 received simvastatin via oral administration and 10 received simvastatin via subcutaneous administration. The other group of 20 mice was divided similarly by route of administration, with placebo given instead of simvastatin. Prior to treatment, investigators placed a monocortical bone defect on the right tibia of each mouse. Within each of the four groups defined by treatment and route of administration, half the mice were sacrificed after 15 days, and the other half were sacrificed after 30 days. After sacrifice, each mouse was examined to determine the percentage of reossification occurring at the center of the bone defect.

4.2.2 Example 4.2.2

Chang and colleagues describe an experiment to investigate how gene transfer of platelet-derived growth factor (PDGF) is related to bone integration around oral implant sites (Chang et al., 2010). The experiment consisted of four treatment groups: a control group receiving adenovirus gene vector encoding luciferase (Ad-Luc), one group receiving Ad-mediated PDGF-B (Ad-PDGF-B), one group receiving a lower dose of PDGF-BB, and one group receiving a higher dose of PDGF-BB (Fig 4-2). A total of 82 animals were assigned to one of the four treatment groups, and each animal was sacrificed at 10, 14, or 21 days after treatment, leading to six to eight animals in each of the 12 groups defined by treatment and time of sacrifice. After sacrifice, several outcomes related to osseointegration were collected on each animal.

4.2.3 Example 4.2.3

Schwarz and colleagues describe an experiment studying the difference in bone regeneration around implant sites using particulated (BOG) or block (BOB) natural bone, both of which are biocoated with either rhGDF-5 or rhBMP-2 (Schwarz et al., 2008). The experiment studied a total of eight dogs, each of which had several teeth extracted from each quadrant. Three standardized, box-shaped defects were surgically placed in the extraction region of each quadrant and allowed to heal. Four of the six defects in the maxilla of each animal were randomly assigned to either BOG or BOB in combination with either rhGDF-5, or rhBMP-2, with the remaining two sites assigned to BOG alone or BOB alone (Fig 4-3). Similar assignments were given to the six sites in the mandible of each animal. Four of the animals were sacrificed after 3 weeks of submerged healing, with the remaining four animals sacrificed after 8 weeks of submerged healing. Outcomes measured on each of the 48 sites included the defect length, the width of the new ridge at various points along the defect

4.2 Illustrative Examples

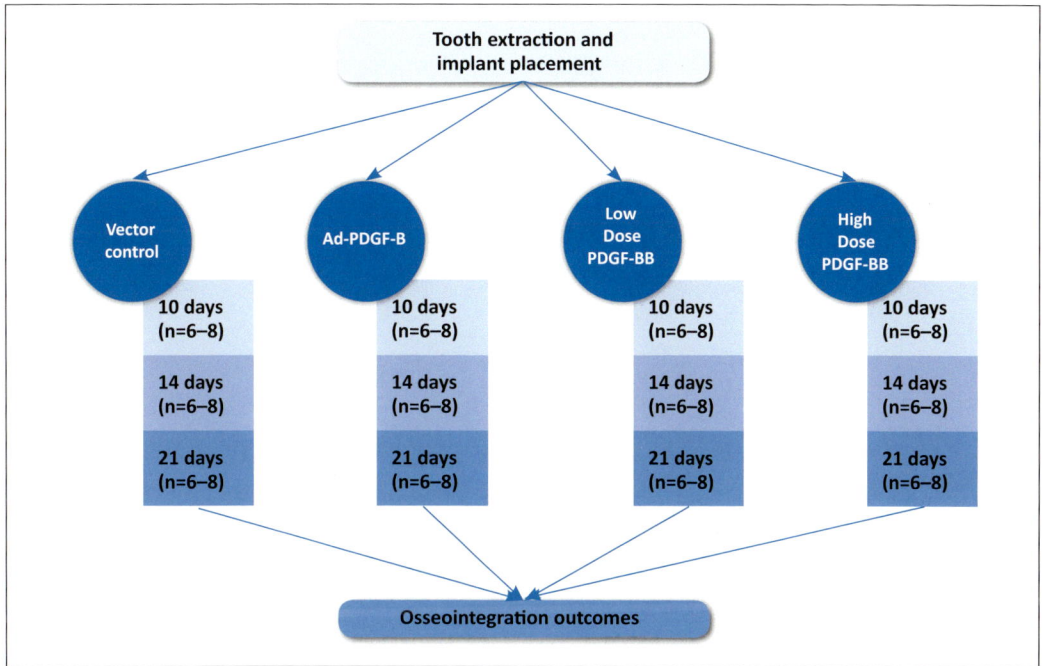

Fig 4-2 Schematic of study design used in Example 4.2.2.

length, the total bone fill area, and the proportions of mineralized tissue, nonmineralized tissue, and remaining BOG or BOB in the bone fill area.

4.2.4 Example 4.2.4

Huh and colleagues describe an experiment to examine the stability of miniplates used to bridge mandibular defects after osteotomy (Huh et al., 2006). Sixteen female dogs were each given a 15 mm excision of the mandible that was eventually resected. Four dogs were randomly assigned to each of four experimental conditions that varied by the number (one or two) of plates used, the type of screws (mono- and/or biocortical) used to attach the plate(s), and the borders of the mandible (superior and/or inferior) to which the plates were attached (Fig 4-4). The dogs were given regular diets and examined after 6 weeks for five different binary outcomes: plate exposure, plate fracture, plate bending, screw loosening, and infection.

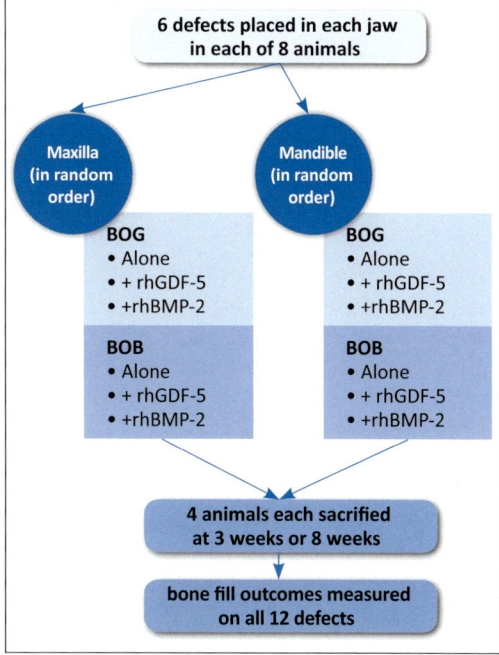

Fig 4-3 Schematic of study design used in Example 4.2.3.

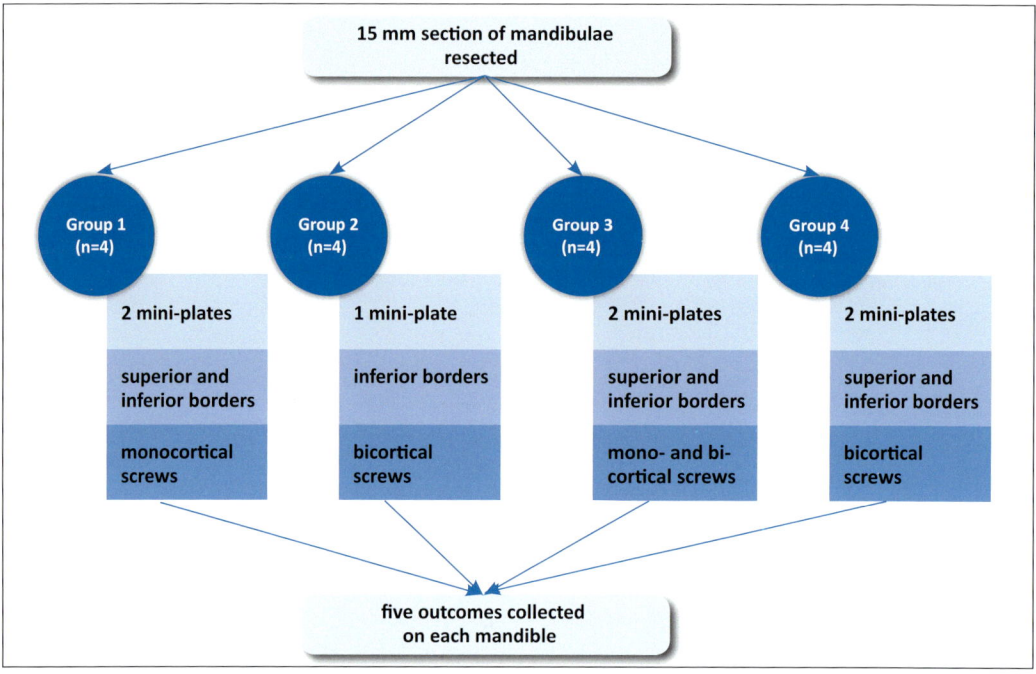

Fig 4-4 Schematic of study design used in Example 4.2.4.

4.3 Issues in Experimental Design

4.3.1 Specifying Hypotheses

Any scientific question of interest must be expressed as a pair of hypotheses under consideration. The alternative hypothesis is what the investigator hopes to show is true; the null hypothesis is everything contrary to the alternative hypothesis. In order for these hypotheses to be testable, the hypotheses must be expressed as explicitly as possible and must be stated in reference to measurable quantities comprising the data being collected. For example, statistical comparison of the alternative hypothesis "Simvastatin is necessary for bone reformation" versus the null hypothesis "Simvastatin is not necessary for bone reformation" is not possible as the hypotheses are devoid of specific and measurable quantities. First, "necessary" is a subjective and nonquantitative term. Second, there are several biological parameters that could be measured to assess bone reformation. The hypotheses should instead refer directly to the biologic parameter that will be examined in the experiment. Third, bone reformation is a process that occurs over time. The hypotheses must state the point in time after implant when bone formation will be assessed. After clarifying these three issues, a better alternative hypothesis would be "the average percentage of reossification of the bone defect center 30 days after implant differs between mice receiving simvastatin and mice receiving placebo". The corresponding null hypothesis would be "the average percentage of reossification of the bone defect center 30 days after implant is the same for mice receiving simvastatin and mice receiving placebo".

4.3.2 Sample Size Considerations

From a statistical standpoint, there are four quantities that need to be specified *before* an experiment commences. These four quantities will determine n, the sample size, or number of independent units that need to be studied in any preclinical experiment. The first two quantities, usually represented by the Greek letters α and β, are error probabilities that quantify acceptable rates of incorrect conclusions. The first error probability, α, is known as type I error or false positive rate, and quantifies the probability that an experiment will make a positive conclusion (reject the null hypothesis) when a negative conclusion (fail to reject the null hypothesis) should have been reached.

The second error probability, β, is known as the type II error or false negative rate, and quantifies the probability that an experiment will lead to a negative conclusion (fail to reject the null hypothesis) when a positive conclusion (reject the null hypothesis) should have been reached. It is also common for studies to be designed around the desired *power* of the experiment, which is simply $1 - \beta$, the desired true positive rate of the experiment.

Historically, and for mostly undocumented reasons, the values $\alpha = 0.05$ and $\beta = 0.20$ are the error rates set in most preclinical experiments. However, these values should be viewed as benchmarks that can be varied depending on the requirements of the experiment. When using the standard values $\alpha = 0.05$ and $\beta = 0.20$, we make the implicit judgment that a false positive conclusion, i.e., concluding a significant result exists when none truly does, is four times as "bad" as a false negative conclusion, i.e. failing to conclude a significant result exists when it actually does. In the early discovery phase of preclinical research, an investigator may be comfortable with a higher false positive rate, such as $\alpha = 0.10$, so as to increase the probability of finding even mildly interesting signals in the data. These findings will then be examined more stringently in later stage experiments to remove the false positive findings. It is during these later confirmatory phases of preclinical research where an investigator may also wish to limit the probability of false negative findings to a more stringent level of, perhaps, $\beta = 0.10$.

Once an investigator determines appropriate levels of type I and type II errors, the next quantity to specify is the quantitative difference between the two null and alternative hypotheses. The Greek letter Δ typically denotes this difference. With regard to the hypotheses stated in Section 4.3.1, Δ would quantify the difference in rates of reossification between mice receiving simvastatin and mice receiving placebo that investigators feel is large enough so as to be clinically interesting and warrant further research. For example, if investigators felt that a difference of 10 percentage points would warrant clinical research into the use of simvastatin with bone healing, then the sample size would be determined using a value of $\Delta = 0.10$.

The final quantity that is needed for determining sample size is denoted by the Greek letter σ, and describes how much the data are expected to vary about their average. If the data are approximately normally distributed around the mean, then a majority of the data will be within 2σ of the mean. Of the four quantities necessary for sample size calculations, variance is the one quantity that is a (fixed) characteristic of the data and is not up to the discretion of the investigators. As a result, the variance must either be known, or a rough estimate must be determined from pilot data or an existing publication prior to commencing with a sample size calculation.

Although specific sample size formulae and rules of thumb have been created for a variety of settings (for examples, see van Belle, 2008 and Whitley and Ball, 2002), the necessary sample size is typically proportional to $(\sigma/\Delta)^2$, where the constant of proportionality is a function of the error rates α, β, as well as the number of groups being compared and type of data being collected. Thus, when designing a study, it is more useful to express Δ in units relative to σ, rather than the absolute value of Δ by itself. More importantly, the value of Δ by itself is insufficient for determining a sample size until it is accompanied by a value for σ. As an example, imagine an experiment designed to compare two treatment groups assuming the standard false positive and false negative values of $\alpha = 0.05$ and $\beta = 0.20$, respectively. In this example, the constant of proportionality is 16, i.e., each group should consist of approximately $16(\sigma/\Delta)^2$ independent units, for a total of $32(\sigma/\Delta)^2$ independent units studied in the entire experiment. Thus, for an effect size Δ equal to one standard deviation, i.e. $\sigma/\Delta = 1$, a total of 32 independent units, divided equally between the two groups, must be studied. It is often not appreciated that the sample size increases quickly with small increases in Δ or small increases in σ due to the exponent of two in the computation. Specifically, halving of Δ or doubling of σ, i.e., $\sigma/\Delta = 2$, causes the necessary sample size to quadruple.

Investigators should also recognize that existing sample size formulae were generated from specific hypothetical settings that were likely much simpler than the current experiment is. As a result, generic sample size formulae can provide rough approximations to the necessary sample size, but a more precise sample size estimate requires statistical simulation of the experiment at hand. These simulations can sometimes be time-consuming to both conceptually develop and physically program. As a result, generating appropriate sample size estimates can take anywhere from a few minutes to a few days, depending on the complexity of the experiment.

It should also be noted that many preclinical experiments are precursors to larger, hypothesis-confirming experiments. As such, the smaller preclinical experiment is designed primarily to both develop reasonable hypotheses for later study, as well as study the feasibility of performing experiments to address these hypotheses. These smaller experiments are often termed "pilot studies". In these experiments, the number of independent units that will be studied is most often determined by the amount of monetary, human, and/or time resources that can be devoted to the experiment, rather than from a specific sample size calculation. It is frequent to see published results from experiments of $n = 5$ independent units per group, which often is sufficient to detect extremely large effect sizes. However, it should be emphasized that this value of n was not developed to address a specific hypothesis, nor was it developed to maintain specific rates of false positive and false negative errors. As a result, any statistical tests applied to data from a pilot study suffer from both low power and higher than desired false positive (type I) errors. These weaknesses do not necessarily invalidate results from pilot studies, but they weaken greatly the strength of evidence that pilot data can provide in support of a hypothesis.

It cannot be emphasized strongly enough that sample size and the quantities needed to compute sample size are issues to be addressed *before* the experiment is executed. Once the experiment is completed, the data will lead to either a significant or a nonsignificant result. Using the data after the fact to determine what the power of the experiment would have been or what the correct sample size should have been are exercises in futility and provide no evidence of the merit or lack thereof for the completed experiment.

It is a common misconception that if an experiment fails to produce a significant result, i.e., the P value is too large, it follows that the experiment has shown the null hypothesis to be true. However, such a conclusion can *never* be reached, as hypothesis testing is designed to either reject or fail to reject the *alternative* hypothesis only. Furthermore, a P value is highly dependent upon the sample size of the experiment. Thus, an insignificant P value is not evidence of the null hypothesis being true, but is rather evidence of an insufficient sample size to determine the veracity of the alternative hypothesis. If a large P value was evidence of a true null hypothesis, then all preclinical experiments would require no more than two independent units, as such an experiment would always produce a large P value. However, such an experiment is never done, precisely because it would fail to provide any worthwhile evidence for any hypothesis because the sample size is too small.

4.3.3 The Necessity of Replications

Preclinical experiments often take triplicate ($m = 3$) measures of each independent unit and use the mean of those three values as the single value from each sample that will be used in the statistical analysis. However, little thought is often given to whether replication is necessary, and if so, how many times each independent unit should be measured in order to provide "good" data. The answer to these questions is based on two quantities: σ_a^2, the among-sample variability, or the amount of variability that inherently exists among different independent units, and σ_w^2, the within-sample variability, or the amount of variability produced when inaccurately measuring the same independent unit repeatedly (Singer et al., 2007). Furthermore, the impact of σ_a^2 and σ_w^2 is determined by their magnitudes relative to each other.

We let the non-negative quantity, $q = \sigma_w^2/\sigma_a^2$, denote the amount variability produced when measuring the same independent unit repeatedly relative to the variability produced when measuring two different independent units. When $q = 0$, this implies that $\sigma_w^2 = 0$, meaning there is no variability among repeated measures on the same independent unit, which further implies that we get the same value every time we measure the independent unit. This is the (nearly always unrealistic) situation when replication is useless ($m = 1$), as every time we measure the independent unit, we get exactly the same value, which produces no additional information regarding the independent unit. As q moves in value away from zero, replication will become necessary, as every time we measure the independent unit, we get a different value. As q continues to increase, the need for replication and number of replications continues to increase as well.

The need for replication becomes apparent when examining the variance of the mean of the replications for each independent unit (which, for brevity, we refer to as the replication mean), which will comprise the data that will be analyzed. If m replications are averaged together, the replication mean has variance $\sigma^2 = \sigma_a^2 + \sigma_w^2/m = \sigma_a^2 (1+q/m)$. Since m appears in the denominator, each additional replication serves to reduce the variance of the replication means. The number of necessary replications (m) will depend upon the amount of between- and within-sample variability, as well as the level of variability necessary for the desired power and resulting sample size of the experiment.

For example, let us assume that the variability among values from different independent units has a value of $\sigma_a^2 = 0.8$, while variability among replications of the sample independent unit has a value of $\sigma_w^2 = 0.6$. These values of σ_a^2 and σ_w^2 lead to a total variance of $\sigma^2 = 0.8 + 0.6/m$ for the replication mean for each independent unit. Suppose our sample size has been determined with a value of $\sigma^2 = 1$, so that the replication mean for each independent unit must have a variance of 1.0 in order for the experiment to have sufficient power to support the alternative hypothesis being examined. We would therefore need three replications ($m = 3$) for each sample in order to maintain the variability among the replication means to 1.0. However, suppose that the replications are rather easy to measure accurately and σ_w^2 is only 0.2. Due to the small amount of variability among replications, only one replication for each independent unit is needed in order to maintain the desired level of variation. However, if σ_w^2 was 2.0 instead, then $m = 10$ replications would be required, which is probably unfeasible for most experiments. The only solution to maintain the desired power of the experiment would be to increase n, the number of independent units.

However, there is no one-to-one trade-off between n and m. Specifically, if the budget for the experiment requires a reduction in the number of independent units studied, the power of the study cannot be maintained by simply proportionally increasing the number of replications per independent unit. For example, suppose that we plan an experiment of 20 animals and each animal will be analyzed twice. Further suppose each animal costs 2,000 and each replicate sample per animal costs 500, so that the entire experiment costs 20 × (2,000 + 500 × 2) = 60,000. Although we could lower the entire cost of the experiment to 40,000 if we measured four replications (double the number of replications) on each of 10 animals (halve the number of animals), this new design does not have the same statistical power as the original design. Using an approximate sample size calculation, it can be seen that with four replications per animal, the experiment would require 17 animals, which although less than the original 20, is much larger than the suggested value of 10.

4.3.4 Use of a Split-mouth Design

Replication is a useful study design technique to adequately control, and hopefully reduce, the amount of noise in an experiment. As described in Section 4.3.3, replication assumes that each independent unit is measured more than once, but always under the same experimental condition, i.e., treatment group.

A split-mouth design is related to the idea of replication, in that the end goal is to reduce the amount of noise in the experiment. Like replication, each independent unit is measured several times in a split-mouth design. However, unlike replication, each measurement of the independent unit is made from a different experimental condition. Example 4.2.3 is one example of an experiment using this design. In a standard design, each independent unit (dog) would have been randomly assigned to a single treatment group and possibly measured more than once. One weakness of such a design is that the variability between independent units may be rather big, making it difficult to identify differences among the treatment groups unless a large number of independent units are studied.

As an alternative to the standard design, the investigators in Example 4.2.3 randomly assigned each of the six treatment groups to a separate region in the mouth of each independent unit, thereby reducing the number of independent units required for the experiment. Such a design is known as a split-mouth design and was first suggested for use in clinical trials in 1968 by Ramfjord *et al.*, although the concepts discussed are equally applicable to preclinical experiments. Although there are possible benefits to be realized from a split-mouth design, namely reducing the number of independent units required for the experiment, there are necessary assumptions and requirements underlying the validity of a split-mouth design. Unless investigators can provide sufficient evidence that the necessary assumptions and requirements hold for their current experiment, the validity of any results produced from the experiment will be greatly suspect. We now describe these assumptions in greater detail; for further discussion, see Hujoel (1998) and Lesaffre *et al.* (2009).

First, the regions of the mouth in each independent unit must be randomly assigned to the treatment groups so that no treatment group is assigned to the same region of the mouth in a majority of the independent units. Randomization helps to ensure that any differences seen between the treatment groups can be explained solely by the treatment groups and not by the regions of the mouth.

Second, in the absence of treatment, the outcome measure must be relatively stable and uniformly distributed throughout the mouth. Otherwise, there is a possibility of one or more of the treatment groups being assigned disproportionately to areas with more severe, or harder to measure, outcomes, thereby making it unclear if any results seen are truly due to differences among the treatments or differences among the outcomes assigned to the treatments.

Third, the effect of each treatment being evaluated must be localized, thereby removing the possibility of any "spill-over" or "carry-over" effect within the mouth. For example, suppose we have a study in which treatments A and B are randomly assigned to the maxilla and mandible of each experimental unit. If it is discovered that treatment B has systemic, rather than local, effects on the outcome to be collected from each jaw, it will be impossible to compare the two treatments with each other, since we cannot determine the effect of treatment A on the outcome separately from the effect of treatment B on the outcome.

Fourth, it is of utmost importance to ensure that faulty or immeasurable outcomes are avoided as much as possible, and ideally, will be avoided completely. A split-mouth design, by definition, requires a comparison among outcomes from the same experimental unit. Faulty or missing outcomes for an experimental unit reduce the contribution that unit can make to the eventual findings of the study. For example, suppose again that we have treatments A and B randomly assigned to the maxilla and mandible of each independent unit. If the outcome from the mandible of an independent unit is lost or unable to be measured, then the corresponding outcome from the maxilla has nothing to which it can be compared. As a result, that experimental unit contributes no information to the experiment, thereby reducing the sample size of the experiment by one unit, as well as the overall power of the experiment.

Fifth, the analysis of data from a split-mouth design must be analyzed with methods that account for the fact that some outcomes belong to the same experimental unit (mouth). Basic statistical methods, such as those described in Sections 4.4.1 to 4.4.3, assume that each outcome is independent, i.e., the outcomes from the same mouth are mistakenly assumed to come from different mouths. The impact of this mistake is to use statistical methods that are less powerful and make it less likely to find a significant result if one truly exists.

4.4 Issues in Statistical Analysis

4.4.1 *t* tests and Analysis of Variance (ANOVA)

A *t* test is a statistical test for comparing two experimental conditions in which each independent unit belongs to only one of the experimental conditions and all units in an experimental condition are not related to any members of the other experimental conditions. Furthermore, the outcome measured on each experimental condition is continuous. In this setting, the *t* test is sometimes referred to more accurately as a two-sample or independent-samples *t* test.

The null (alternative) hypothesis for the *t* test is that the mean outcome in one experimental condition is equal (not equal) to the mean outcome in the other experimental condition. To determine whether or not the null hypothesis will be rejected in favor of the alternative hypothesis, the sample mean of the outcomes in each experimental condition is computed, as well as the sample standard deviation of the outcomes in each experimental condition. The difference in the two sample means is our signal, and a pooled average of the two standard deviations is our noise. We divide the signal by the noise to create our statistic, which can be viewed as a score. The larger the magnitude of the score (we do not care which group has the larger mean, so a score of, say, −5 is equivalent to a score of +5), the more likely we are to reject the null hypothesis and conclude that the experimental conditions have different means.

However, a large score could also be observed simply by chance when the two experimental conditions are equal (null hypothesis is true).

Thus, we ask ourselves, if the two groups are truly not different from each other, what is the probability of observing our score or any score higher in magnitude? This is the P value. If the P value is "small enough", then we conclude that our results are in conflict with null hypothesis, and so we reject the null hypothesis. If the P value is not "small enough", then we conclude that our results are not in conflict with the null hypothesis and we fail to reject the null hypothesis (but do not accept the null hypothesis). "Small enough" is defined as being less than the desired type I error rate (α), which is typically set at 0.05.

If more than two experimental conditions are to be compared, we use analysis of variance (ANOVA), which is simply a generalization of the two-sample t test. In other words, one could use ANOVA to compare two experimental conditions, and doing so would be identical to using a two-sample t test. When comparing more than two groups, the null hypothesis is that all of the groups have the same mean outcome, while the alternative is that at least two of the groups have different mean outcomes. As with the t test, ANOVA compares the differences between the sample means of the experimental conditions and compares this difference to an estimate of the noise, or variability, seen in the data. The resulting test to determine whether or not to reject the null hypothesis is called an F test. If the F test concludes that we should reject the null hypothesis, we conclude that at least two of the groups (and possibly more) have different mean outcomes.

However, the F test in ANOVA supplies no information regarding *which* or *how many* groups differ. Thus, if we use ANOVA to compare several groups and find there is a difference, we would then compare the means of every possible pair of groups using a two-sample t test to determine which groups truly differ from each other. These t tests are commonly referred to as *post hoc* tests, as they are done after the results of the primary F test are known.

Note that the statistical theory behind t tests and ANOVA assumes that the outcomes from each experimental condition have a normal distribution. Thus, many investigators mistakenly believe that t tests cannot be used with non-normal or skewed data. In reality, t tests and ANOVA are very insensitive to modestly skewed data, meaning that the results (P values) produced from t tests and ANOVA are valid and acceptable in most realistic settings, regardless of normality. Furthermore, although one can assess normality of their data, either by plotting the data, or by doing a formal statistical test of normality, these assessments are fraught with error and perform poorly unless one has an amount of data that is much larger than what is collected in most experiments.

The examples presented in Sections 4.2.1 and 4.2.2 are both experiments in which two-sample t tests and ANOVA would be appropriate analysis methods. The experiments of Anabinder et al. contained eight independent groups of animals, depending on the agent given, route of administration, and time of sacrifice. These eight groups could be compared using ANOVA, while comparisons of any two of the groups could be done using a two-sample t test.

4.4.2 Rank (Nonparametric) Tests

If the amount of skewness is felt to be more than what is desired, there are counterparts to the two-sample t test and ANOVA that can be used to compare the experimental conditions. Generally speaking, the experimental conditions are now being compared with respect to their medians, rather than their means because the data have skewed distributions. Rather than analyzing the outcomes directly, each outcome is first replaced by its rank among all the data, i.e., the lowest value in the data is given a rank of 1, the next lowest value is given a rank of 2, etc. With heavily skewed data, the ranks tend to be much less skewed than the original data. Thus, we can apply t tests or ANOVA to the ranks rather than the original observations to assess differences among the experimental conditions. A *t* test (when comparing two groups) applied to the ranks is formally known as a Wilcoxon rank sum test or a Mann-Whitney U test, while ANOVA (when comparing more than two groups) applied to the ranks is formally known as a Kruskal-Wallis test.

As stated in Section 4.4.1, *t* tests and ANOVA are rather insensitive to modest skewness that may be apparent in the data. As a result, investigators should realize that the *P* value that results from using a *t* test or ANOVA will differ very little from the *P* value that results from using the corresponding rank-based approach. Thus, although the authors in the examples presented in Sections 4.2.1 and 4.2.2 chose to use *t* tests and ANOVA to analyze their data, they could have instead chosen instead to use rank tests, with little change to the conclusions they reached.

4.4.3 Chi-squared Tests and Fisher's Exact Test
Similar to a *t* test or ANOVA, a chi-squared test is used for comparing multiple experimental conditions in which each independent unit belongs to only one of the experimental conditions and all units in an experimental condition are not related to any members of the other experimental conditions. However, unlike a *t* test or ANOVA, a chi-squared test is used when the outcome measured on each experimental condition is now categorical rather than continuous. The number of possible categories that each outcome can take should be limited to a small number, say four or five; when there are only two possible categories, the categorical outcome is said to be binary.

In this setting, the null hypothesis states that all groups have the same distribution of outcomes among the possible categories, while the alternative hypothesis states that the groups have differing distributions of outcomes among the possible categories, i.e., one experimental condition may tend to have a majority of outcomes in one category while another experimental condition may tend to have a majority of outcomes in a different category. Thus, if we reject the null hypothesis, we conclude that the number of outcomes that fall into each category is dependent on, or associated with, the experimental condition to which each outcome belongs. Thus, a chi-squared test is more precisely referred to as a chi-squared test *of association*.

A chi-squared test of association, when rejecting the null hypothesis, concludes that experimental conditions differ with regard to the distribution of units among the possible categories. As such, this conclusion is rather unspecific, as it does not specify *how* the distributions differ from each other. For example, suppose we have an experiment consisting of two groups of 15 animals each. After two weeks, we examine each of the 30 animals for bone growth, categorized as low, moderate, and high. We find that one group has five animals falling into each of the three categories of bone growth. A chi-squared test of association would make the same conclusion whether (a) the other group had 1, 2, and 8 animals, with low, moderate, and high bone growth, respectively, or (b) the other group had 8, 1, and 2 animals with low, moderate, and high bone growth, respectively. However, results (a) and (b) tell distinctly different stories with regard to how the groups differ from each other. Thus, although a chi-squared test of association is useful for determining if differences exist among the experimental conditions, the test should be supplemented with a summary of the data to determine how the experimental conditions differ.

The *P* value generated for a chi-squared test is an approximation that tends to perform poorly in experiments with small samples of data. Specifically, when some experimental conditions have few or no outcomes in one or more of the categories, the *P* value may be lower than it should be. The example given in the previous paragraph is an example of such a situation in which a chi-squared test may be inappropriate, as one of the groups has only one or two outcomes in two of the categories. Fisher's exact test is a test that is often used as

Osteology Guidelines for Oral and Maxillofacial Regeneration

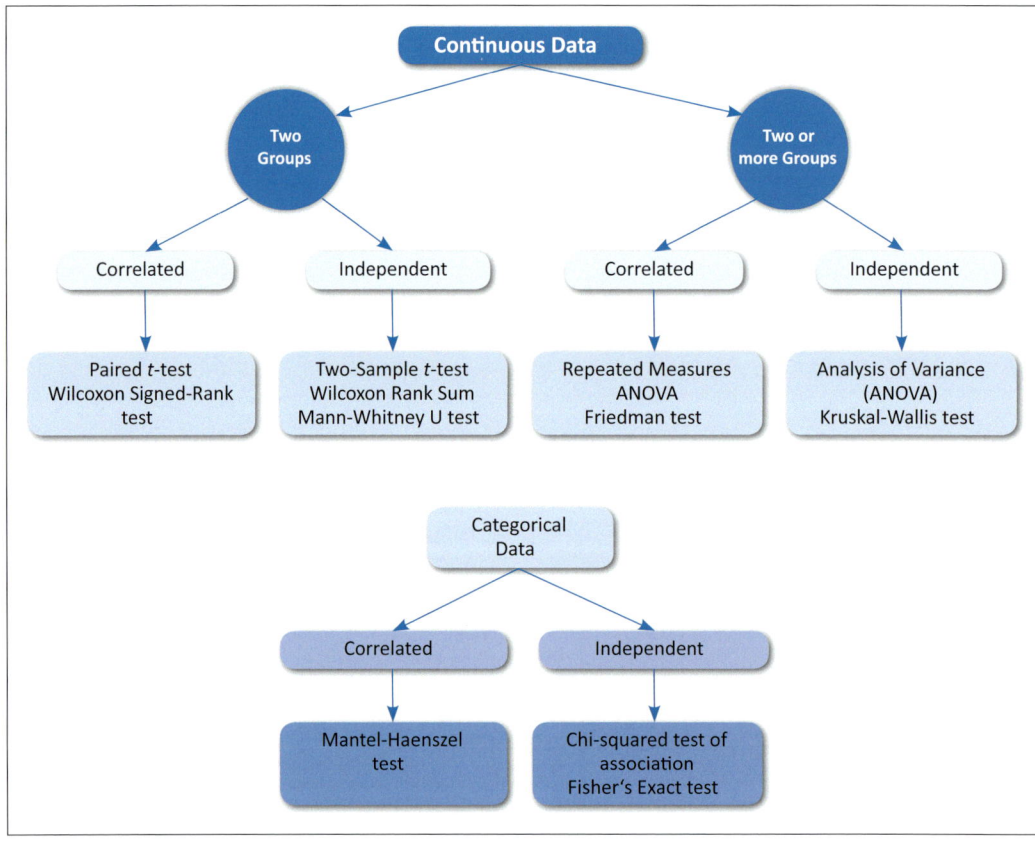

Fig 4-5 Flow chart of statistical methods useful with preclinical data.

a replacement for the chi-squared test. However, as with *t* tests and ANOVA and their rank-based counterparts, the results from Fisher's exact test and a chi-squared test rarely differ enough to substantially affect the overall conclusions of the experiment.

The data collected from the experiment in Example 4.2.4 would be suitably analyzed with chi-squared tests of association, with the caveat that a single categorical outcome, such as any plate exposure or any screw loosening, were measured on each animal. One could then compare the proportions of animals with any plate exposure or the proportions of animals with any screw loosening among the four experimental conditions. However, the investigators in this experiment instead chose to compare the proportions of plates that were exposed and the proportions of screws that loosened among the four treatment groups. Given that some animals had more than one plate and/or more than one screw, not all of the plates or all of the screws are independent units, and a chi-squared test is inappropriate for analysis of these proportions. The correct analysis method for this experiment will be discussed in the next section.

4.4.4 Extensions for Non-independent Data

The statistical methods described in Sections 4.4.1 to 4.4.3 all assume that a single outcome is collected from each independent unit. Put another way, each outcome collected in an experiment must have no relationship with all other outcomes collected in the experiment. This assumption of statistical independence is crucial to the validity of the P values that result from the methods in Sections 4.4.1 to 4.4.3. If the assumption of independence is violated, then the variability (noise) among the experimental conditions is underestimated, which leads to test statistics that are too large and P values that are too small. As a result, an experiment is more likely to conclude a significant difference exists among the experimental conditions, even if one does not exist, leading to an inflated rate of type I errors, or false positive findings.

For experiments in which some dependence between experimental outcomes exists, i.e., two teeth of each experimental unit are studied, both jaws of each experimental unit are studied, or each experimental unit is measured under two or more experimental conditions, simple extensions exist for the methods presented in Sections 4.4.1 to 4.4.3. A two-sample t test would be replaced with a paired t test, while ANOVA would be replaced with repeated measures ANOVA. The Wilcoxon rank sum test would be replaced with a Wilcoxon signed-rank test, and the Kruskal-Wallis test would be replaced with the Friedman test. A chi-squared test of association would be replaced with a Mantel-Haenszel test. Many of these approaches are also simplified versions of more general methods for non-independent data known as linear and generalized linear mixed models (LMMs and GLMMs) and generalized estimating equations (GEEs) (Omar *et al.*, 1999). Figure 4-5 presents a flowchart that shows what tests are appropriate for different types of data.

References

1. Anabinder AL, Junqueira JC, Mancini MNG, Balducci I, da Rocha RF, Carvalho, YR (2006). Influence of simvastatin on bone regeneration of tibial defects and blood cholesterol level in rats. *Braz Dent J* 17:267–274.
2. Chang PC, Seol YJ, Cirelli JA, Pellegrini G, Jin Q, Franco LM *et al*. (2010). PDGF-B gene therapy accelerates bone engineering and oral implant osseointegration. *Gene Ther* 17:95-104.
3. Huh JY, Choi BH, Zhu SJ, Jung JH, Lee SH, You TM *et al*. (2006). Bridging mandibular continuity defects with miniplates: an experimental study. *Oral Surg Oral Med Oral Pathol Oral Radiol Endod* 102:307–311.
4. Hujoel P (1998). Design and analysis issues in split-mouth clinical trials. *Community Dent Oral Epidemiol* 26:85–86.
5. Lesaffre E, Philstrom B, Needleman I, Worthington H (2009). The design and analysis of split-mouth studies: What statisticians and clinicians should know. *Stat Med* 28:3470–3482.
6. Omar RZ, Wright EM, Turne RM, Thompson SG (1999). Analyzing repeated measurements data: a practical comparison of methods. *Stat Med* 18:1587–1604.
7. Ramfjord S, Nissle R, Shick R, Cooper H (1968). Subgingival curettage versus surgical elimination of periodontal pockets. *J Periodontol* 39:167–175.
8. Schwarz F, Rothamel D, Herten M, Ferrari D, Sager M, Becker J (2008). Lateral ridge augmentation using particulated or block bone substitutes biocoated with rhGDF-5 and rhBMP-2: an immunohistochemical study in dogs. *Clin Oral Implants Res* 19:642–652.
9. Singer JM, Pedroso-de-Lima AC, Tanaka NI, Gonzalez-Lopez VA (2007). To tripicate or not to triplicate? *Chemometr Intell Lab Syst* 86:82–85.
10. van Belle G (2008). Statistical rules of thumb, 2nd ed. Oxford: Wiley-Blackwell.
11. Whitley E, Ball J (2002). Statistics review 4: sample size calculations. *Crit Care* 6:335–341.

CHAPTER 5

Screening Models for Tissue Engineering

Myron Spector, Khalid Al-Hezaimi, and Marc L. Nevins

5.1 General Overview

5.1.1 Roles of Screening Models in the Development of Devices for Oral and Maxillofacial Regeneration

In vivo tests of the tissue response to implants represent just one facet of the evaluation of candidate implant materials/devices. The myriad tests included under the heading of "biocompatibility" reflect the wide variation in the different components to the host response to implants. Implantation tests can be employed to assess the efficacy of devices (functional effectiveness of devices) as well as the safety of the materials of fabrication. The term "biocompatible" is employed to describe a wide variety of (generally *in vivo*) findings, from a benign tissue response to a biomaterial in an animal model to the successful clinical implementation of a medical device. Moreover, the term is also often used to generally describe biomaterials which have met certain standards of safety and efficacy in select situations. While there is convenience in using the term "biocompatibility" to convey a general assessment of a biomaterial or medical device, its nonspecific use can be misleading. Its use should be qualified with respect to the specific conditions under which the biomaterial/device is being evaluated. The device should be considered biocompatible only in the context of the criteria used to assess the acceptability of the tissue response in relation to the required function of the device.

This chapter will deal with select protocols that have been found to be of value for the initial *in vivo* screening of implants. While most of these implants comprise nonresorbable biomaterials, they can be adapted for use with scaffolds for tissue engineering and regenerative medicine and for tissue-engineered constructs. Preclinical tests required for qualification of the device for human trial are generally directed toward the evaluation of the device in animal models – often using large animals – that approach the specific clinical application in which the device is to be used. Because these preclinical test protocols, which are the subjects of other chapters in this book, are expensive and time-consuming, it is important to prescreen the device in less complex animal experiments, which can provide an indication whether the next step of preclinical testing is warranted.

Experiments involving the implantation of materials into animal tissues date back to the early 1800s. The level of interest in devising more effective chronic implantation protocols has increased significantly during the last 20 years. This is due to:
- The need for new materials with properties that satisfy the ever-increasing functional demands of implant devices
- The availability of new candidate implant materials, especially the large number of tissue engineering products
- The increasing awareness of the complexity of the biological response to biomaterials.

Most recently there has been an increased awareness that standardized screening protocols need to be developed. Such standardized protocols are considered by many as essential for "evidence-based medicine" and to facilitate the requirements of federal regulatory agencies. The elements of the screening protocol include the:
- Species: gender and age
- Site of implantation
- Shape of the implant
- Period of implantation
- Method of evaluation of the tissue response
- Criteria for determining if the response in the animal model is potentially harmful to the human host.

The problematic aspects of this type of testing include:
- Identification of an experimental animal and site of implantation that will serve as an adequate model of the human response
- The selection of a shape of implant and site of implantation that will adequately distinguish the response elicited by the chemical formulation of the specimen from tissue responses to the implant shape, mechanical trauma associated with the very presence of the implant, and the wound healing processes
- The selection of criteria to determine if the animal response can be used to predict whether the material can be safely used in the human host.

Despite these challenging aspects of implantation testing, there has been no disputing the implementation of screening protocols to assist in the initial determination of the safety and potential efficacy of candidate implant materials.

Tissue engineering concepts for oral and maxillofacial regeneration require appropriate models to test osteogenic devices. A strategic approach to preclinical testing is needed to determine the *in vivo* performance of material devices for oral wound healing. There is a significant complexity to the healing *in vivo* compared with the *in vitro* environment. There is the need for various studies on a particular biomaterial, biologic agent or device including safety and efficacy studies in multiple models prior to proceeding to Phase I human clinical trials.

There are multiple factors that affect osseous bone healing that are best evaluated in the *in vivo* environment, including biomechanical, cellular, and vascular mechanics that comprise the healing process. The models chosen to assess a particular device should mimic the environment in which the device will be used therapeutically. One should choose a "critical-size defect" that will not spontaneously regenerate, to best characterize the contribution of the device to healing. Tissue engineering devices can be screened in various preclinical animal models to determine their potential. Depending on the knowledge base and previous data on a product one can choose the appropriate model to screen the potential of a new device. For new technology it is advised to begin with small animal models which can provide early data in a relatively fast and cost-effective way. The research can then progress to large animal wound systems that simulate more closely the human wound and therapeutic environment, more closely associated with the planned clinical application of the device.

The goal of this chapter is to provide a stepwise "roadmap" for evaluating potential biomaterials to be utilized for bone healing such as: osteoconductive or osteoinductive systems, either passive or bioactive scaffolds, and biomimetic systems. It is necessary to demonstrate adequate safety and efficacy prior to moving to more complex preclinical models, and it is advised to gather adequate data from small animal models prior to investing economically in large animal model research.

5.1.2 Historical Perspective on Implantation Protocols

While a chronological review of the implant literature can be instructive in revealing how an understanding of the tissue response to materials evolved, it can also be confounding. Tissue responses observed in experimental studies have varied considerably with the animal model, site of implantation, and shape of the implant. For example, while no adverse response was elicited by a cobalt-chrome specimen implanted in bone, fibrosarcoma was found adjacent to films of the same material implanted in subcutaneous sites in the rat. Results of this type evidence the need for some degree of standardization of screening protocols. Only a few studies reported in the literature have had as their objective the development of an implantation protocol to be used in the assessment of the safety of candidate implant materials. Most implantation investigations have had as their focus the tissue response elicited by specific materials. The choice of the site of implantation was most often determined by the projected use of the material. Little rationale beyond the availability and ease of handling was generally given for the choice of animal model. Routine histopathological examination of tissue adjacent to the implant material was most often the method of evaluation of the biologic response. Generally very little discussion was directed toward the influence of implantation time or size and shape of the implant on the biologic response. In addition, little mention was made of the criteria that might be appropriate for interpreting the changes observed in the host tissue adjacent to the implant. Nevertheless these studies have generated the data which serve as the foundation for an understanding of subacute tissue responses to biomaterials. The protocols that we now accept as standardized screening tests are those specific protocols which have been "validated" through repeated use by different groups. Their utility has been demonstrated in the consistent results that they generate.

5.1.3 Determinants Underlying the Tissue Response to Implants

Determinants of the tissue response to biomaterials, and the subsequent assessment of biocompatibility, reside in the intrinsic wound healing process in the particular tissue or organ into which the biomaterial has been implanted. This wound healing process, initiated by the surgical trauma of implantation, can be modulated by: the physical presence of the device, and its porosity and modulus of elasticity; and the chemical composition of the material and agents released by the biomaterial. The tissue response to a biomaterial is, therefore, a characteristic of the host tissue's wound healing process as well as being a characteristic of the biomaterial. There is often an implication that a biomaterial which displays a favorable (biocompatible) response in a particular test (i.e., tissue) has met the condition of biocompatibility for all applications in which it may be used. In light of the above, the tissue response to the same biomaterial might be quite different depending on the tissue in which it is implanted. Biocompatibility is not, therefore, an invariant property of a biomaterial.

5.2 Models for Bone and Soft Tissue Implants

5.2.1 Extraoral Bone Defects
Screening protocols have been employed for decades to assess the osseous response to the chemical make-up, pore structure, and surface features (at the nanometer, micrometer, and millimeter scales) of implants. These studies have been directed to evaluate the degree to which implants fabricated from certain biomaterials and with surface features become osseointegrated, and the amount of bone that forms within surface and internal pores (i.e., "bone ingrowth") of porous implants. The results, quantitatively, can be influenced by the type of bone into which the implant is placed, e.g., cortical versus cancellous, based on the available pools of osteoprogenitor cells available to participate in the bone regeneration process.

5.2.2 Advantages of the Circumscribed Defect Model in Long Bones
One of the first protocols to be used systematically (Melcher and Irving, 1962) to compare the osseous response to a variety of biomaterials involved implantation into cylindrical (circumscribed) defects through the cortex and into the medullary canal of the femoral diaphysis of rats (Melcher and Irving, 1962), rabbits, and dogs (Spector et al., 1976).

One of the advantages of this model is that the response of both cortical and cancellous bone to the implant can be evaluated. In addition, for larger animals, such as dogs, goats, and sheep, six implants can be implanted into each femur. Moreover, an option to harvesting all of the implants at the time of sacrifice is to biopsy select implants at various time periods post-implantation (Spector et al., 1976). These aspects of the consideration of the critical-size defect model have been under scrutiny over the past years (Horner et al., 2010; Reichert et al., 2009).

5.2.3 Surgical Procedure in the Circumscribed Defect Model in Long Bones
A longitudinal incision is made in the skin overlying the lateral aspect of the femur. The thigh muscles are separated and the lateral aspect of the femur is exposed. The holes are produced with a slow-speed power (e.g., dental drill) or hand drill, operated under ample irrigation for cooling. The diameter of the holes and depth are adjusted to the diameter of the femur. For example, for rats the hole diameter is 2 mm, and for dogs the holes are 4 to 6 mm in diameter. The medullary cavity is exposed, the wound irrigated with saline, and the implants inserted with a press-fit. In order to assure a proper interference fit of the cylindrical implant in the hole, a fluted reamer precision-machined to match the diameter of the implant can be used after the hole is prepared with the twist drill. After insertion of the implant the soft tissues are closed over the hole.

If the plan is to biopsy select implants prior to sacrifice, a trephine with a diameter 1 to 2 mm larger than the diameter of the implant can be used to remove the implant with a collar of surrounding bone. One difficulty with this procedure is that the bone regeneration process is generally so rapid and complete that it is difficult to precisely identify the location of the implants in the diaphysis. One option is to use a custom-designed drill guide to ensure reproducibility of the location and size of the defect and subsequent boring of the material within the defect after the designated implantation time (Orr et al., 2001). The drill jig is held onto the bone with two stainless steel guidewires and the guide hole used to locate the drill bit at the desired site of implantation. After the hole is drilled the jig is removed but the two stainless steel pins are left in the bone. At the time of the harvest, the corresponding recovery jig is fixed on the two stainless steel pins. The hole in the recovery jig is sized to accept the trephine used to core bore the implant and surrounding bone from the site of implantation.

5.2.4 Methods of Evaluation of the Circumscribed Defect Model in Long Bones

The circumscribed bone implant protocol lends itself to several methods of evaluation, including: mechanical testing, micro-computed tomography (CT), microradiography, and histology. The resected samples can be trimmed to enable mechanical test of the push-out strength (Chang *et al.*, 2010a; Chang *et al.*, 2010b). The bone surrounding the implant can be supported in a jig in a mechanical test machine and a plunger placed on the implant to enable a compressive load to be applied to push the sample out of the bone. The load to failure can be divided by the estimate of the implant–bone interfacial surface area to yield the interfacial shear strength. Specimens of the implant and surrounding bone which remain undecalcified can be (formalin) fixed immediately after resections from the bone or after mechanical testing and dehydrated and embedded in a plastic embedding resin. Sections approximately 100 μm can then be sawn from the blocks. These sections can be placed on high resolution X-ray film or digitized plate to yield contact radiographs with less than 1 mm resolution of bone features (i.e., microradiography). The 100 μm sections can subsequently be ground to about 40 μm and surface stained (e.g., with toluidine blue) and examined under a light microscope for "ground section histology". Alternatively the samples resected from the bone can be fixed, decalcified, dehydrated, and embedded in paraffin for histological evaluation.

These same methods of evaluation can be employed for implants in other sites, which are described below.

5.2.5 Mandibular Symphyseal Defect Model and Ramus Trephine Defect Model

Extraoral incisions are utilized to access the mandible for the use of the mandibular symphysis or the ramus for implantation. The ramus trephine defect creates a through-and-through defect due to the limited thickness of the ramus bone. The use of a trephine drill creates a critical-size defect that will not heal spontaneously, but which fills spontaneously with fibrous tissue. This defect lends itself to early testing for osteogenic response to a biomaterial implant.

For implantation into the ramus, an oblique incision is made over the ramus and the tissues are elevated to access the bone surface with full thickness blunt dissection. The defect is then created utilizing a trephine with rotary instrumentation. The implant is placed *in situ* and then the site is closed in two layers: first the muscle layer with internal absorbable sutures, and then the surface incision is sutured.

5.2.6 Calvarium Standardized Defect Model

Numerous studies have employed defects in the calvarium as the site in which to screen biomaterials for the bone response that they elicit, principally because the diameter of the critical-size defect is smaller than in long bone sites. Another advantage is that multiple defects can be produced in the same surgical field. An incision is made through the scalp to expose the periosteum, which is then elevated and retracted to expose the bone. Defects can be produced with standardized trephine burs, using continuous saline irrigation for cooling. The biomaterials can then be placed into the defects (Cooper *et al.*, 2010).

5.3 Models for Bone and Soft Tissue Implants

5.3.1 Soft Tissue Sites for Implantation – The Ectopic Bone Model

Several soft tissue sites of implantation have been proposed for screening protocols. The paravertebral muscle has been proposed because of its advantage of being large enough to host at least three implants per muscle (Coleman et al., 1974). In addition, this muscle provides a homogeneous implant environment and is easily accessible surgically. The disadvantage of the paravertebral muscle, however, is that it is mechanically active.

Sites in the subcutaneous tissue of rats and rabbits, and in the paravertebral muscles of the back of rabbits (Coleman et al., 1974), are sites frequently used to evaluate the soft tissue response to implants. For these procedures, the animals are positioned such that the operative site on the back of the animal can be shaved, and the skin cleaned and prepared for the sterile procedure. Sterile drapes are placed around the surgical area and attached to the skin with staples; 1 cm long incisions are made on each side of the spine, approximately 1.5 to 2 cm from the midline. Two subcutaneous pockets, one rostral and one caudal with 2 cm spacing, are made in each incision by blunt dissection. Four implant sites are thus prepared on the back of each animal and have also been demonstrated for other small animals such as mice and rats (Jin et al., 2008).

For intramuscular sites in rabbits, four longitudinal incisions about 1 cm long are made on the back of the animal. One superior and one inferior incision, located by the thoracic 9 to 11 and lumbar 3 to 4 spinous processes, are placed 1.2 to 2 cm apart on each side of the spine. The subcutaneous tissue and fascia are incised, and the tissues retracted to expose the underlying muscle. The muscle incision is sutured using 3-0 resorbable suture, and the skin incisions are closed using 4-0 interrupted suture.

5.3.2 Ectopic Bone Models for Screening of Osteogenic Molecules

Such ectopic bone models are useful for the screening of osteogenic molecules for proof-of-concept studies for bone regeneration (Anusaksathien et al., 2004). Figure 5-1 to Figure 5-5 provide examples of using such constructs with a variety of different carrier devices (e.g., polymeric or ceramic) for characterization macroscopically, histologically or using micro-CT. Further, in addition to the evaluation of pure bone wound healing models in the ectopic sites, more recently the evaluation of bone-tooth-ligament constructs can also be assessed with a variety of imaging methods (Park et al., 2010). The specifics for these animal models are described elsewhere (Anusaksathien et al., 2004; Park et al., 2010).

5.4 Recommended Practices for *in vivo* Screening from Standards-Writing Organizations

The development of standardized screening protocols is of obvious importance and has been the subject of previous reports in the literature extending over the past few decades. One such review (Coleman et al., 1974) proposed that certain basic criteria should be met by any implantation study.

- The elimination and/or standardization of variables which might affect the tissue reaction to the material.
- Adequate controls to eliminate the variability of the reaction due to unusual or unique individuals in the test population.
- Test animals should be relatively inexpensive and easily cared for.
- Implantation sites should be easily accessible surgically, provide a homogeneous environment for the implant, and be mechanically inactive as possible (unless mechanical trauma is being studied).

Fig 5-1 Engineering of hard tissues (bone or cementum) in three-dimensional polymer scaffolds. (a) Images depict microscopic structure of poly(lactic-*co*-glycolic acid) (PLGA) scaffold and cells seeded into the scaffold. The polymer scaffold exhibits open-pore structures allowing cell penetration and attachment. A representative phase contrast image depicts the polymer seeded with cells transduced with a control vector 48 hours after transduction. The fluorescent image shows the corresponding cells expressing green fluorescent protein (GFP) in the scaffold. (b) Diagram depicts transduced with adenovirus encoding growth factor transgenes, or no treatment, 24 hours after transduction. The transduced cells were seeded into polymer scaffolds and implanted into immunodeficient (severe combined immunodeficiency [SCID]) mice. PDGF, platelet-derived growth factor. Reprinted from Anusaksathien *et al.* (2004), with permission from the American Academy of Periodontology.

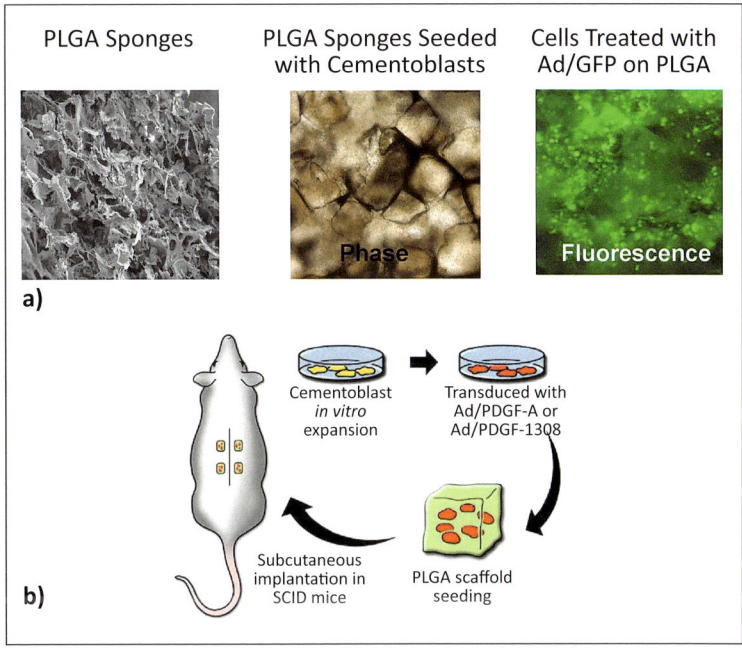

Fig 5-2 Macroscopic appearance and size of retrieved tissue engineered implants. (a) Standardized image shows the macroscopic appearance of polymer-cell implants following gene transfer of Ad/GFP, Ad/PDGF-A, AD/PDGF-1308 or NT, at 3 and 6 weeks post implantation. The bar represents 10 mm. (b) Histomorphometric analysis of the peri-implant areas (mm²). GFP, green fluorescent protein; PDGF, platelet-derived growth factor; NT, no treatment. Reprinted from Anusaksathien *et al.* (2004), with permission from the American Academy of Periodontology.

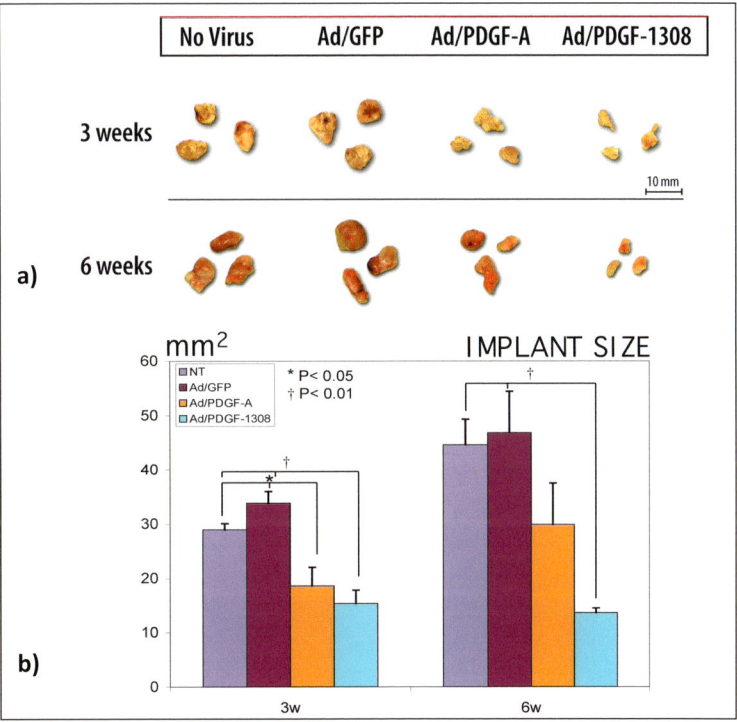

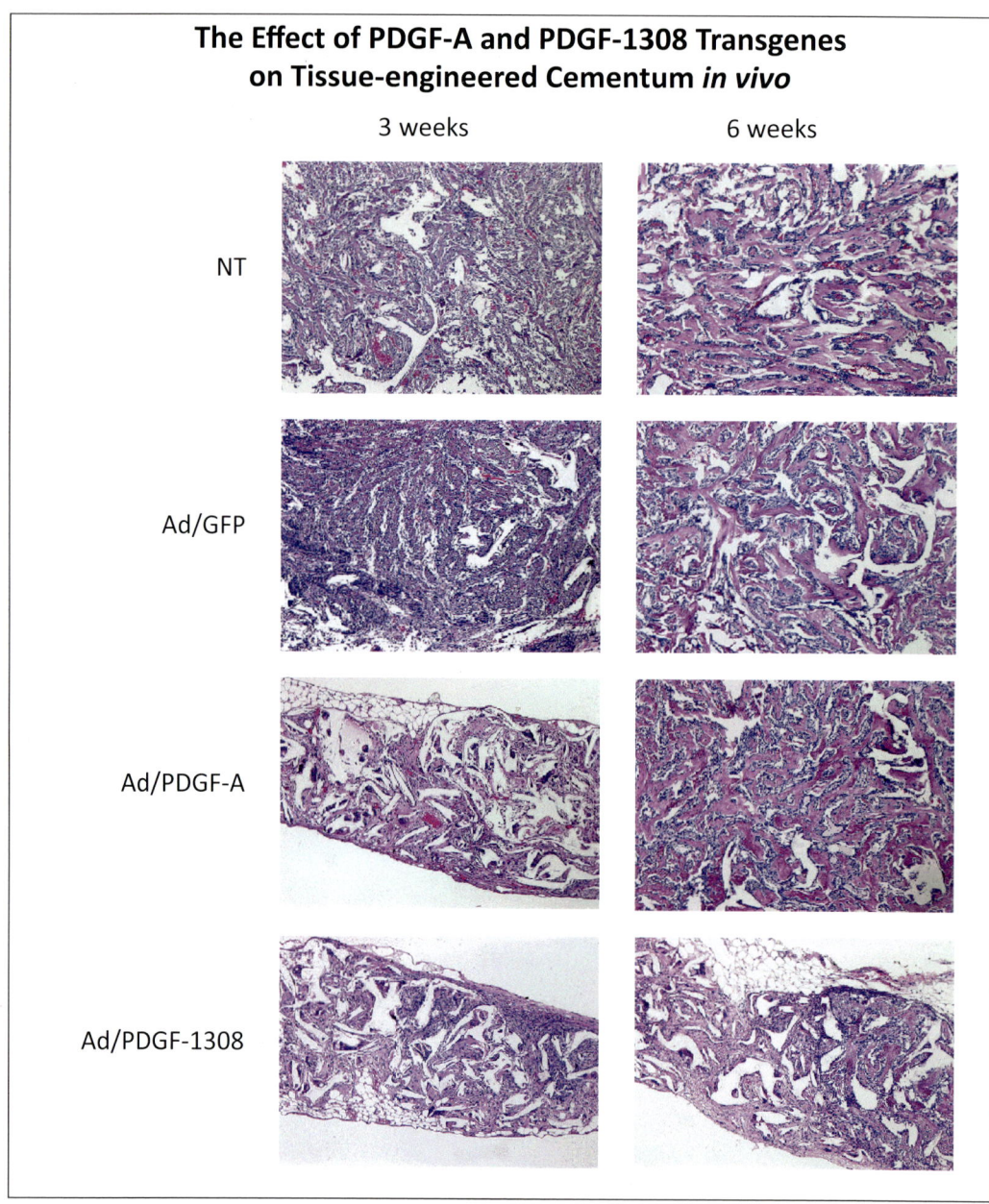

Fig 5-3 The effect of growth factor transgenes on tissue-engineered mineralized structures at 3 and 6 weeks *in vivo*. Mineralization was minimal to none in the Ad/PDGF-A and Ad/PDGF-1308 treated implants, whereas immature mineral formation was present in the NT and Ad/GFP implants at 3 weeks (left panels). Mineral formed was laced-like, with no hematopoietic or fatty tissue. At 6 weeks, mineral formation progressed in all groups, except the Ad/PDGF-1308 specimens, where minimal mineral formation was noted (right panels). (Hematoxylin and eosin, ×100 magnification). GFP, green flourescent protein; PDGF, platelet-dervied growth factor; NT, no treatment. Reprinted from Anusaksathien *et al.* (2004), with permission from the American Academy of Periodontology.

5.4 Recommended Practices for *in vivo* Screening from Standards-Writing Organizations

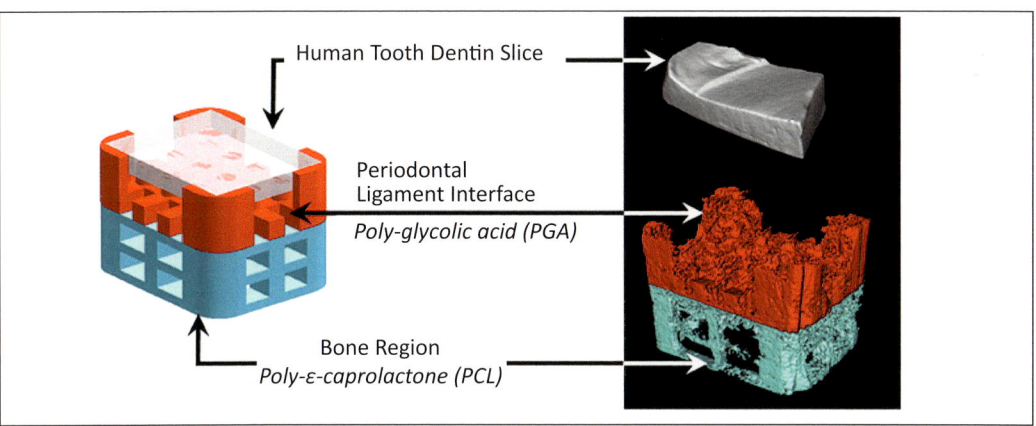

Fig 5-4 Schematic illustration of the modeling and dimensions of hybrid scaffold shows the procedure of polymeric architecture manufacturing for *ex vivo* engineering of tooth-ligament-bone constructs. After acid-treatment of human tooth dentin slices, the complex with a polymer-casted hybrid scaffold and a human tooth dentin slice was made using fibrin gel with or without cells. The right panel is the three-dimensional micro-CT scanned and reconstructed hybrid scaffold and a dentin slice. Reprinted from Park *et al*. (2010), with permission from Elsevier.

- Proper sterile and pyrogen-free techniques should be used during implantation.
- Experimental design should be such that results are reproducible within experimental limits.
- Ideally the results should be quantitative rather than purely qualitative.

Over the years, several organizations have sought to develop standardized test protocols which include as one of their components recommended practices for assessing the long-term (chronic) tissue response. At the time that the protocols were developed the intent was to screen permanent biomaterials for their "biocompatibility", but some of these same screening tests could be adapted for use with tissue engineering products. Some of these organizations have discontinued their support of standards-writing activities.

5.4.1 US Pharmacopeia

The United States Pharmacopeia (USP; www.usp.org/aboutUSP/) is "a non-governmental, official public standards-setting authority for prescription and over-the-counter medicines and other healthcare products manufactured or sold in the United States. USP sets standards for the quality, purity, strength, and consistency of these products – critical to the public health. USP's standards are recognized and used in more than 130 countries around the globe."

In 1967 the USP adopted an implantation protocol first proposed by Lawrence *et al*. (1963), as part of their classification scheme for plastic containers. While most chronic tests include implantation times of longer than 30 days, the USP implantation protocol has a 3-day minimum duration. The standard protocol published by the USP includes a description of the specimen size and shape and implantation and evaluation procedure. This protocol (along with the other USP *in vitro* procedures) is a frequently used test for screening candidate implant materials.

5.4.2 American Dental Association

In 1972 the American Dental Association (ADA) Council on Dental Materials and Devices published standardized laboratory procedures for screening materials and devices (Council on Dental Materials and Devices, 1972). The stand-

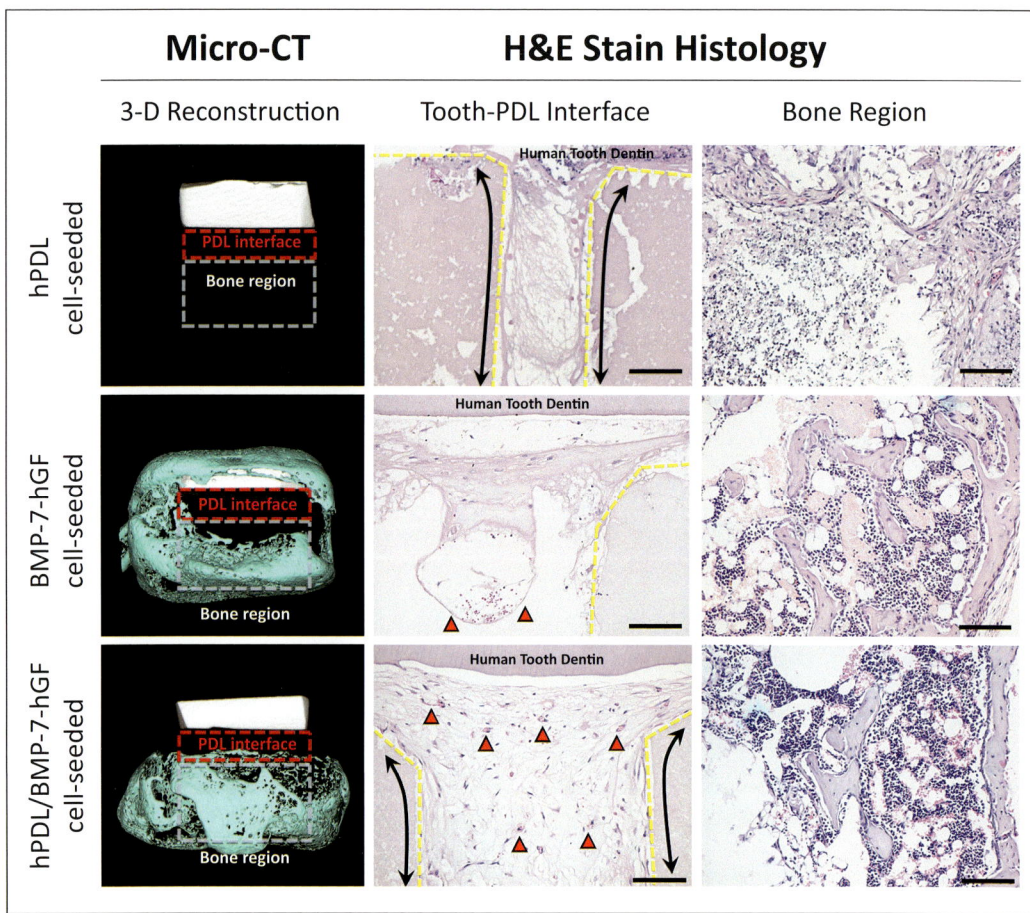

Fig 5-5 **Tissue-engineered tooth-ligament-bone constructs.** Three-dimensional reconstructed colorized micro-CT images and hematoxylin and eosin (H&E) stained histologic slices of tooth-ligament-bone constructs. The mineralized tissue (blue) was formed around the hybrid scaffolds and there was no ankylosis or bone fusion to the dentin surface (white). Red and blue dashed-line boxes were represented with periodontal ligament (PDL) interface and bone region, respectively. H&E stained histologic slices show the PDL interface and bone region tissues to evaluate fibrous tissue orientation along the column-like structures in the PDL interface, which were designed with a perpendicular direction to the dentin surface. The yellow dashed line is the borderline of channel-type PDL architecture and the black-arrowed lines represent the fibrous cell/tissue directionality following the wall of PDL interface structure. Red triangles indicate the blood vessels and yellow triangles point to the cementum-like tissue layer or cell deposition for cementogenesis on the dentin surface. Scale bar: 125 mm. Reprinted from Park et al. (2010), with permission from Elsevier.

ard protocols included short- and long-term implantation tests. Chronic implantation protocols included in the ADA-approved standards utilized subcutaneous as well as osseous tissue as the site of implantation. The standards provided details of the specimen preparation and implantation and evaluation procedure. While the test protocol is not often employed currently, it is an example of the type of standardized test that can be employed for a wide range of biomaterials. In the subcutaneous protocol that was initially adopted, test materials were placed into 10 mm long Teflon tubes having an inside diameter of 1.3 mm. Tubes were inserted into pockets made in the subcutaneous tissue of each of the four dorsal quadrants of guinea pigs. Short-term tests had a 2-week duration, while the long-term tests are terminated after 12 weeks. At least four specimens at each time period needed to be evaluated histologically. The tissue reaction to the test material as viewed at the ends of the Teflon cylinders is compared with the "control reaction" adjacent to the midsection of the tube. The tissue reaction at the 2- and 12-week periods was classified as:

- No to minimal tissue reaction
- Moderate tissue reaction
- Severe tissue reaction.

The classification was based on the degree of inflammation and types of cells present. Materials which caused no-to-slight reactions were considered acceptable for usage tests in humans, those which elicit moderate reactions need further testing to establish the irritant components before usage tests, and those which cause severe reactions are considered unacceptable. In the standard recommended practice for implantation in bone, test specimens were placed into cylindrical Teflon cups. The cups were open at one end and had an outer surface containing a spiral ridge or treads. The cylinder was 2 mm long with an inner diameter of 1.3 mm and an outer diameter of 2 mm. Holes were drilled in the distal ventral symphyseal region of the mandibles of guinea pigs. One test cup was implanted in each half of the mandible with the open end toward the spongy bone. The periods of evaluation were 4 and 26 weeks. Forty specimens were to be evaluated at each time period. At necropsy, segments of bone including the test cups were decalcified and embedded in paraffin. The interface area at the opening of the cup between the test material and bone was to be evaluated for:

- Presence or absence of necrosis and inflammation
- The intensity of inflammation
- Resorption and possible replacement of the test material
- Presence or absence of bone, osteolytic, osteosclerotic, or osteoclastic activity.

The protocol outlined the criteria to be used in classifying the reaction as mild, moderate, or severe. The ADA-approved standards also included (Laing et al., 1967) tests to determine the mucous membrane and pulp irritation of materials.

5.4.3 American Society for Testing and Materials (ASTM)

The ASTM is a voluntary standards-writing organization which develops and approves standards by consensus. In 1972 the society approved a standard recommended practice for experimental testing for biological compatibility of metals for surgical implants. The standard was developed by the F4 subcommittee on surgical implants. The chronic implantation protocol described in the standard was essentially derived from some of the earlier investigations conducted by Laing et al. (1967). Cylindrical test specimens of metal are implanted in muscle or bone and the tissue reaction compared with control specimens implanted in the same animals.

5.4.4 International Standards Organization (ISO)

The ISO includes about 80 member bodies, each representing a national standards institute or bureau. In 1972, a technical committee (TC 150) was founded to consider standards relating to surgical implants. Constituent subcommittees and working groups have subsequently developed standards for a wide variety of implant materials and devices.

5.5 Summary

The screening of tissue engineering products is an essential step in the assessment of the potential utility of the constructs. There is an array of standardized test protocols employing bone and soft tissue implant sites which can be performed before the products are evaluated in models to determine their efficacy.

Acknowledgment

MS was supported by the Department of Veterans Affairs.

References

1. Anusaksathien O, Jin Q, Zhao M, Somerman MJ, Giannobile WV (2004). Effect of sustained delivery of PDGF or its antagonist (PDGF-1308) on tissue-engineered cementum. *J Periodontol* 75:429–440.
2. Chang P, Lang NP, Giannobile WV (2010a). Evaluation of functional dynamics during osseointegration and regeneration associated with oral implants. *Clin Oral Implants Res* 21:1–12.
3. Chang P, Seol Y, Kikuchi N, Goldstein SA, Giannobile WV (2010b). Functional apparent moduli as predictors of oral implant osseointegration dynamics. *J Biomed Mater Res* B 94:118–126.
4. Coleman DL, King RN, Andrade JD (1974). The foreign body reaction: a chronic inflammatory response. *J Biomed Mater Res* 8:199–211.
5. Cooper GM, Mooney MP, Gosain AK, Campbell PG, Losee JE, Huard J (2010). Testing the critical size in calvarial bone defects: revisiting the concept of a critical-size defect. *Plast Reconstr Surg* 125:1685–1692.
6. Council on Dental Materials and Devices (1972). Recommended standard practices for biological evaluation of dental materials. *J Am Dent Assoc* 84:382–387.
7. Horner EA, Kirkham J, Wood D, Curran S, Smith M, Thomson B et al. (2010). Long bone defect models for tissue engineering applications: criteria for choice. *Tissue Eng Part B Rev* 16(2):263–271.
8. Jin Q, Wei G, Lin Z, Lynch SE, Ma PX, Giannobile WV (2008). Nanofibrous scaffolds incorporating PDGF-BB microspheres induce chemokine expression and tissue neogenesis in vivo. *PLoS ONE* 3:e1729.
9. Laing PG, Ferguson AB, Hodge ES (1967). Tissue reaction in rabbit muscle exposed to metallic implants. *J Biomed Mater Res* 1:135–149.
10. Lawrence WH, Mitchell JL, Guess WL, Autian J (1963). Toxicity of plastics used in medical practice. I. Investigation of tissue response in animals by certain unit packaged polyvinyl chloride administration devices. *J Pharm Sci* 52:958–963.
11. Melcher AH, Irving JT (1962). The healing mechanism in artificially created circumscribed femoral defects in the albino rat. *J Bone Joint Surg Br* 44:928.
12. Orr TE, Villars PA, Mitchell SL, Hsu HP, Spector M (2001). Compressive properties of cancellous bone defects in a rabbit model treated with particles of natural bone mineral and synthetic hydroxyapatite. *Biomaterials* 22:1953–1959.
13. Park CH, Rios HF, Jin Q, Bland ME, Flanagan CL, Hollister SJ et al. (2010). Biomimetic hybrid scaffolds for engineering human tooth-ligament interfaces. *Biomaterials* 31:5945–5952.
14. Reichert JC, Saifzadeh S, Wullschleger ME, Epari DR, Schütz MA, Duda GN et al. (2009). The challenge of establishing preclinical models for segmental bone defect research. *Biomaterials* 30:2149–2163.
15. Spector M, Flemming WR, Kreutner A, Sauer BW (1976). Bone ingrowth into porous high-density polyethylene. *J Biomed Mater Res* 7:595.

CHAPTER 6

Soft Tissue Regeneration

Daniel S. Thoma, Ronald E. Jung, and Christoph H.F. Hämmerle

6.1 General Overview

6.1.1 Background

Soft tissue augmentation is a well-established procedure in a variety of disciplines in dentistry. It is indicated in partially and fully edentulous patients to augment areas with a lack of or a reduced width of keratinized tissue, as well as to increase soft tissue volume around dental implants and teeth in conjunction with dental reconstructions. For the latter, a certain amount of keratinized tissue has been considered necessary to maintain periodontal health and to prevent gingival recession (Nabers, 1966; Sullivan and Atkins, 1969). It has also been concluded that for the maintenance of gingival health 2 mm of keratinized gingiva is adequate (Lang and Löe, 1972).

With respect to dental implants, the discussion on the need for a grafting procedure to increase the width of keratinized tissue is somewhat contradictory in the literature. Several studies have suggested associations between an adequate width of keratinized tissue, higher survival rates of dental implants, health of the peri-implant mucosa, and an improved esthetic outcome (Adell *et al.*, 1986; Artzi *et al.*, 1993; Langer, 1996; Schrott *et al.*, 2009).

Soft tissue grafting procedures are also performed to augment soft tissue volume in partially edentulous patients. These procedures have been proposed to surgically correct localized alveolar defects, as preprosthetic site development, as ridge preservation procedures, and to improve the outcome of single-tooth implants (Seibert, 1983a; Studer *et al.*, 2000; Jung *et al.*, 2004; Prato *et al.*, 2004).

6.1.2 Current Treatment Concepts and Limitations

The use of autogenous tissue is associated with a variety of disadvantages including surgical difficulties, limitations with respect to the quality and quantity of tissue that can be retrieved, lack of color match with the surrounding tissue, prolonged healing time at the donor site and therefore an increased patient morbidity (Farnoush, 1978; McGuire and Nunn, 2005; Griffin et al., 2006; Soileau and Brannon, 2006; McGuire et al., 2008).

To overcome these limitations related to the use of autogenous tissue, various techniques and materials, predominantly of allogenic origin, have been developed. Acellular dermal matrix grafts (ADMGs) were among the first products introduced in dentistry. ADMGs were originally developed for covering full thickness burn wounds (Wainwright, 1995) and were later used in dentistry to increase the width of keratinized tissue, to deepen the vestibular fornix, and to augment localized alveolar defects (Wei et al., 2000; Batista et al., 2001; Harris, 2003). Even though ADMGs are still in use, results from clinical studies are not convincing due to a high shrinkage rate and histologic findings demonstrating a tissue that is substantially different from the oral mucosa (Wei et al., 2000; Wei et al., 2002). Recently, a cellular component has been added to dermal replacement grafts. The results from various studies suggest that these tissue-engineered grafts may be more favorable in terms of clinical outcomes although they may still be associated with difficult clinical handling (McGuire and Nunn, 2005; McGuire et al., 2008; Nevins, 2010).

In contrast to tissue-engineered products derived from human skin, collagen devices of xenogenic origin have been successfully used in dentistry for guided tissue and bone regeneration (GTR and GBR) (Hämmerle and Jung, 2003). These collagen devices are characterized by a hemostatic effect, early wound stabilization, chemotactic properties to attract fibroblasts, and semipermeability (Postlethwaite et al., 1978). A high degree of anastomosis in the vasculature in the regenerated tissue has been reported to be induced by the collagen membrane after subcutaneous implantation in rats (Schwarz et al., 2006).

Recently, a prototype membrane with characteristics similar to the most commonly used resorbable collagen membrane was developed with an additional indication for GTR procedures in periodontal defects. These prototype membranes will allow to further influence the healing cascade, reduce scar retraction, and will serve as a replacement for autogenous tissue to increase the width of keratinized tissue. Results from a randomized controlled clinical trial have demonstrated that this newly developed collagen matrix is as effective and predictable as the gold standard, the connective tissue graft, for attaining a band of keratinized tissue (Sanz et al., 2009).

6.1.3 Animal Models

Based on the different needs, animal models vary for devices/grafts intended to be used for augmentation of keratinized tissue and soft tissue volume. In the two-dimensional augmentation of keratinized tissue, successful integration into the surrounding tissue, degradation and replacement by connective tissue, color match with the surrounding tissue, and stability of the width of the augmented area are desirable. The histologic outcomes should be characterized by the absence of elastic fibers (as this is typical for the alveolar mucosa), an epithelium–connective tissue interface exhibiting rete pegs, and by a distinct keratin layer at the epithelial surface (Lozdan and Squier, 1969; Karring et al., 1971). The understanding of the tissue specificity of transplanted oral soft tissue goes back to the early 1970s. A series of animal studies demonstrated that the specificity of the epithelium is determined by the hereditary mechanism rather than by functional adaptation (Karring et al., 1971). In addition, the connective tissue of a transplanted free gingival graft appears to originate from the periodontal ligament, whereas the epithelium is most likely proliferated from the surrounding tissue (Karring et al., 1975).

The differentiation of the proliferated epithelium is then induced by the periodontal connective tissue (Karring et al., 1975).

Historically, the methods to augment keratinized tissue included: an apically positioned flap (APF) (Friedman, 1962); an APF in combination with autogenous tissue (Edel, 1974); and an APF in combination with allogenic tissue (Yukna and Sullivan, 1978). Therefore, for keratinized tissue positive control groups may include an APF and/or an APF in combination with a free gingival graft (FGG). Sites not undergoing treatment can serve as the negative control group.

For soft tissue volume grafting, three main parameters have to be evaluated clinically and by histologic and histomorphometric analyses when testing an artificial or autogenous graft: (1) successful integration of the device/graft into the surrounding tissue, (2) ability to degrade and being replaced by soft connective tissue, and (3) three-dimensional volume stability over time. Currently, autogenous soft tissue grafts, mainly the subepithelial connective tissue graft (SCTG), are considered as treatment of choice for soft tissue volume augmentation (Seibert, 1983a; Studer et al., 2000). Therefore, positive control groups may include the SCTG. Sham-operated sites and sites without any treatment may serve a negative control groups.

Since soft tissue augmentation surgeries were and are still performed using autogenous soft tissue grafts, available animal models are scarce. Early models used to determine the tissue specificity after auto-transplantation of oral soft tissues have limitations; they were not developed to observe two- and three-dimensional changes of width and thickness of augmented tissues (Karring et al., 1971; Karring et al., 1975). In other models, the palate in dogs served as defect site for the implantation of tissue-engineered mucosal substitutes (Ophof et al., 2004; Ophof et al., 2008). This animal model allows study of tissue integration, re-epithelialization, and revascularization of grafts. However, the palate appears to heal very slowly and no information can be derived with respect to the extent of the regenerated keratinized tissue (Ophof et al., 2008).

Soft tissue regeneration procedures have recently gained attention as new materials have been developed. However, with respect to allogenic devices and preclinical experiments, there is little information as well. This may have at least two reasons. First, allogenic devices have a long tradition in dermatology and were considered as transplants in some countries. This allowed transfer of information from extraoral usage into the oral cavity and probably prevented performance of additional preclinical research. Second, tissue-engineered allogenic devices include living cells from humans. Possible cross-over effects and subsequent auto-immunologic reactions can be expected when these devices are used in animal models.

Very recently, a variety of collagen-based and extracellular matrix-derived matrices of xenogenic origin have been developed for oral soft tissue augmentation and have also been tested in preclinical models and clinical studies (Badylak, 2002; Nevins et al., 2010; Thoma et al., 2010). For this purpose, new animal models specifically designed to evaluate devices for oral soft tissue augmentation (keratinized tissue and soft tissue volume) have been developed.

With respect to soft tissue volume augmentation, there is also a lack of suitable techniques for the measurement of volume changes (Thoma et al., 2009). Several methods have been described for noninvasive measurement of volume changes in the oral cavity. The techniques range from simple clinical observation (Allen et al., 1985) and two-dimensional measurements using a periodontal probe (Batista et al., 2001) to complicated volumetric assessments using the Moiré projection method (Studer et al., 2000). The use of different techniques impairs any comparison of volumetric outcomes between studies. In a recent study (Thoma et al., 2010), a three-dimensional optical method has been used to detect volume changes over time. The applied technique showed high reproducibility and excellent accuracy for measuring volume changes in a methodologic study (Windisch et al., 2007). A variety of studies have demonstrated that this method offers great advantages in being easy to apply, noninvasive, and precise (Windisch et al., 2007; Fickl et al., 2009; Strebel et al., 2009; Schneider et al., 2011). A broader use of this technique may be desirable in the future and will allow comparison of volume measurements between different studies.

It is expected that within the coming years the number of available models will continuously increase. The suggested animal models for soft tissue regeneration may potentially undergo changes and further refinements in the future.

6.2 Keratinized Tissue – Pig Model

6.2.1 Aim
The aim of this animal model is to evaluate and compare the tissue integration, the local tolerance, and the clinical performance of experimental devices to increase the width of keratinized tissue by macroscopic and microscopic analysis.

6.2.2 Advantages/Disadvantages
Defect sites that are close to the clinical situation characterize the advantages of this animal model. Sites with a reduced amount of keratinized tissue around teeth are augmented. In addition, a variety of clinical and histologic outcome measures can be evaluated:
- Macroscopically (clinically): width of keratinized tissue over time; thickness of keratinized tissue (by using stents); color match with the surrounding tissue; signs of local inflammation or intolerance; contraction of defect sites (two-dimensional); and re-epithelialization.
- Microscopically (histologically): histological and histomorphometric measurements.

The disadvantages include possible growth of the animals during the study period resulting in difficulties in performing the clinical measurements and that markings serving as reference points may disappear.

6.2.3 Timing
The experiment is characterized by one surgical procedure. Tooth sites with a reduced amount of keratinized tissue are scheduled for augmentation surgery. On the day of surgery, the width of the keratinized tissue is increased using test and control groups. Follow-up time points are scheduled at 1 and 6 months. This allows studying the healing of the performed augmentation procedures over time with a variety of clinical and histologic parameters that can be analyzed (Fig 6-1).

6.2.4 Surgical Procedures
The surgical procedures performed in this experiment have a long tradition in mucogingival surgery and do not require special training. Surgical procedures to increase the width around dental implants and teeth are indicated for a variety of reasons and have gained further attention in recent years. This is predominantly due to the fact that a minimal amount of keratinized tissue has been considered necessary to maintain periodontal health and to prevent gingival recession around teeth (Nabers, 1966; Sullivan and Atkins, 1969). Surgical procedures to increase the width of keratinized tissue around dental implants have been proposed based on reports of higher survival rates of dental implants, health of the peri-implant mucosa, and an improved esthetic outcome (Adell et al., 1986; Artzi et al., 1993; Langer, 1996; Schrott et al., 2009). The proposed surgical procedures include an apically positioned flap or vestibulo-

6.2 Keratinized Tissue – Pig Model

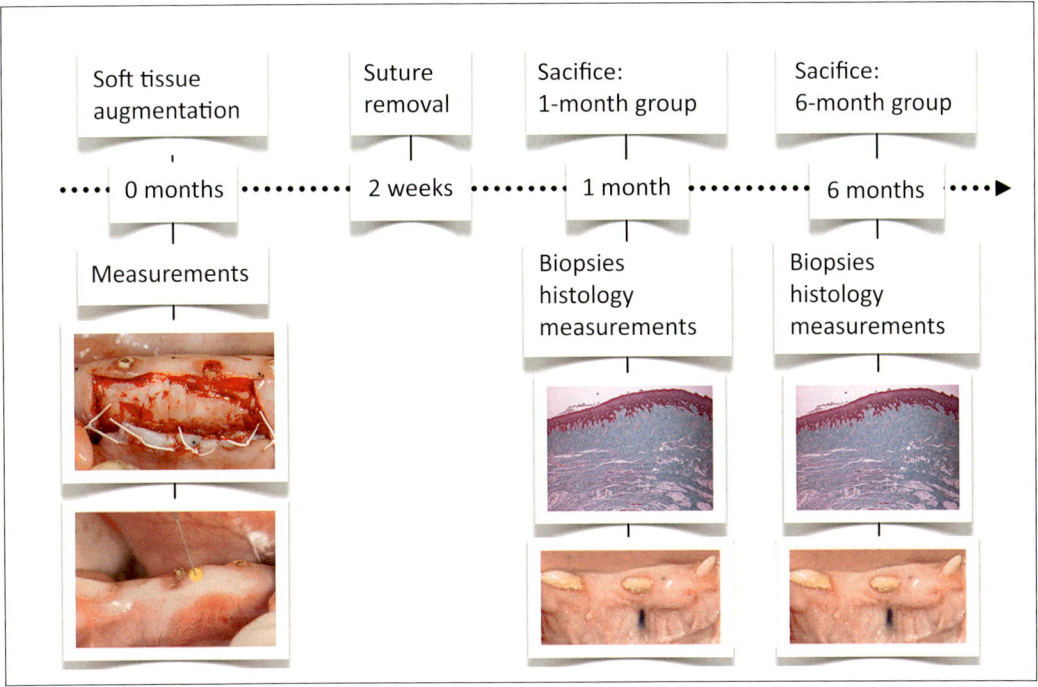

Fig 6-1 Timing of surgical phase and sacrifice time points.

plasty procedure (Thoma et al., 2009). These procedures are characterized by a displacement of the mucogingival junction in a further apical direction. The increased distance between the original position of the mucogingival junction and the position after flap positioning is allowed to allow to heal by secondary intention or covered with an artificial or autogenous graft (Jung et al., 2011).

6.2.5 reparation

On the day of surgery, each animal is anesthetized using atropine for tranquillization, induction with tiletamine-zolazepam and then sodium thiopental, followed by inhalation of an O_2–N_2O isoflurane (1–4%) mixture. A preoperative injection of a local anesthetic is administered.

Prior to the surgery, the width and thickness of the keratinized tissue are measured using a periodontal probe. In order to reproducibly repeat the measurements (width of keratinized tissue, contraction of sites) at a later stage, four tattoo points are placed coronally, apically, mesially, and distally to each defect site. In addition, impressions are taken from each hemi-mandible using polyether impression material (Fig 6-2a). Individual acrylic stents are then fabricated and used to repeatedly perform measurements of the tissue thickness at five sites per defect area (Figs 6-2b and 6-2c).

6.2.6 Detailed Methodology

In each animal, two standardized gingival defects (1 cm vertical × 3 cm horizontal distance) are created bilaterally on the buccal side of the mandible. A horizontal incision is made in the keratinized gingiva 2 mm coronal to the mucogingival line (Fig 6-3a). Subsequently, two releasing incisions are made into the vestibular mucosa defining the lateral borders of the defect (Fig 6-3b). To elevate the flap, a split-thickness flap is elevated, creating a standard-

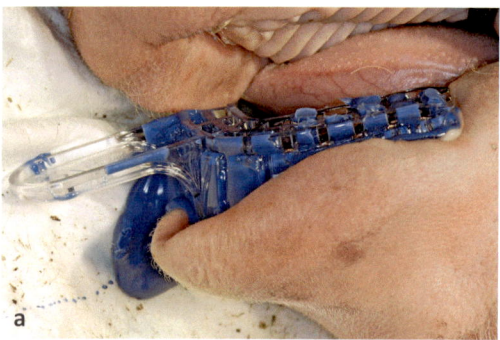
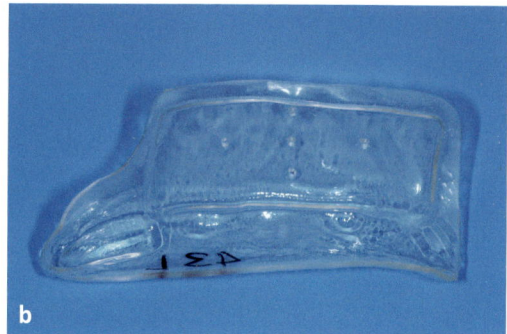
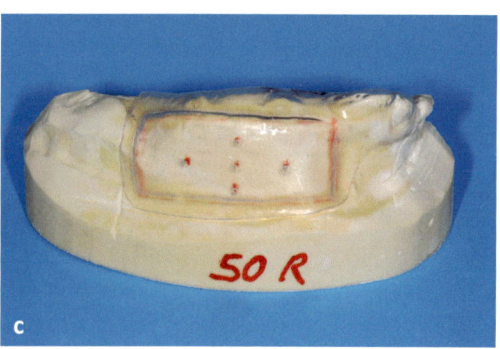

Fig 6-2 (**a**) Impression taken prior to surgery to produce a surgical stent for repeated and standardized measurements of soft tissue thickness. (**b**) Individualized acrylic stent. (**c**) Individualized acrylic stent on plaster model (which represents the clinical situation prior to the surgery).

ized soft tissue defect (1 cm vertical, 3 cm horizontal distance) (Figs 6-3c, 6-3d, and 6-3e). The horizontal border of the mucosal flap is sutured to the underlying periosteum by interrupted single sutures (Fig 6-3f). The denuded defect area in each hemi-mandible is randomly covered with one experimental device/graft of the exact same size as the defect (Fig 6-3g). Subsequently, the device is securely stabilized and held in place by horizontal mattress sutures. The other defect (contralateral side of mandible) is left untreated and serves as control (Fig 6-3f). The apical margin of the device is fixed to the periosteum by interrupted single sutures.

6.2.7 Post-operative Care

Prophylactic antibiotic treatment with spiramycin and metronidazole is initiated on the day of surgery and continued for 10 days thereafter. Each animal receives carprofen for analgesia for 3 days. The sutures are removed 14 days following surgery. The animals are fed a soft diet for the remainder of the study.

6.2.8 Endpoint Measurements

Clinical Observations and Measurements
At 1 month, photographs are taken of the defect sites (Figs 6-4a and 6-4b). The thickness and width of the keratinized gingiva are measured using a periodontal probe and individualized stents (Figs 6-2b and 6-2c). The defect sites are checked for signs of inflammation or local intolerance. The re-epithelialization of the defect sites is evaluated on the photographs by digital planimetry using an overlaid grid with 289 intersections and a 0.5 mm distance between them. The re-epithelialization is then

6.2 Keratinized Tissue – Pig Model

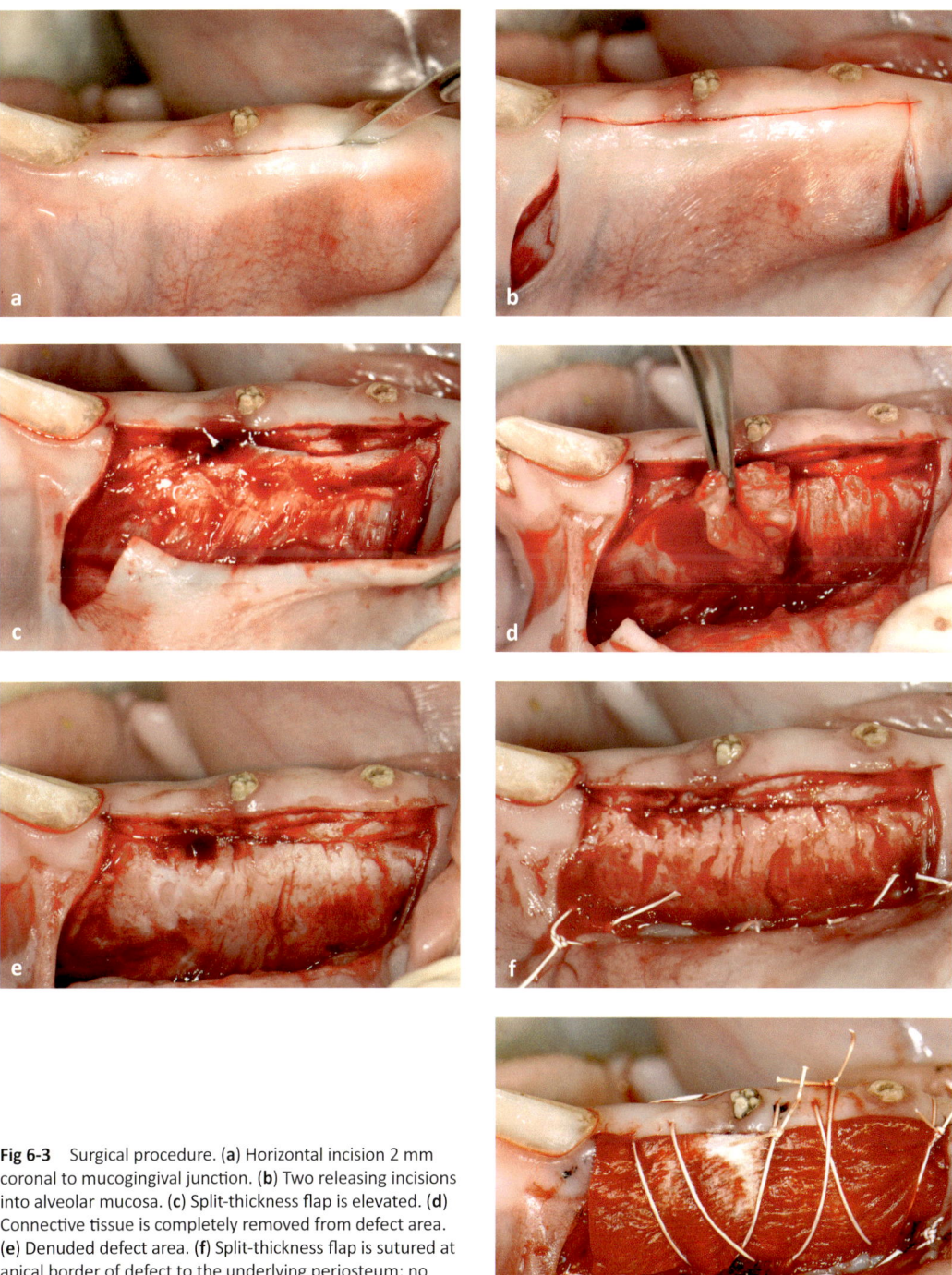

Fig 6-3 Surgical procedure. (**a**) Horizontal incision 2 mm coronal to mucogingival junction. (**b**) Two releasing incisions into alveolar mucosa. (**c**) Split-thickness flap is elevated. (**d**) Connective tissue is completely removed from defect area. (**e**) Denuded defect area. (**f**) Split-thickness flap is sutured at apical border of defect to the underlying periosteum; no further treatment is applied in the control group. (**g**) Device/graft is sutured in the defect area.

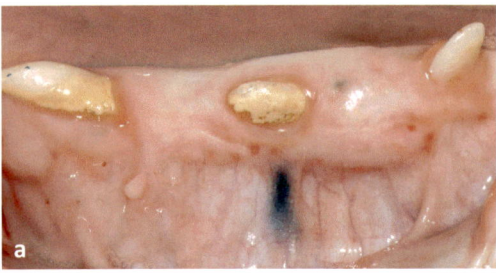
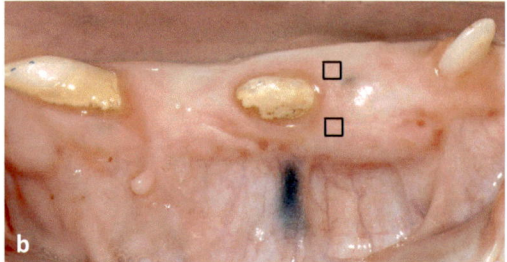

Fig 6-4 Follow-up. (**a**) Clinical situation at 6 months demonstrating fully healed gingival tissue and gain in keratinized tissue. (**b**) Same site as in (a) showing the zones (squares) used for measurements of color differences between augmented tissue and host tissue.

expressed in percentage of the entire grafted area. The contraction of each defect site is evaluated by measuring the gap between the horizontal and vertical tattoo points (height × length in mm). In addition, biopsy samples can be harvested from some or all of the animals.

At 6 months, the same macroscopic observations and measurements are performed as at 1 month (Figs 6-4a and 6-4b). Subsequently, the animals are euthanized. The soft tissues are resected together with the underlying bone and the adjacent intact gingival tissue. The coronal border of each biopsy sample is identified by means of a suture thread.

Histological Processing and Analysis
After fixation, each sample is decalcified, dehydrated in alcohol solutions of increasing concentration, cleared in isoparaffin H, and embedded in paraffin. Embedded samples are cut at 5 μm into three blocks (anterior, medial, and posterior according to the corono-apical axis) using a microtome. One section per block is prepared and stained with Masson's trichrome.

All histologic sections are evaluated using a light microscope for qualitative and semiquantitative histologic analysis.

Color Match
For colorimetric analysis, the clinical photographs taken at baseline (prior to surgery) and after surgery at 1 and 6 months are digitized. The images are then assessed and analyzed according to standard colorimetric parameters (Commission Internationale de l'Eclairage [CIE] Lab; L = lightness, a = chroma along red-green axis, and b = chroma along yellow-blue axis). Two areas, one from the defect site and one from the adjacent keratinized tissue, are chosen for comparison (Fig 6-4b). The colorimetric difference between the two areas (ΔE) are calculated according to the following equation: $\Delta E = [(L_{Graft} - L_{Adjacent\ tissue})^2 + (a_{Graft} - a_{Adjacent\ tissue})^2 + (b_{Graft} - b_{Adjacent\ tissue})^2]^{1/2}$ (Jung et al., 2004).

6.2.9 Statistical Analysis Plan

Statistical analyses are performed to compare test devices and control sites at baseline, and at 1 and 6 months. Summary statistics (mean, standard deviation, minimum, and maximum) are used to describe the quantitative parameter. The groups are compared at each time point with analysis of variance (ANOVA). Summary statistics (frequency and percentage) are used to describe the ordinal parameter. The groups are compared at each time point by site with the chi-squared test of association for independent data and with the Cochran Mantel-Haenszel test for dependent data. For all tests a P value lower than 0.05 is considered as statistically significant.

6.2.10 Materials, Consumables, Equipment

Operating room: A purpose-designed room for experimental animals in accordance with the requirements of the FDA "Good Laboratory Practice" (GLP) Regulations.

Animals: Seghers Hybrid pigs, more than 2 years old, weighing between 50 and 61 kg.

Anesthesia:
- Tranquilization by atropine
- Induction by tiletamine-zolazepam, then thiopental sodium followed by inhalation of a O_2–N_2O isoflurane (1–4%) mixture
- Preoperative injection of a local anesthetic is administered.

Surgery:
- Standard surgical instrument kit for mucogingival surgery
- Test devices/graft disinfectant
- Non-resorbable sutures
- Polyether impression material
- Master casts out of dental stone
- Acrylic material for individualized stents
- Ink for tattoo points.

Postoperative care:
- Antibiotic treatment with spiramycin and metronidazole
- Analgesia with carprofen.

Analyses:
- Histology and histomorphometry:
  - Decalcification
  - Dehydration in alcohol solutions of increasing concentration
  - Embedding in paraffin
  - Microtome
  - Staining with Masson's trichrome
  - A stereoscope with a video camera
  - An automated image analysis system.
- Color measurements:
  - An image analysis program.
- Clinical measurements:
  - Re-epithelialization
    Using photographs and an overlaid grid with 289 intersections and a 0.5 mm distance between them
  - Thickness
    Acrylic stents (see above) and a periodontal probe
  - Width of keratinized tissue
    Periodontal probe or a caliper.

6.3 Soft Tissue Volume – Dog Model

6.3.1 Aim

The aim of this animal model is to histologically and volumetrically evaluate a potential device for soft tissue volume augmentation. For that purpose, single-tooth gaps with chronic ridge defects are created in a dog model.

6.3.2 Advantages/Disadvantages

This animal model is characterized by chronic ridge defects that are close to the clinical situation in single tooth gaps. Three defects sites can be prepared in each hemi-mandible and allow a variety of treatment modalities to be included. The use of chronic ridge defects minimizes bone regeneration as a result of the first surgical intervention (tooth extraction). Any volume changes may predominantly be a result of the second surgery (soft tissue augmentation). The tissue regeneration, which takes part following the preparation of the ridge defects, should be completed at the day of the second surgery.

Possible disadvantages include the need for a variety of interventions that are necessary to create the chronic ridge defects and to obtain volumetric measurements. The defect sites are not standardized on the day of soft tissue augmentation surgery (as it would be when using acute defects). Each defect site has an individual shape and form and therefore individual healing potential. In addition, the differentiation between native bone and regenerated

Osteology Guidelines for Oral and Maxillofacial Regeneration

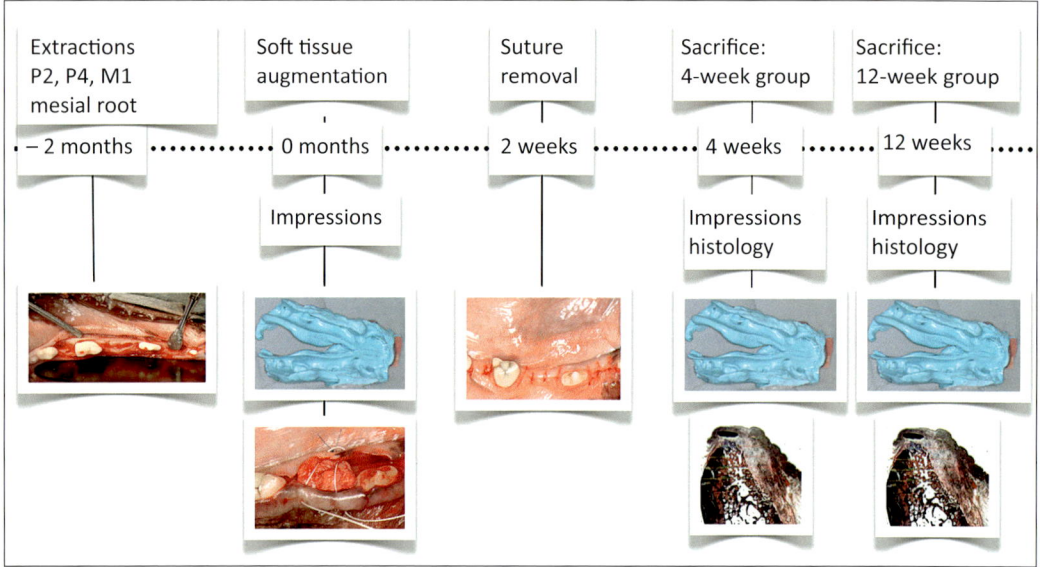

Fig 6-5 Timing of surgical phases 1 and 2, and sacrifice time points.

bone may be difficult in the histologic analysis since two interventions are made (extraction and defect creation, ridge augmentation).

6.3.3 Timing

The experiment is characterized by two surgical procedures. Initially, single-tooth gaps have to be created during surgery 1. Subsequently, a healing period of 2 months allows the defects to heal and to establish chronic ridge defects. During surgery 2, augmentation procedures are performed using test and control grafts as well as a negative control group. The sacrifice time points are scheduled at 4 and 12 weeks. These two time points allow study of the volumetric and histologic changes over time (Fig 6-5).

6.3.4 Surgical Procedures

The soft tissue volume augmentation surgeries described in the following experiment are routinely performed in single-tooth gaps between dental implants and teeth predominantly to obtain an ideal contour for esthetic reasons. The surgical technique itself has been described extensively in the literature with a variety of modifications (Langer and Calagna, 1980; Seibert, 1983a, 1983b; Orth, 1996; Studer et al., 2000; Batista et al., 2001). In brief, a full- or split-thickness flap is elevated in sites with chronic ridge defects (osseous and/or soft tissue). Subsequently, either an artificial or autogenous graft is prepared and cut to fit into the recipient site and placed underneath the buccal flap. Periosteal releasing incisions are performed and help to suture the flap back to the lingual side, preventing compression of the augmented site (Thoma et al., 2010).

6.3.5 Preparation and Surgical Equipment

All surgical procedures are performed under general anesthesia and sterile conditions in an operating room using thiopental sodium solution 4%, 0.4 mL/kg body weight as a premedication. The dogs are placed on a heating pad, intubated, anesthetized with isoflurane 1.5–2%, and monitored with electrocardiography during the surgery.

6.3 Soft Tissue Volume – Dog Model

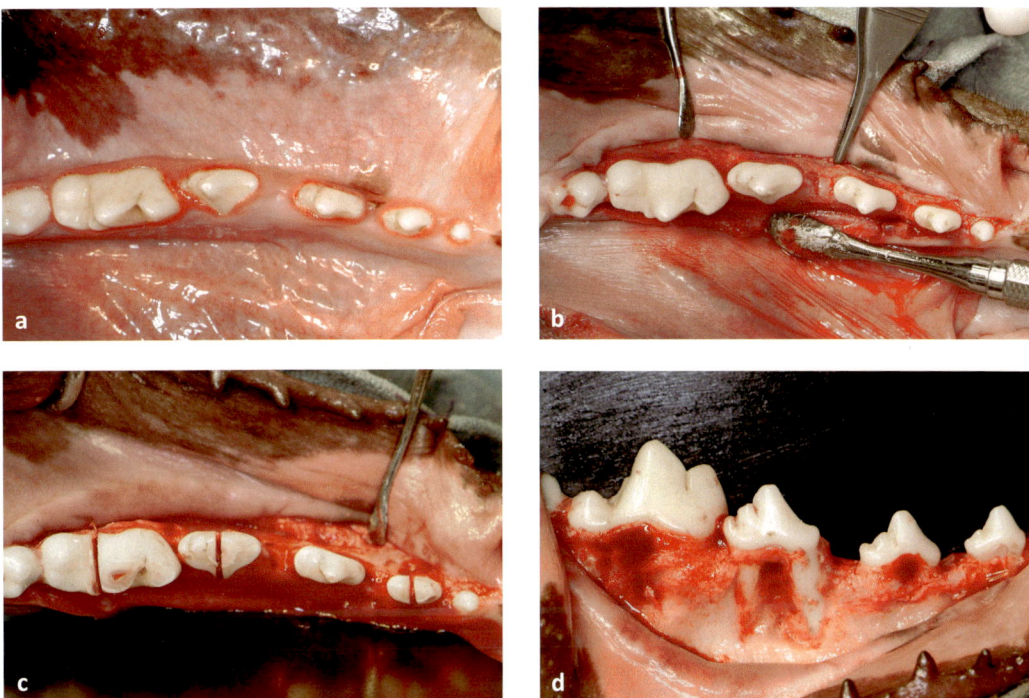

Fig 6-6 (continuation next page) Surgery 1. (**a**) Preoperative situation of a left mandible. (**b**) Sulcular incisions are made around the premolars and M1, and a full-thickness flap is elevated. (**c**) Premolars 2 and 4 (P2, P4), and M1 are sectioned to prevent fracture. (**d**) The buccal bone plate of P2 and P4, and of the distal root of M1 are removed.

6.3.6 Detailed Methodology

Surgery 1 (Tooth Extraction)
Crevicular incisions are made around all mandibular premolars (P) and the first molar (M1) and buccal and lingual flaps are reflected (Figs 6-6a and 6-6b). The teeth are sectioned in order to prevent fractures (Fig 6-6c). Following extraction of all mandibular P2, P4, and the distal roots of M1 (Figs 6-6d and 6-6e), the buccal plate of the extraction sites is removed and the defect sites are enlarged using a round bur (Figs 6-6d and 6-6e). Rubber dam is placed around the mesial root of each M1 on both sides of the mandible. The pulp tissue of the mesial roots is extirpated and the root canals are filled with gutta-percha and a sealer (Figs 6-6f, 6-6g, and 6-6h). The coronal portion of the pulp is filled using a self-curing composite material. Following rinsing with sterile saline, primary wound closure is obtained (Fig 6-6i).

Surgery 2 (Soft Tissue Volume Augmentation)
After a healing period of 2 months, surgery 2 is performed on all dogs under the same operating room conditions as surgery 1. Before starting the surgery, the mandibles are inspected and polyether impressions of the mandibles are made using the individualized trays (Figs 6-7a and 6-7b). Following midcrestal incisions (between M2 and the mesial root of M1; between the mesial root of M1 and P3; between P3 and P1) and sulcular incisions around the mesial root of M1, P3, and P1, full-thickness

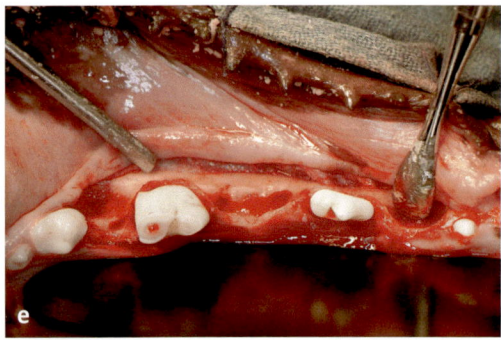
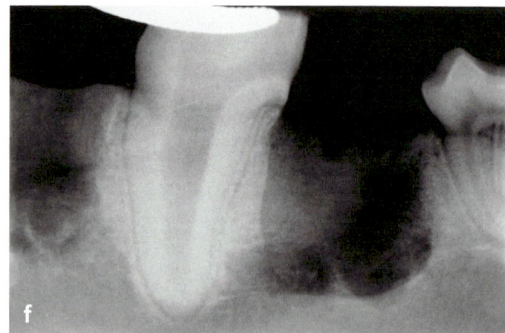
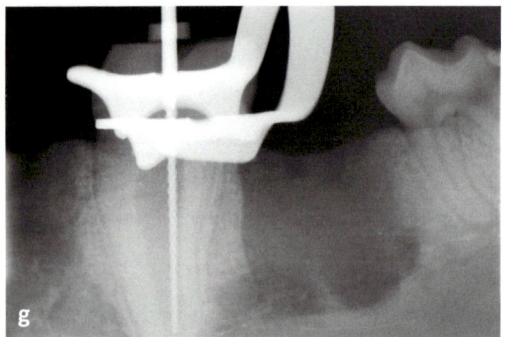
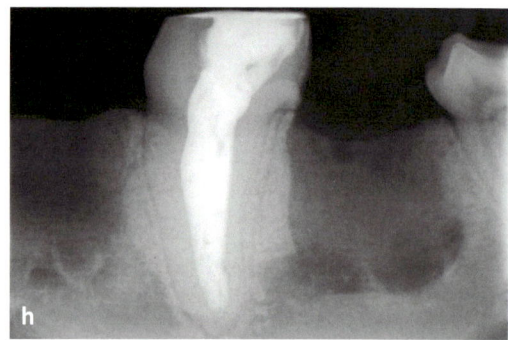
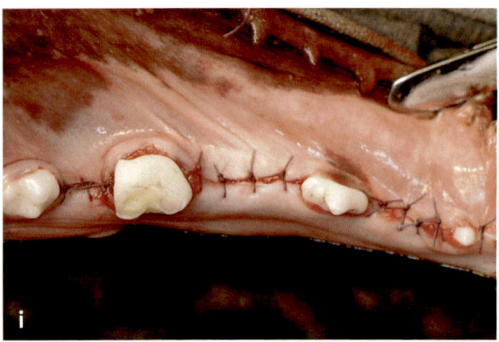

Fig 6-6 (continuation) Surgery 1. (**e**) P2, P4, and the distal root of M1 are removed; the defect sites are enlarged to establish chronic ridge defects. (**f–h**) Root canal treatment of the mesial root of M1. (**f**) Preoperative view. (**g**) Radiograph taken for determining the length. (**h**) Final radiograph taken after root canal treatment; the occlusal access hole has been closed using composite. (**i**) Primary wound closure has been obtained.

mucoperiosteal flaps are elevated over the crest of the ridge (Fig 6-7c). The chronic ridge defects are then inspected and their height, depth, and width measured. A titanium pin is placed on top of the bone crest in the middle of each chronic defect to simplify histologic processing (Fig 6-7c). Periosteal releasing incisions are made to make room for volume augmentation.

The following three treatment modalities are then randomly applied to the defects (Fig 6-8 and Table 6-1):
- Group a: test device/graft
- Group b: an autogenous SCTG (positive control)
- Group c: sham-operated site (negative control)

6.3 Soft Tissue Volume – Dog Model

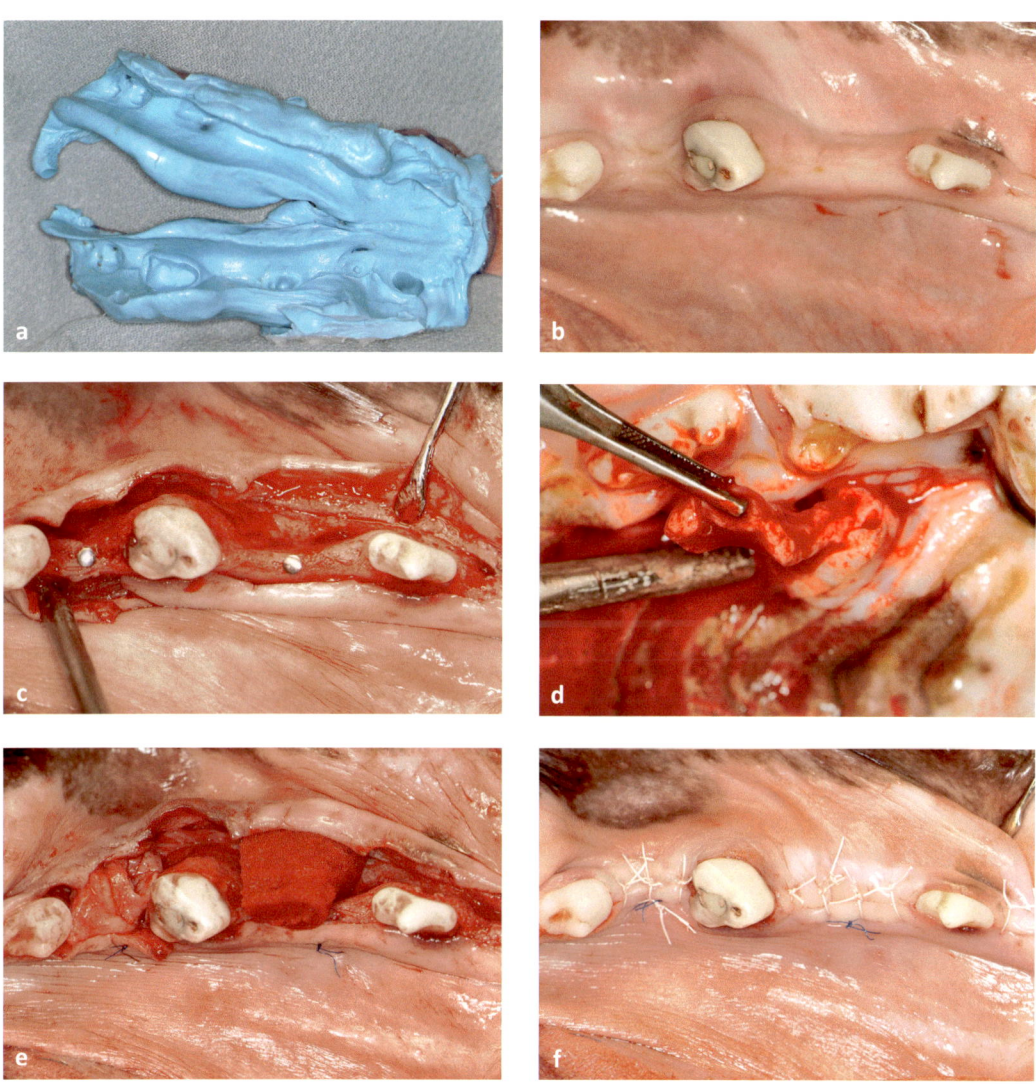

Fig 6-7 Surgery 2. (**a**) Preoperative impression using a polyether impression material. (**b**) Preoperative view after 2 months of healing following surgery 1. (**c**) Full-thickness flaps are raised; titanium pins are placed on top of the bone crest and in the center of the defects. (**d**) A connective tissue graft is harvested from the palate. (**e**) All treatment modalities are placed in the three defect sites (one control site in the mesial defect, the SCTG in the posterior defect, and the test device/graft in the middle defect). (**f**) Primary wound closure is obtained.

Group a: The test device/graft is applied according to the manufacturer's recommendations. It is positioned in the pouch under the elevated buccal flap. A horizontal mattress suture is placed to immobilize the test device, connecting it to the lingual flap.

Group b: The autogenous SCTG is harvested from the palatal vault (Fig 6-7d). A U-shaped incision is made in the lateral part of the palatal vault and a mucoperiosteal flap is elevated. An SCTG is then dissected (dimensions: width 10 mm, length 12 mm, thickness 5 mm). Fatty

Osteology Guidelines for Oral and Maxillofacial Regeneration

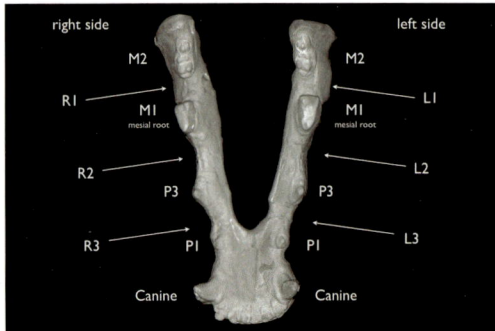

Fig 6-8 Randomization figure; the order of the three treatment modalities is kept in all subsequent dogs, but the positions are changed in a clockwise direction.

tissue, glandular tissue, and remnants of the epithelium are removed. Any bleeding in the palate is controlled by the use of local anesthetic, compression with a sterile gauze, and three to four single sutures. The SCTG is then folded once and positioned in the pouch under the elevated buccal flap. A horizontal mattress suture is made to immobilize the SCTG connecting it to the lingual flap (Fig 6-7e).

Group c: No further treatment is applied to the sham-operated sites (control). The buccal flaps in all sites are repositioned without tension to the lingual part. One horizontal mattress suture is placed over the buccal prominence created by the volume gain through the SCTG, and the test device to stabilize and stretch the grafts toward the vestibular fornix. The flaps are adapted using four to five single sutures to ensure primary wound closure (Fig 6-7f).

6.3.7 Postoperative Care

Surgery 1: For the first 7 to 14 days after extraction, the dogs are fed a soft diet. After a period of 7 to 10 days, the animals are briefly anesthetized with 1 mL/13.6 kg by IV – ketamine 50 mg/mL, xylazine 7.1 mg/mL, acepromazine 2.1 mg/mL, atropine 0.1 mg/mL; the sutures removed and teeth cleaned. At this time, polyether impressions of the mandible are taken from every animal. Master casts out of dental stone are obtained and individualized trays fabricated using light-curing tray material.

Surgery 2: The dogs are maintained on a soft diet for the remainder of the study. The sutures are removed 14 days after surgery 2.

6.3.8 Endpoint Measurements

Volumetric Analysis to Evaluate Soft Tissue Volume Changes
Master casts are made out of dental stone utilizing the preoperative (baseline) and follow-up impressions at 28 days (dogs 1–6) and 84 days (dogs 4–6).

Table 6-1 Randomization table for six dogs and two time points (28 and 84 days).

Endpoint	Dog number	Site					
		Right anterior	Right middle	Right posterior	Left anterior	Left middle	Left posterior
28 days	1	Test	SCTG	Control	Test	SCTG	Control
28 days	2	SCTG	Control	Test	SCTG	Control	Test
28 days	3	Control	Test	SCTG	Control	Test	SCTG
84 days	4	Test	SCTG	Control	Test	SCTG	Control
84 days	5	SCTG	Control	Test	SCTG	Control	Test
84 days	6	Control	Test	SCTG	Control	Test	SCTG

6.3 Soft Tissue Volume – Dog Model

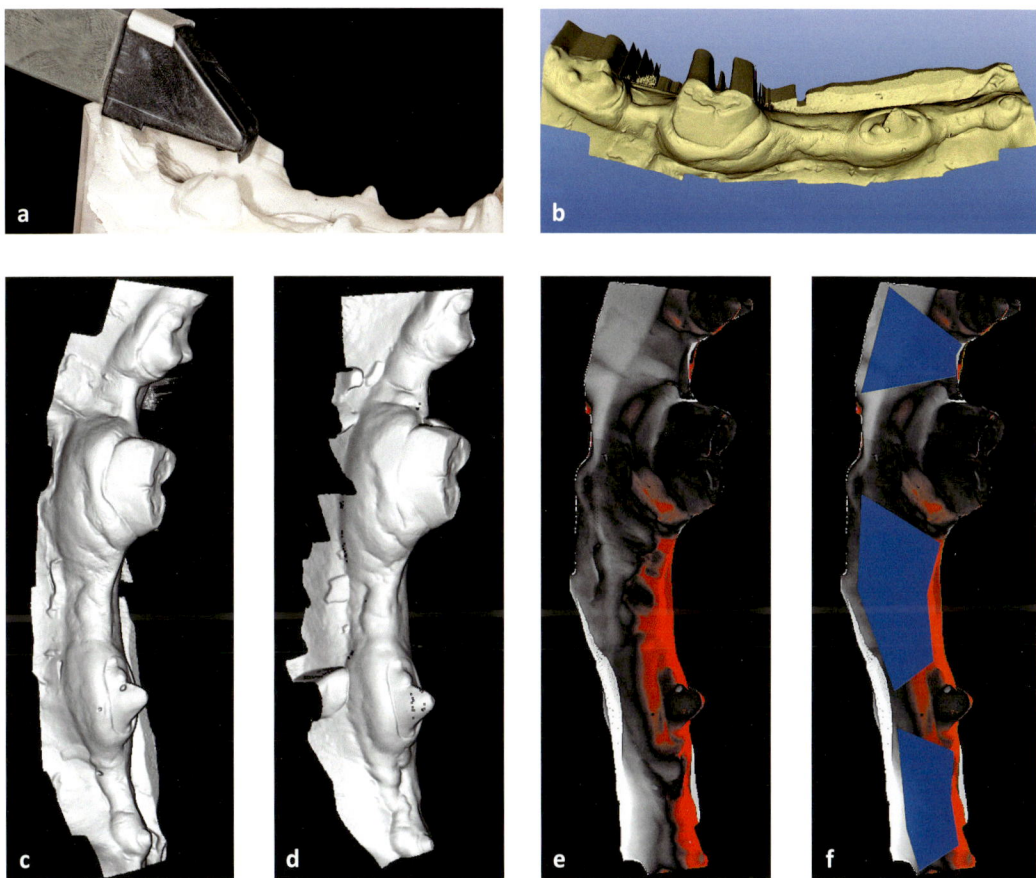

Fig 6-9 Volumetric measurements. (**a**) Master cast is scanned using a digital camera. (**b**) Digitized image of scanned plaster model; this image is transferred into another software program, capable of superimposing digital images. (**c**) Three-dimensional image of initial situation prior to augmentation surgery (baseline). (**d**) Three-dimensional image of clinical situation at sacrifice. (**e**) Superimposed image demonstrating volumetric changes between baseline and sacrifice; white color areas represent a gain in volume; red color areas represent a loss of volume; black areas show volumetric changes <50 μm. (**f**) Superimposed image including the measured areas (region of interest) of all three defects sites in blue color.

For the evaluation of the dimensional changes at the defect sites, the casts are optically scanned with a three-dimensional camera (Fickl et al., 2009; Schneider et al., 2011) (Fig 6-9a). Since the accessible area for the optical scanner is limited to a field of 17 × 14 mm at a time, several overlapping optical impressions from the buccal and the bucco-occlusal direction are taken, including the canine, P1, P3, the mesial root of M1, and M2. The acquired data are then composed into one digital image using CAD/CAM software (Cerec 3D®, Sirona Dental Systems, Bensheim, Germany), encompassing the jaw segments from the canine to the second molar (Fig 6-9b). The obtained digital images of the casts reflecting the different treatment time points (baseline, 28 days, 84 days) are then transferred into another digital imaging software product (Match3D, University of Munich, Munich, Germany) (Figs 6-9c and 6-9d).

These images are superimposed and matched in one common coordinate system (Fig 6-9e). The buccal surfaces of the remaining teeth are used as reference points for the superposition of the different images. Subsequently, a defined area of interest at each defect site is measured and the volume difference between the time points is calculated. Due to an individually variable anatomic situation the measured area varies between the sites, but is kept constant at one site over time. The region of interest exhibits a trapezoid shape and reaches in a bucco-oral dimension from the most coronal aspect of the lingual defect side to roughly 1 cm into the buccal mucosa, and in a mesiodistal dimension from one neighboring tooth (mesial) to the other neighboring tooth (distal) at a distance of 1 mm from the neighboring tooth (Fig 6-9f).

In order to allow a direct comparison of the different sites and the different treatment modalities, the calculated variable Δd is the measured volume difference per measured area (Δd [mm] = Δ vol [mm^3] / area [mm^2]).

The obtained data is statistically analyzed regarding volume alterations in terms of different treatment modalities and time points.

Histological Preparation
The non-decalcified specimens are embedded in methyl methacrylate resin. Radiographic recordings are performed for each site in order to accurately determine cutting planes. From each specimen, one central orofacial section through the augmented defect (reference pin), one mesial (at a distance of 2 mm from the reference pin) and one distal (at a distance of 2 mm from the reference pin) section are prepared for histologic assessment. The longitudinal sections of 50 to 60 μm thickness are obtained by a microcutting and grinding technique adapted by Donath (Donath and Breuner, 1982). Thereafter, the sections are stained with toluidine blue and basic fuchsin.

Descriptive Histology
A qualitative analysis can be performed using a stereoscope, which allows evaluaton of the different components according to the standard nomenclature of the International Society for Stereology (Exner, 1987). Digital images of the sections are acquired and descriptive histology is applied evaluating the following parameters: vascularization of the device/graft, remaining device/graft material, tissue integration of the device/graft, newly formed connective tissue, newly formed bone, and inflammatory reaction.

Histomorphometric Analysis
Computer-assisted histomorphometric measurements are performed using an automated image analysis system, coupled with a video camera mounted on a light microscope.

The following parameters are calculated in all three sections: ridge width at four different levels (1.5 mm, 3.5 mm, 5.5 mm, 7.5 mm below the crest) including measurements of native bone, newly formed bone, and regenerated soft tissue (Fig 6-10).

6.3.9 Statistical Analysis Plan
The volume differences are assessed at 28 and 84 days, relative to the preoperative dimension of the defect inside a defined region of interest. The ridge widths are assessed at 24 and 84 days. Based on the two site values by dog and treatment, the mean values are always used in the statistical description and analysis. Measured parameters are summarized in terms of means and standard deviations. Volume differences and ridge width differences are analyzed with analysis of variance (ANOVA) in order to describe and compare the three treatment modalities. The paired t test is used in order to judge the mean changes within the treatment groups. The level of significance is set at $P < 0.05$.

6.3 Soft Tissue Volume – Dog Model

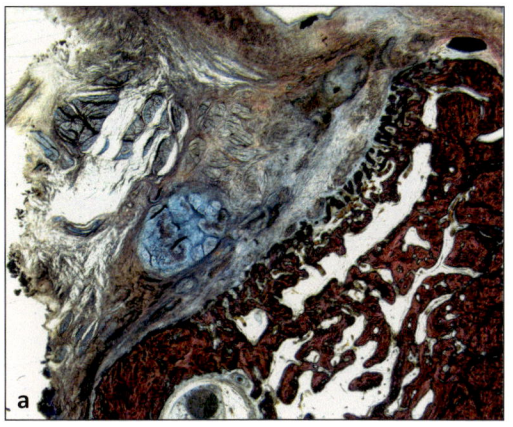
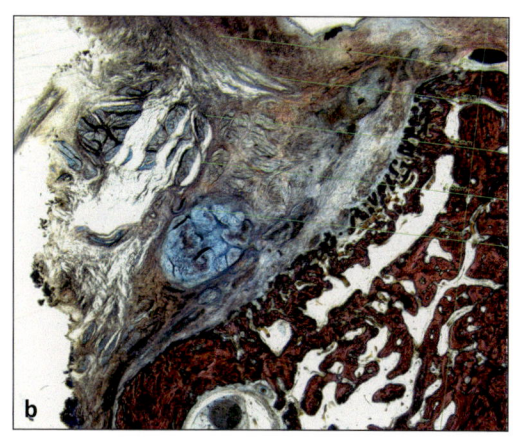
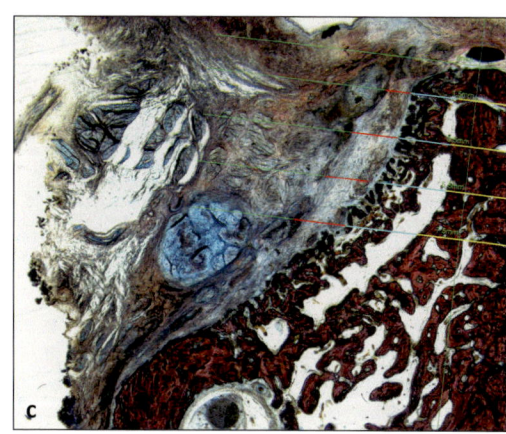

Fig 6-10 (**a**) Representative histologic slide (original magnification ×2.5). Central section through center augmented site (middle defect). (**b**) Same slide including grid used for histomorphometric measurements; measurements are performed at four levels below the bone crest (1.5 mm, 3.5 mm, 5.5 mm, 7.5 mm). (**c**) Calculated measures shown in colors: yellow = old bone; blue = new bone formation; red = newly formed soft tissue.

6.3.10 Materials, Consumables, Equipment

Operating room: a purpose-designed room for experimental animals in accordance with the requirements of the FDA "Good Laboratory Practice" (GLP) Regulations.

Animals: male, large, hound-type dogs, more than 2 years old, weighing between 60 and 70 kg.

Anesthesia:
- Thiopental-sodium solution 4%, 0.4 mL/kg body weight as a premedication
- Isoflurane 1.5–2%.

Surgery 1 (tooth extraction):
- Standard surgical instrument kit for tooth extraction
- Disinfectant
- Non-resorbable sutures
- Standard endo kit for root canal filling of M1 (mesial root)
- Gutta-percha and sealer
- Portable radiographic machine.

Impressions:
- Polyether impression material
- Master casts out of dental stone
- Light-curing tray material for individualized trays.

Surgery 2 (soft tissue augmentation):
- Standard surgical instrument kit for mucogingival surgery
- Disinfectant
- Test devices
- Titanium pins as reference markers
- Non-resorbable sutures.

Postoperative care:
- Antibiotic treatment with spiramycin and metronidazole
- Analgesia with carprofen.

Analyses:
- Volumetric analyses
- 3D camera (Cerec 3 Bluecam®)
- Digital imaging software (Match3D).
- Histology and histomorphometry
- Poly(methyl methacrylate) resin
- Band-saw
- Microtome
- Staining with basic fuchsin and toluidine
- A stereoscope with a video camera
- An automated image analysis system.

References

1. Adell R, Lekholm U, Rockler B, Branemark PI, Lindhe J, Eriksson B et al. (1986). Marginal tissue reactions at osseointegrated titanium fixtures (I). A 3-year longitudinal prospective study. *Int J Oral Maxillofac Surg* 15:39–52.
2. Allen EP, Gainza CS, Farthing GG, Newbold DA (1985). Improved technique for localized ridge augmentation. A report of 21 cases. *J Periodontol* 56:195–199.
3. Artzi Z, Tal H, Moses O, Kozlovsky A (1993). Mucosal considerations for osseointegrated implants. *J Prosthet Dent* 70:427–432.
4. Badylak SF (2002). The extracellular matrix as a scaffold for tissue reconstruction. *Semin Cell Dev Biol* 13:377–383.
5. Batista EL Jr, Batista FC, Novaes AB Jr (2001). Management of soft tissue ridge deformities with acellular dermal matrix. Clinical approach and outcome after 6 months of treatment. *J Periodontol* 72:265–273.
6. Donath K, Breuner G (1982). A method for the study of undecalcified bones and teeth with attached soft tissues. The Sage-Schliff (sawing and grinding) technique. *J Oral Pathol* 11:318–326.
7. Edel A (1974). Clinical evaluation of free connective tissue grafts used to increase the width of keratinised gingiva. *J Clin Periodontol* 1:185–196.
8. Exner HE (1987). A model stereological nomenclature. *Acta Stereologica* 6(Suppl II):179–184.
9. Farnoush A (1978). Techniques for the protection and coverage of the donor sites in free soft tissue grafts. *J Periodontol* 49:403–405.
10. Fickl S, Schneider D, Zuhr O, Hinze M, Ender A, Jung RE et al. (2009). Dimensional changes of the ridge contour after socket preservation and buccal overbuilding: an animal study. *J Clin Periodontol* 36:442–448.
11. Friedman A (1962). Mucogingival surgery: The apically repositioned flap. *J Periodontol* 33:328–340.
12. Griffin TJ, Cheung WS, Zavras AI, Damoulis PD (2006). Postoperative complications following gingival augmentation procedures. *J Periodontol* 77:2070–2079.
13. Hämmerle CH, Jung RE (2003). Bone augmentation by means of barrier membranes. *Periodontol 2000* 33:36–53.
14. Harris RJ (2003). Soft tissue ridge augmentation with an acellular dermal matrix. *Int J Periodontics Restorative Dent* 23:87–92.
15. Jung RE, Siegenthaler DW, Hämmerle CH (2004). Post-extraction tissue management: a soft tissue punch technique. *Int J Periodontics Restorative Dent* 24:545–553.
16. Jung RE, Hürzeler MB, Thoma DS, Khraisat A, Hämmerle CHF (2011). Local tolerance and efficiency of two prototype collagen matrices to increase the width of keratinized tissue. *J Clin Periodontol* 38:173-179.
17. Karring T, Ostergaard E, Löe H (1971). Conservation of tissue specificity after heterotopic transplantation of gingiva and alveolar mucosa. *J Periodontal Res* 6:282–293.
18. Karring T, Lang NP, Löe H (1975). The role of gingival connective tissue in determining epithelial differentiation. *J Periodontal Res* 10:1–11.
19. Lang NP, Löe H (1972). The relationship between the width of keratinized gingiva and gingival health. *J Periodontol* 43:623–627.
20. Langer B (1996). The regeneration of soft tissue and bone around implants with and without membranes. *Compend Contin Educ Dent* 17:268–270, 272 passim; quiz 280.
21. Langer B, Calagna L (1980). The subepithelial connective tissue graft. *J Prosthet Dent* 44:363–367.
22. Lozdan J, Squier CA (1969). The histology of the mucogingival junction. *J Periodontal Res* 4:83–93.
23. McGuire MK, Nunn ME (2005). Evaluation of the safety and efficacy of periodontal applications of a living tissue-engineered human fibroblast-derived dermal substitute. I. Comparison to the gingival autograft: a randomized controlled pilot study. *J Periodontol* 76:867–880.
24. McGuire MK, Scheyer ET, Nunn ME, Lavin PT (2008). A pilot study to evaluate a tissue-engineered bilayered cell therapy as an alternative to tissue from the palate. *J Periodontol* 79:1847–1856.
25. Nabers JM (1966). Free gingival grafts. *Periodontics* 4:243–245.

References

26. Nevins M, Nevins ML, Camelo M, Camelo JM, Schupbach P, Kim DM (2010). The clinical efficacy of DynaMatrix extracellular membrane in augmenting keratinized tissue. *Int J Periodontics Restorative Dent* 30:151–161.
27. Nevins ML (2010). Tissue-engineered bilayered cell therapy for the treatment of oral mucosal defects: a case series. *Int J Periodontics Restorative Dent* 30:31–39.
28. Ophof R, Maltha JC, Von den Hoff JW, Kuijpers-Jagtman AM (2004). Histologic evaluation of skin-derived and collagen-based substrates implanted in palatal wounds. *Wound Repair Regen* 12:528–538.
29. Ophof R, Maltha JC, Kuijpers-Jagtman AM, Von den Hoff JW (2008). Implantation of tissue-engineered mucosal substitutes in the dog palate. *Eur J Orthod* 30:1–9.
30. Orth CF (1996). A modification of the connective tissue graft procedure for the treatment of type II and type III ridge deformities. *Int J Periodontics Restorative Dent* 16:266–277.
31. Postlethwaite AE, Seyer JM, Kang AH (1978). Chemotactic attraction of human fibroblasts to type I, II, and III collagens and collagen-derived peptides. *Proc Natl Acad Sci U S A* 75:871–875.
32. Prato GP, Cairo F, Tinti C, Cortellini P, Muzzi L, Mancini EA (2004). Prevention of alveolar ridge deformities and reconstruction of lost anatomy: a review of surgical approaches. *Int J Periodontics Restorative Dent* 24:434–445.
33. Sanz M, Lorenzo R, Aranda JJ, Martin C, Orsini M (2009). Clinical evaluation of a new collagen matrix (Mucograft prototype) to enhance the width of keratinized tissue in patients with fixed prosthetic restorations: a randomized prospective clinical trial. *J Clin Periodontol* 36:868–876.
34. Schneider D, Grunder U, Ender A, Hämmerle CHF, Jung RE (2011). Volume gain and stability of peri-implant tissue following bone and soft tissue augmentation: 1-year results from a prospective cohort study. *Clin Oral Implants Res* 22:28-37.
35. Schrott AR, Jimenez M, Hwang JW, Fiorellini J, Weber HP (2009). Five-year evaluation of the influence of keratinized mucosa on peri-implant soft-tissue health and stability around implants supporting full-arch mandibular fixed prostheses. *Clin Oral Implants Res* 20:1170–1177.
36. Schwarz F, Rothamel D, Herten M, Sager M, Becker J (2006). Angiogenesis pattern of native and cross-linked collagen membranes: an immunohistochemical study in the rat. *Clin Oral Implants Res* 17:403–409.
37. Seibert JS (1983a). Reconstruction of deformed, partially edentulous ridges, using full thickness onlay grafts. Part I. Technique and wound healing. *Compend Contin Educ Dent* 4:437–453.
38. Seibert JS (1983b). Reconstruction of deformed, partially edentulous ridges, using full thickness onlay grafts. Part II. Prosthetic/periodontal interrelationships. *Compend Contin Educ Dent* 4:549–562.
39. Soileau KM, Brannon RB (2006). A histologic evaluation of various stages of palatal healing following subepithelial connective tissue grafting procedures: a comparison of eight cases. *J Periodontol* 77:1267–1273.
40. Strebel J, Ender A, Paqué F, Krähenmann M, Attin T, Schmidlin PR (2009). In vivo validation of a three-dimensional optical method to document volumetric soft tissue changes of the interdental papilla. *J Periodontol* 80:56–61.
41. Studer SP, Lehner C, Bucher A, Scharer P (2000). Soft tissue correction of a single-tooth pontic space: a comparative quantitative volume assessment. *J Prosthet Dent* 83:402–411.
42. Sullivan HC, Atkins JH (1969). The role of free gingival grafts in periodontal therapy. *Dent Clin North Am* 13:133–148.
43. Thoma DS, Benic GI, Zwahlen M, Hämmerle CH, Jung RE (2009). A systematic review assessing soft tissue augmentation techniques. *Clin Oral Implants Res* 20(Suppl 4):146–165.
44. Thoma DS, Jung RE, Schneider D, Cochran DL, Ender A, Jones A et al. (2010). Soft tissue volume augmentation by the use of collagen based matrices – a volumetric analysis. *J Clin Periodontol* 37:659–666.
45. Wainwright DJ (1995). Use of an acellular allograft dermal matrix (AlloDerm) in the management of full-thickness burns. *Burns* 21:243–248.
46. Wei PC, Laurell L, Geivelis M, Lingen MW, Maddalozzo D (2000). Acellular dermal matrix allografts to achieve increased attached gingiva. Part 1. A clinical study. *J Periodontol* 71:1297–1305.
47. Wei PC, Laurell L, Lingen MW, Geivelis M (2002). Acellular dermal matrix allografts to achieve increased attached gingiva. Part 2. A histological comparative study. *J Periodontol* 73:257–265.
48. Windisch SI, Jung RE, Sailer I, Studer SP, Ender A, Hämmerle CH (2007). A new optical method to evaluate three-dimensional volume changes of alveolar contours: a methodological in vitro study. *Clin Oral Implants Res* 18:545–551.
49. Yukna RA, Sullivan WM (1978). Evaluation of resultant tissue type following the intraoral transplantation of various lyophilized soft tissues. *J Periodontal Res* 13:177–184.

Preclinical Protocols for Periodontal Regeneration

Hector F. Rios and William V. Giannobile

7.1 General Overview

The periodontium represents the tooth-supporting apparatus and can be described as a dynamic tissue complex, sensitive to a variety of factors, and with an inherent capacity that allows the translation of mechanical stimuli into biochemical signals that govern its homeostasis (Burger et al., 1995; Duncan and Turner, 1995; Marotti, 2000; Marotti and Palumbo, 2007; Bonewald and Johnson, 2008). Its structure and function during remodeling and healing is determined by the orchestration of important bioactive proteins (platelet-derived growth factor [PDGF], vascular endothelial growth factor [VEGF], epidermal growth factor [EGF], fibroblast growth factor [FGF], bone morphogenetic proteins [BMPs], insulin-like growth factor 1 [IGF-1], transforming growth factor β-1 [TGF-β1], etc. (Long et al., 2002; Sato et al., 2002; Tsuji et al., 2004; Yang et al., 2006), thus resulting in an increased adaptive potential that protects and maintains the integrity of its four fundamental components: the alveolar bone, the periodontal ligament (PDL), the cementum, and the gingiva (Fig 7-1).

In humans, the detrimental changes that the tooth-supporting tissues undergo are primarily the result of inflammatory periodontal diseases that undermine and disrupt the functional and structural integrity of the alveolar bone, the PDL, and the cementum. The restoration of the original structure, properties, and function of these tissues represents a therapeutic advantage and the most ideal and desired outcome of periodontal therapy. Unfortunately, altered healing often disrupts the normal restoration of the periodontium and as a result different clinical compromised outcomes can be identified. Today, the available preclinical research models serve as the foundation of successful periodontal regenerative therapies. These *in vivo* animal models represent a valuable approach to elucidate the key factors or devices that promote periodon-

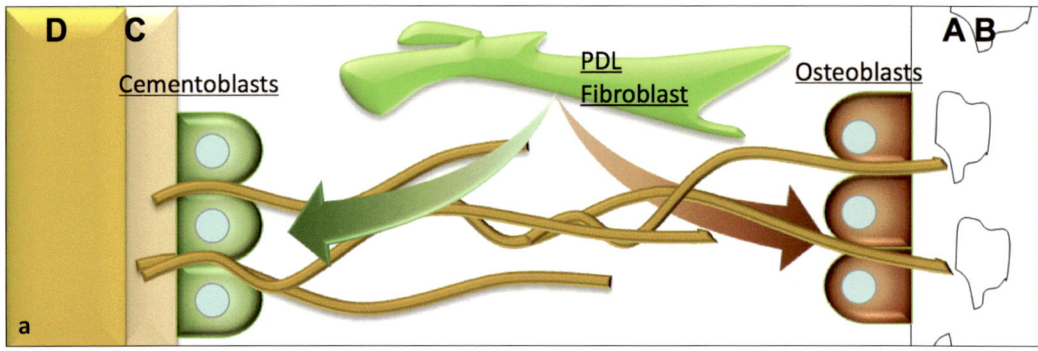
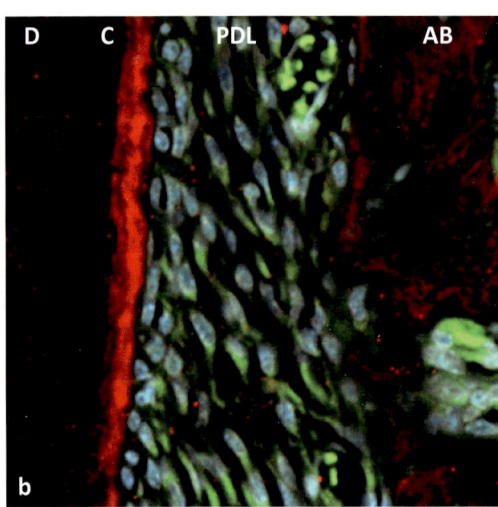

Fig 7-1 (a) The mature periodontium contains undifferentiated stem cells that retain the potential to differentiate into osteoblasts, cementoblasts, and fibroblasts. The PDL fibroblasts are important regulators of the periodontal integrity. (b) These subpopulations of fibroblasts (green) have the ability to prevent/regulate the invasion of bone (red) and cementum (red) into the PDL space and therefore maintain its structural homeostasis and regulate its remodeling potential. D, dentin; C, cementum; AB, alveolar bone.

tal regeneration and are critical for evaluating the biologic responses before human clinical trial testing.

Preclinical animal models allow the implementation of investigations for determination of the safety and efficacy of regenerative devices and biologics for periodontal repair. In this chapter we provide an overview of the commonly used preclinical animal models for the study of reconstructive procedures to promote bone and soft tissue repair of tooth-supporting periodontal defects. Steps are provided on the animal management for evaluation of outcome measures using descriptive histology, histomorphometry, three-dimensional imaging, and safety assessments. The use of these key measures of periodontal regeneration should aid investigators in the selection of appropriate surrogate endpoints to be utilized in the clinical arena, which are not practical or ethical in humans. These methods will prepare investigators and assist them in identifying endpoints that can then be adapted to human clinical trial planning.

7.2 Small Animal Models for Periodontal Regeneration

Rodents are the most commonly used animal models in biomedical research. Rats are cost-effective, easy to handle, and allow for the

7.2 Small Animal Models for Periodontal Regeneration

Table 7-1 Advantages and disadvantages of small animal models (mice, rats)

Advantages	Disadvantages
Gives a proof of concept in a short interval	Small size, surgical microscopes required
Relatively low cost	Spontaneous healing
Known age	Narrow healing window
Known genetic background	Different anatomic structures compared to humans
Controllable microflora	Different histopathologic features
Ease of handling and housing	Different host responses compared with humans

standardization of experimental conditions in genetically similar individuals. Rats are suitable to study the effect of systemic diseases and pharmacologic therapies on tissue destruction and regeneration (Graves et al., 2008), and to evaluate physiologic alterations related to aging (Benatti et al., 2006). In addition, tissue destruction and regeneration in an immunodeficient background can be investigated in this model (Klausen, 1991). However, surgery and the evaluation of study endpoints are challenging because of the animals' small size. Moreover, the rodent dentition undergoes continuous tooth eruption, including bone and cementum apposition, which has to be considered in planning a study (Belting et al., 1953) (Table 7-1).

7.2.1 Fenestration or Dehiscence Periodontal Regeneration Model

Rats are not susceptible to developing natural periodontitis. However, chronic inflammation that leads to periodontal destruction can be induced by placing a cotton or silk floss ligature in the sulci around the molars (Jin et al., 2007). Chronic inflammation can also be achieved by repeated intragingival injection of bacterial lipopolysaccharide eliciting the release of proinflammatory cytokines by the host (Park et al., 2007; Rogers et al., 2007). Both models are suitable to evaluate the pathogenesis of periodontitis and therapeutic strategies to modulate disease progression (Graves et al., 2008). Studies on reconstructive therapies, however, require surgically created periodontal defects, as originally described by Melcher (1970).

The Rat Model
The *Rattus* (Rat) species have being recommended to use for this particular model. The fenestration periodontal wound defect model is widely employed and is accepted as an appropriate one to test periodontal wound healing in small animals. This model provides isolation from the oral environment, due to the extraoral approach, and thus can prevent negative effects such as contamination, and infection by saliva and other microorganisms.

> **Box 7-1 Aims of the Rat Model**
> The rat fenestration periodontal wound defect model is primarily adapted to determine the therapeutic efficacy of key factors, material or devices, and provide proof of principle before proceeding to a larger animal model.

7.2.2 Advantages/Disadvantages of the Presented Model

Advantages:
- Proof-of-concept in a short timeframe
- Well-contained defect
- No gingival tissue ingrowth.

Disadvantages:
- Narrow healing time window
- Technically challenging (small size)

- Rapid repair as kinetic healing model
- Not a "natural disease" model.

7.2.3 Timing

Recommended study evaluation time ranges from 2 to 6 weeks to capture early healing events and wound maturation. The early healing process follows the conserved sequence of wound healing that is initiated by blood coagulation and immigration of neutrophils and monocytes for wound debridement and bone resorption. This microenvironment favors the proliferation and migration of mesenchymal progenitors, which can originate from the PDL or the host bone (Lekic et al., 1996a,b). After 10 days, a thin cementum layer with a connective tissue attachment can be observed, in particular on the apical side of the teeth where the cementum is thicker compared with the narrow coronal region (King et al., 1997). Bone formation starts from the bone margins (Rajshankar et al., 1998). In young rats (King et al., 1997) periodontal regeneration is complete after 1 month, while geriatric animals at 18 months of age show a delayed healing capacity (Benatti et al., 2006). It is therefore crucial to select the appropriate time point to determine the therapeutic efficacy of a candidate molecule, material, or device.

7.2.4 Preparation

Animals require an acclimatization period of approximately 2 to 7 days after arrival in a new housing facility. The surgical area should be conducive to an aseptic surgery, and must not be used for any other purpose during the time of the surgery. Ideally, the surgical area can be located within the housing facilities, therefore limiting stress and potential health hazards to the animals. Disinfectants such as sodium hypochlorite, chlorine dioxide, dimethyl ammonium chloride, or glutaraldehyde-based solutions can be used to clean and disinfect the surgery area, although some may not be as effective at eliminating all contaminants. Animals and instruments must also be prepared in a way to prevent contamination and ensure success of the survival surgery.

Animal preparation for rodent surgery

Following anesthesia, ophthalmic ointment (lubricant) must be applied to the eyes of the animal receiving anesthetic to prevent drying. Incision sites must be cleared of hair if the incision is >1 cm, using clippers, a razor, or a depilatory agent. Hair removal should be performed in a separate location to avoid surgical area contamination. Skin must then be disinfected with three alternating scrubs of povidone-iodine topical antiseptic, and warm, sterile saline, water, or 70% ethanol (ethanol is less desirable) scrubbing in an outward and spiral direction. All instruments should be cleaned and sterilized (e.g., autoclaved) prior to surgery. Disinfection/sterilization of multiple sets of instruments should be carried out for successive surgeries. Following use, instruments should be thoroughly cleaned before sterilization. Hot bead sterilization is a fast, dry method to prevent cross contamination between animals during surgery. Alternative sterilization methods may incorporate the use of glutaraldehyde or chlorine dioxide immersion followed by a sterile water or saline rinse. Aseptic techniques and sterile environments are critical to animal survival and positive experimental results. Effective drug dosage may vary from animal to animal according to body weight, metabolism, and age. There are no exact calculations to relate the effective dose between animal and humans. Dosage can be determined by previous study results, published literature, and veterinary guidelines. Surgeons should also undergo appropriate preparation including, but not limited to, handwashing, wearing sterile gloves, gowns, and masks for each animal's surgical procedures.

7.2.5 Surgical Procedures

For the rat periodontal fenestration defect (King et al., 1997; Jin et al., 2004; Huang et al., 2005), an extraoral buccal approach should be used. After a flap is raised by extraoral access to expose the mandibular alveolus, the distal and buccal roots of the first molar and the mesial root of the second molar are denuded, includ-

7.2 Small Animal Models for Periodontal Regeneration

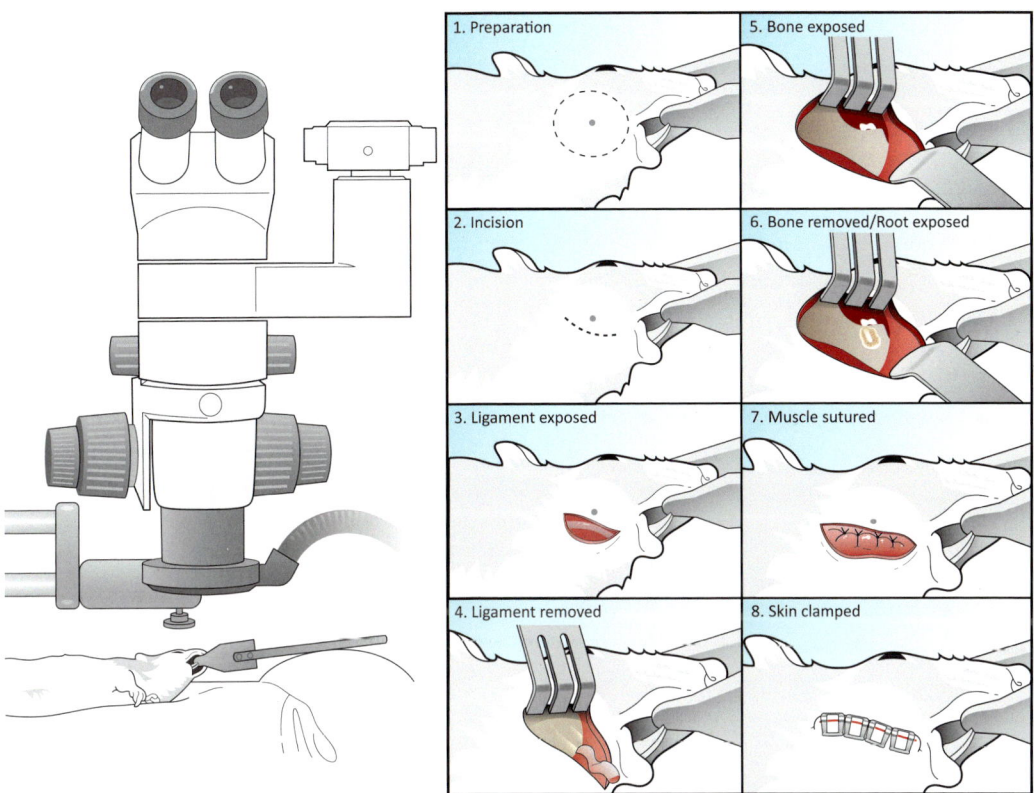

Fig 7-2 Surgical scope. Appropriate magnification with an external light source is essential to overcome the dimensional limitations of the rat fenestration defect model. (**1**) Preparation. Iodine disinfection should be performed together with proper isolation of the surgical site. Soft tissue and hard tissue landmarks should be identified prior to initiating any incision. (**2**) Incision. Incision is designed to expose in an anterior-posterior direction the surface of the masseter muscle. (**3**) Ligamentous line. After the initial cutaneous incision is completed, the operator should identify a ligamentous line that follows the trajectory of the lower border of the mandible. (**4**) Ligament removed. The dissection of the masseter muscle leads to the exposure of an anterior ligament that covers the area of the first molar in a more lateral position. This ligament should be removed to ensure proper access to the buccal plate at the level of the first molar. (**5**) Bone exposure. The periosteum should be elevated in the area of interest with proper flap reflection. (**6**) Defect creation. High-speed burs (no. 4 and ¼) are used to initiate the delineation of the defect and ensure proper cementum removal. (**7**) Muscle sutured. After the regenerative agent or construct is delivered to the defect site, proper would closure is first ensured by single interrupted sutures approximating the masseter muscle to its original position. (**8**) Skin clamped. Surgical staples are utilized to close the cutaneous incision and protect the surgical site. Proper wound stabilization should be maintain for 2 weeks.

ing the superficial dentin. New medical formulations (NMF) can be delivered into the fenestration defects ($3 \times 2 \times 1$ mm) and secured by flap repositioning. The surgery should be performed under a magnifying stereoscope ($\times 2$ to 10) to allow proper identification of anatomic landmarks and site preparation (Fig 7-2):

1. After preparing the animal for surgery, proper identification of epithelial and hard tissue landmarks should guide the operator for the initial incision.
2. A superficial incision is first used to expose the masseter muscle and gain access to a ligamentous landmark that extends in a pos-

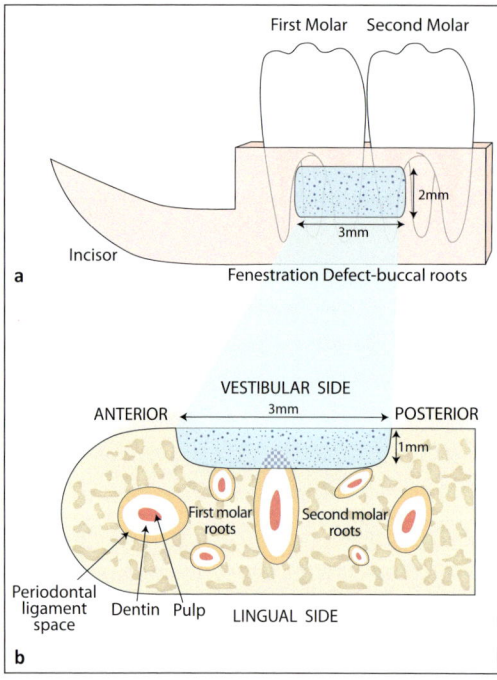

Fig 7-3 (a) The fenestration defect is created on the buccal surface of the mandibular alveolar bone. Distal and buccal roots of the first molar and the buccal root of the second molar are exposed. (b) Novel regenerative therapeutics (light blue) are delivered into the defect. The coronal section of the alveolar bone shows the defect outline. The cemental layer, superficial dentin, and the PDL are removed. At 3, 10, 21, and 35 days post surgery tissue samples are harvested and bone and cementum regeneration are evaluated. Reproduced from Pellegrini et al. (2009), with permission from SAGE Publications.

teroanterior direction approximating the lower border of the mandible. At this time it is also important to separate the skin from the muscle around the incision line to allow proper closure and space for the use of surgical staples at the end of the surgery.

3. A scalpel incision can be made under this ligamentous line on the masseter muscle to expose the rat mandibular bone (buccal plate). In some cases, the parotid gland duct (Stenson's) can be involved, causing postsurgical buccal swelling. This swelling can affect tissue regeneration as it produces mechanical pressure to the surgical area. Swelling can be eliminated by surgical removal of the parotid gland in those rare cases.

4. A distinct ligament is usually covering the area lateral to the first molar; this should be dissected to ensure proper flap refection and adequate surgical access.

5. Once the bone is exposed and access to the first molar region is gained, the operator will be able to distinguish a more opaque and bulbous bone region with a tear-like shape, which is characteristic of the buccal plate.

6. The target defect creation area is the distal root of the mandibular first molar. Buccal roots of the first and second molars can be included in the surgical defect. Using a round bur with high-speed instrumentation, one can create a bony defect of 3 × 2 × 1 mm size (Fig 7-2; Fig 7-3 and Fig 7-4). Initiate access with a no. 4 round bur and once roots become visible, continue with a ¼ bur to complete the osteotomy and remove the cementum. During bone and cementum removal, it is difficult to irrigate with saline due to the small defect size, thin bone, and cementum. Special care should be taken to not generate heat damage at the surgical site, as it prevents a normal healing process. The PDL, cementum, and

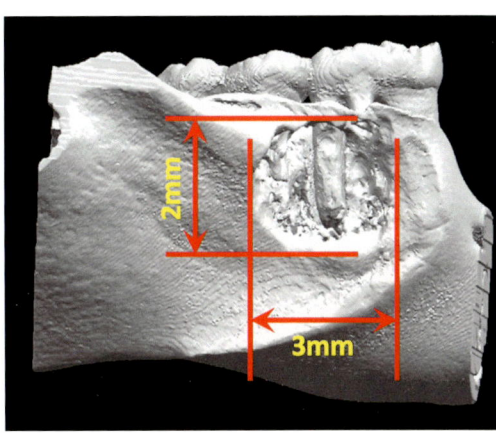

Fig 7-4 Micro-computed tomography image of the created defect area. Within the 2 × 3 mm window, the distal root of the first molar is usually located in the center of the defect and at a depth of ~1 mm. One very small ledge of crestal bone remains coronally to maintain the integrity of the ridge and prevent communication with the oral cavity.

superficial dentin can be removed by a combination of hand instrumentation and careful use of rotatory instruments.
7. After applying test agent(s) or regenerative devices into the created defect area, the muscle is first repositioned using resorbable sutures.
8. Once proper muscle approximation and closure is ensured, the skin is repositioned by surgical clips.

7.2.6 Anesthesia

Rats can be anesthetized with a combination of ketamine and xylazine via intraperitoneal (IP) injection, lasting for 45–90 minutes.

Rat anesthetics and analgesics: A combination of ketamine (IP, 40–90 mg/kg) and xylazine (IP 5–10 mg/kg) can be used as a general, injectable anesthesia for oral procedures. For prolonged anesthesia, supplement with one-third dose of ketamine only. IP injections should be performed using a 20–27-gauge needle that is inserted into the lower left abdominal quadrant with the animal in a head-down position. Buprenorphine (subcutaneous, 0.01–0.05 mg/kg) can be used for 8–12 hours for post-operative pain relief; or for 24-hour pain management, 5 mg/kg ketoprofen (subcutaneous) may be selected. Anesthesia depth is typically monitored by the loss of response to external stimuli, such as a limb pinch.

All animals should be provided an external heat source (e.g., recirculating water blanket, microwaveable heating packs, or self-regulating heating pad) in indirect contact with the animal to prevent hypothermia during the entire anesthesia and recovery period.

7.2.7 Postoperative Care, Including Analgesics and Wound Management

Following surgery, rats may be administered analgesia for pain, and antibiotics for infection control within the surgical site. Analgesics, such as buprenorphine, (0.01–0.05 mg/kg subcutaneous or IP) should be administered for at least 24 hours after the periodontal defect surgery. Antibiotics can be dispensed via the water supply, although normal chow should be readily available. Antibiotics may be added to the drinking water in order to reduce the incidence of infection following oral surgery. Ampicillin 268 mg/L may be added to a 5% to 10% dextrose solution. Colored water bottles should be used with light-sensitive antibiotics.

Animals should be mobile and feed freely following surgical recovery. Animal recovery time will vary with type of anesthesia, and dose of anesthesia, and may also vary between animals of similar sex, size, body mass, and genetic background. During the recovery process, all animals should be housed individually. Animals should be treated and monitored according to the animal surgery guidelines given by their institution in accordance with regulations and in compliance with animal housing authorities. For example, if biohazardous materials, such as viral vectors, are applied the animal must be kept in a biohazard facility until viral shedding has completed. If biologic hazardous agents are used such as viral vectors, each virus will have a specific shedding period for which it can be considered contagious, and contact should be limited during this period. For example, adenovirus should be considered biohazardous for at least 72 hours following application/inoculation.

7.2.8 Endpoint Measurements

The distal root of first molar is the main target for histologic and histomorphometric evaluation. Even though the fenestration defect may not be of critical size, this model provides a reasonable proof-of-concept approach over a short time interval. Moreover, isolation from oral environment excludes the negative variables resulting from bacterial contamination with caged animals. Based on this model, cementum and bone regeneration have been evaluated following the delivery of BMPs in a collagen carrier (King and Hughes, 2001; Talwar et al., 2001; Huang et al., 2005) and PDGF gene therapy (Jin et al., 2004), as well as other growth factors, genes, and cells (King and Hughes, 1999, 2001; Talwar et al., 2001; Jin et al., 2003; Jin et al., 2004; Zhao et al., 2004; Huang et al., 2005).

At study endpoints animals can be sacrificed and the tissues harvested for analysis. Experimental endpoints are determined by previous studies, published literature, and/or may be based on the properties of biologic materials themselves. If the molecules of interest act early in the healing process, the endpoints should be selected accordingly in order to capture important healing events. Euthanasia methods, such as carbon dioxide asphyxiation, should be selected according to institutional guidelines. A secondary method should be employed in order to confirm animal death prior to resuming tissue collection. Harvested samples should be fixed to prevent degradation without damaging the tissues.

Potential endpoints are the dimension and extension of new cementum, PDL, and bone in the defect region. The length of new cementum and PDL extension can be measured from the original notch. The area of new bone can be measured through histomorphometric analysis.

7.2.9 Statistical Analysis Plan

When considering the use of preclinical animal models, it is important to specify the appropriate sample size that will be required to minimize the risk of having false positive and false negative errors. In general, pilot studies or available scientific literature are used to assist in establishing a proper power analysis prior to the execution of the experiments (see Section 4.3.2 for more details).

In the fenestration/dehiscence periodontal regeneration model, often more than two groups are defined. Commonly, a no-treatment-control, a vehicle-control, and an experimental/treatment group are included. In addition, the parameters are often assessed at different time points that range from 2 to 6 weeks. The mean values are always used in the statistical description and analysis. Measured parameters are summarized in terms of means and standard deviations. Since more than two experimental conditions are to be compared, it is recommended to use analysis of variance (ANOVA) for the evaluation of parametric data in order to reject or accept the null hypothesis. If the result of the ANOVA reflects that there is a difference among the groups, a post hoc analysis is performed to identify where specifically the differences lie (please see Section 4.4 for more details). For the determination of the P value, the type I error rate is often set at 0.05. However, this value should be dictated by the requirements of the experiment.

7.2.10 Materials, Consumables, Equipment

- Visualizing microscope such as a magnifying stereoscope (×2 to 10).
- Initial incision: Surgical blade (#11, 15), periosteal elevator (Pritchard).
- Defect creation: Bur (¼, 4 round bur), low-speed and high-speed handpiece with engine and chisel.
- Surgical retractors, periodontal probe, 17/23 dental explorer.
- Small, sharp, hand instrument such as Gracey curette.
- Wound closure: Needle holder (Crile-Wood), suture material (resorbable), scissors (LaGrange double curved), and metal staples.
- Anesthesia; will vary with animal model.
- Sterile, sanitizable, surgical area with proper ventilation.
- External heat source(s).
- Hot-bead instrument sterilizer.
- Sterile, clean cages for post-surgery animal recovery.
- Staple remover.
- Tissue harvesting: Scissors, round disk and low speed engine for tissue harvesting.
- Optical microscope with imaging analysis apparatus. Ideally, a high-definition charge-coupled device (CCD) color camera capable of taking microscopic images is recommended.
- Micro-computed tomography (CT) for additional three-dimensional analysis.

7.3 Large Animal Models for Periodontal Regeneration

Once the experimental agent has been demonstrated to be efficacious in rodent models, preclinical research is often expanded to large animals prior to human studies, although this sequence is not a Food and Drug Administration (FDA) or European Medicines Agency (EMA) regulatory requirement. Given that most rodent osseous defect models do not represent critical-size defects or a well characterized compromised wound-healing situation, large animals usually validate a move to consideration of clinical applications. These large models include dogs, sheep, pigs, and nonhuman primates. Large animals allow for the study of novel constructs or agents in critical-size defects that, by definition, do not heal spontaneously during the lifetime of the animal (Hollinger and Kleinschmidt, 1990). Another advantage of large animal models is that higher-order animals generally more closely simulate the anatomic, physiologic, and pathologic conditions found in humans (Schectman et al., 1972; Attström et al., 1975; Brecx et al., 1985; Hollinger and Kleinschmidt, 1990).

Consequently, preclinical studies involving dogs and nonhuman primates are generally preferred by regulatory bodies for demonstration of the safety and efficacy. It is recognized that different rates of bone healing occur when large and small animal models are compared (Frost, 1964; Roberts et al., 1987). Thus, critical-size defects of the periodontium or alveolar ridge are generally challenging to create in rodents (much more rapid and complete repair) vs. large animals (slower repair and not as complete). Furthermore, the anatomic similarities (especially for nonhuman primates) and defect size characteristics favor the consideration of large animals over small animals prior to more definitive studies in humans (Table 7-2).

Table 7-2 Advantages and disadvantages of large animal defect models

Advantages	Disadvantages
Surgical Acute-Chronic	**Surgical Acute**
Short time to be created – less expensive	Do not reproduce inflammatory/ infective conditions
Standardized morphological characteristics	Spontaneous partial regeneration (monkey)
Do not regenerate spontaneously (chronic)	Surgical chronic
	Soft tissues compromised
Class II–III furcation	Variable amount of connective tissue regeneration
Bilateral similar defect	
Horizontal defect allows an estimation of the origin of the newly formed tissue	
Solid database describing healing (dog)	
Minimal palatal recession (monkey)	
Ligature-induced	**Ligature-induced**
Microbiologic features similar to humans	Nonpredictable disease development
Morphologic features similar to humans	Nonstandardized defect morphology (dog)
Do not regenerate spontaneously	Require time to be created and expensive
Can make similar lesions as control in contralateral defects	

7.3.1 Canine Natural Periodontal Lesions

Dogs are very commonly used as a large animal for periodontal research because they have many similarities to humans, such as characterization of microbiologic and periodontal pathogenesis. Their premolars have two roots, allowing for creation of critical-size, supraalveolar furcation defects. Furthermore, dogs are generally friendly and cooperative, making care and management easy (Attström et al., 1975). In canine models, periodontal defects can either be created surgically (Wikesjö et al., 1994; Giannobile et al., 1998; Shirakata et al., 2007), involve ligatures around teeth (Martuscelli et al., 2000; Nociti et al., 2001), or develop naturally (Lynch et al., 1991; Lekovic et al., 1998) (Fig 7-5).

7.3.2 Animal Model: *Canis lupus familiaris* – Beagle (Specific Animal Species)

Dogs spontaneously develop periodontitis following accumulation of bacterial plaque and calculus (Lindhe et al., 1975). Similar to humans, elevated levels of *Bacteriodes asaccharolyticus* and spirochetes, and an increased proportion of Gram-negative anaerobes are found in dental plaque (Syed et al., 1981).

> **Box 7-2 Aims of the Dog Model**
> Natural periodontal lesions have been used to test the effects of biologics such as growth factors and barrier membranes on periodontal regeneration (Lynch et al., 1991; Giannobile et al., 1994; Lekovic et al., 1998).

7.3.3 Advantages/Disadvantages of the Presented Model

Advantages:
- Similar to humans
- Similar pathogen-associated microbiota
- Similar healing to humans
- Represents a chronic defect model.

Disadvantages:
- Difficult to predict the shape and extension of the lesions
- Difficult to control or predict the onset of disease activity
- Animals are difficult to locate (typically retired breeders) and are not readily available.

7.3.4 Timing

Spontaneous lesions typically manifest after 4 to 6 years. To achieve periodontal tissue destruction within 2 years, dogs are fed a soft diet. The clinical hallmarks of the disease are changing attachment level, marginal alveolar bone loss, and apical shift of the dentogingival epithelium. The severity of periodontal lesions decreases from the first to the fourth premolar followed by the first molar. Premolars have two roots and can thus develop furcation lesions (Page and Schroeder, 1981).

7.3.5 Surgical Procedures

1. The naturally occurring defects can be accessed and debrided by a regular periodontal surgical approach.
2. Candidate molecules or constructs can be placed into these natural lesions representing Class II–III furcation defects.
3. The elevated mucoperiosteal flap is repositioned and primary closure achieved by using resorbable sutures.

At 2 weeks after open flap debridement, formation of long junctional epithelium lining the root until the base of the instrumented surface is detectable. Connective tissue with randomly oriented fibers fills the majority of the defect volume. At 5 weeks 15% of new bone and 9% of new attachment can be observed. However, in naturally occurring periodontal disease, it is difficult to predict shape and

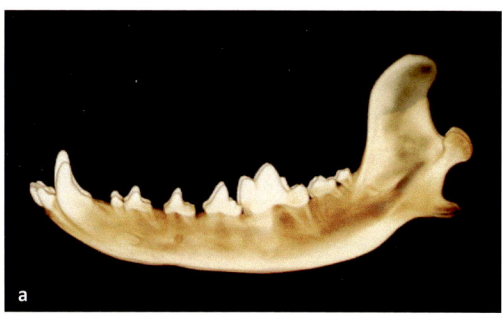

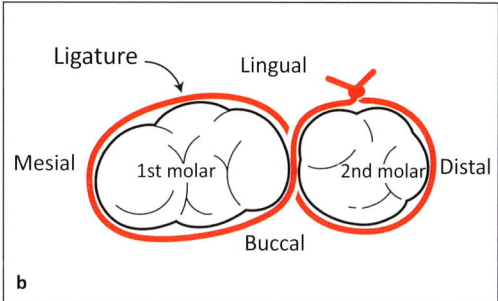

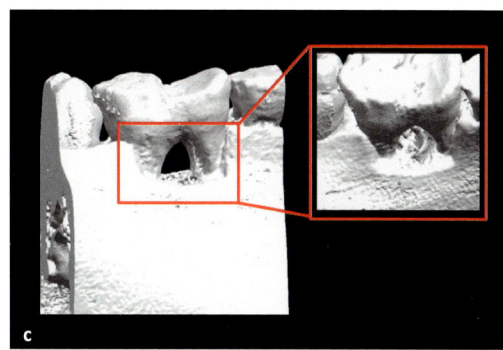

Fig 7-5 Periodontal lesions in dogs may develop naturally; be induced by placing a silk suture into the sulci (animals are normally kept on a soft diet to promote plaque accumulation); or simply created surgically.

extension of the lesions, as well as the onset of tissue destruction (Lindhe *et al.*, 1975). These characteristics limit the use of natural periodontal lesion models for preclinical studies. On the other hand, the pathogenesis of natural periodontal lesions in dog closely resembles the human situation.

7.3.6 Preparation

Animals require an acclimation period of approximately 1 week after arrival in a new housing facility. The surgical area should be easily sanitizable, and undergo careful preparation to ensure the aseptic surgical technique is carried out according to government and institutional guidelines. Ideally, the surgical area can be located within the housing facilities, but should be separated from human occupancy areas, therefore limiting stress and potential health hazards to the animals. Disinfectants such as the ones mentioned for previous models can be used to clean and disinfect the surgery area, although some may not be effective at eliminating all contaminants.

Animals and instruments must also be prepared in a way to limit or prevent contamination and ensure success of the survival surgery. Surgeons should undergo appropriate preparation in a room separate from the operating areas, including, but not limited to surgical staff, wearing sterile gloves, gowns, caps, shoe covers, and masks for each animal's surgical procedures.

The presurgical oral hygiene phase is especially necessary for canine and nonhuman primates to obtain a healing response following surgery by ensuring biofilm removal, and to begin with healthy periodontal tissues. Scaling and root planing procedures should be performed in an area separate from the surgical operating room to prevent contamination, and can be carried out approximately 10 days prior to surgery.

7.3.7 Anesthesia

Prior to anesthesia, canines greater than 10 weeks of age should be fasted for at least 6 hours, with the exception of water. Canines should be sedated using a combination of buprenorphine, acepromazine, and glycopyrrolate (BAG) as a presedative approximately 30 to 60 minutes prior to propofol administration for induction. The canine will then be intubated, and maintained under general anesthesia with isoflurane delivered through a volume-regulated aspirator (Giannobile *et al.*, 1998). Intravenous fluids, such as Ringer's solution (10 mL/kg/h), should be administered during surgery. Local infiltration anesthesia, for example lidocaine hydrochloride with epinephrine, is helpful to limit bleeding at and near to the surgical site. All animals should be provided an external heat source, preferably a recirculating water blanket, to prevent hypothermia during the entire anesthesia and recovery period.

Animals should be monitored until alert and active, and adequate homeostasis is achieved. While the animal is semiconscious it should be monitored every 15 minutes, and then monitored every hour until fully conscious. Once conscious, the animal must be monitored twice daily until fully recovered from the surgical procedure. Recovery should be carried out in a quiet, temperature-controlled, designated recovery area separate from the normal cage. Carprofen every 12 to 24 hours and/or buprenorphine every 8 to 12 hours can be administered for postsurgical pain relief. Antibiotics such as penicillin G benzathine (50,000 U/kg) should be administered subcutaneously on the day of surgery and every 5 days for up to 2 weeks.

7.3.8 Postoperative Care, Including Analgesics and Wound Management

Oral Hygiene Maintenance
For hygiene control, the treatment sites are to be cleaned with 0.1–0.2% chlorhexidine gel for 3

weeks following surgery. After the 3-week period, canines will receive a supragingival debridement and prophylaxis every 2 weeks. Every effort should be made to maintain optimal oral hygiene for each animal. Acepromazine (0.03–0.25 mg/kg intramuscularly, intravenously, or subcutaneously) may be used as a tranquilizer prior to oral hygiene measures, if necessary.

Diet and Miscellaneous

The animals are to be given a soft chow diet for up to 2 weeks following all surgical procedures to minimize trauma to the periodontium, until dry chow can be tolerated. Sutures must be removed between 10 to 14 days post-surgery, under anesthesia if necessary. Surgical records should be kept in the animal housing area for 3 to 7 days following anesthesia and/or surgery.

7.3.9 Endpoint Measurements

At study endpoints animals can be sacrificed, and tissues harvested for analysis. Experimental endpoints are determined based on previous studies, published literature, and/or may be based on the biologic material properties themselves. If the molecule of interest acts early in the healing process, endpoints should be selected accordingly in order to capture important healing events involving the compound of interest. Euthanasia methods, such as barbiturate overdose, should be selected according to institutional guidelines. A secondary method should be employed in order to confirm animal death prior to tissue collection. Harvested samples should be immediately fixed to prevent degradation or damage occurring to the tissues.

Histomorphometric endpoints include the following parameters:
- Area or height of newly formed bone, cementum and complete new attachment formation
- Osseous defect fill
- Root resorption
- Ankylosis.

7.3.10 Statistical Analysis Plan

A proper power analysis should be performed prior to the execution of the experiments (see Section 7.2.9). Similarly to the previously discussed rat model, in the canine and nonhuman primate models, more than two groups are often compared. Therefore, the differences among the various groups are evaluated by ANOVA and appropriate *post-hoc* analysis when necessary (see Section 7.2.9). The level of significance is set at $P < 0.05$ but could be adjusted based on the requirements of the experiment. Please see Section 4.3.2 for discussion on nonparametric data.

7.3.11 Materials, Consumables, Equipment

- Initial incision: Surgical blade (#11, 15), periosteal elevator (Pritchard).
- Surgical retractors, periodontal probe, 17/23 dental explorer.
- Small, sharp, hand instrument such as Gracey curette.
- Sharpening stone.
- Wound closure: Needle holder (Crile-Wood), suture material (resorbable), scissors (LaGrange double curved), and metal staples.
- Anesthesia.
- Sterile, sanitizable, surgical area with proper ventilation.
- External heat source(s).
- Hot-bead instrument sterilizer.
- Sterile, clean cages for postsurgical animal recovery.
- Tissue harvesting: Scissors, round disk and low speed engine for tissue harvesting.
- Optical microscope with imaging analysis apparatus.
- Micro-CT for additional three-dimensional analysis.

7.4 Intrabony or Furcation Periodontal Regeneration Model

7.4.1 Animal Model *Canis Lupus Familiaris* – Beagle

Canis lupus familiaris (Beagle) is very commonly used as a large animal for periodontal research it has many similarities to humans, such as microbiologic and periodontal pathogenesis characterization. Premolars have two roots, allowing for creation of critical-size, supraalveolar furcation defects. Furthermore, dogs are generally friendly and cooperative, making care and management easy (Attström *et al.*, 1975).

> **Box 7-3 Aim(s) of the Animal Model**
> Surgical periodontal defects have been largely used to evaluate periodontal regeneration following placement of membranes (Wikesjo *et al.*, 2003b), promoting biologics such as bone morphogenetic proteins (Giannobile *et al.*, 1998; Wikesjö *et al.*, 2003c; Wikesjö *et al.*, 2004), PDGF (Park *et al.*, 1995), and biomaterials (Sorensen *et al.*, 2004; Chen *et al.*, 2006).

7.4.2 Advantages/Disadvantages of the Presented Model

Surgical periodontal defects require a short time to be created, have standardized anatomic characteristics, morphologic similarity with the challenging human class III furcation defects, and do not heal spontaneously. However, acute periodontal defects fail to reproduce the inflammatory conditions occurring in the periodontal disease.

Advantages:
- Defects are rapidly created
- Standardized anatomical characteristics
- Similar morphology to human class III furcation defects
- Do not heal spontaneously.

Disadvantages:
- Fail to reproduce the microbiological and inflammatory condition
- Represents more of an acute defect model
- Lesions are immediately treated with the experimental factor before wound closure.

7.4.3 Timing

In general, the surgically created periodontal defect model requires a duration that ranges from 2 to 8 weeks. According to the conserved process of wound healing, the clot is replaced by granulation tissue. At the end of the first week, a cellular and fibrous-rich connective tissue gradually replaces the granulation tissue progressing along the root surface to the center of the defect. Woven bone formation starts at 2 weeks and later undergoes remodeling. Cementum formation also starts at about 2 weeks after surgery, characterized by organized collagen fibers adjacent and perpendicular to the root. Concomitant with the formation of cementum, the formation of a PDL is also observed, both originating from the bottom of the furcation (Matsuura *et al.*, 1995; Araujo *et al.*, 1997; Araujo *et al.*, 1999). After 12 to 20 weeks maturation of the periodontium is indicated by intrinsic and extrinsic fibers. Acute periodontal defects heal with a substantial connective tissue repair, a short junctional epithelium, and a minimal amount of new bone, cementum, and attachment, limited at the apical region. Chronic periodontal defects heal spontaneously with a longer junctional epithelium and some connective tissue repair, but still limited bone and cementum formation.

7.4.4 Surgical Procedures

- Surgically created defects can be made to the same size or shape to compare test groups and controls (5 mm in apico-coronal height at the furcation fornix region). The defects are typically created around the second, third, and fourth mandibular premolars (Fig 7-6).

7.4 Intrabony or Furcation Periodontal Regeneration Model

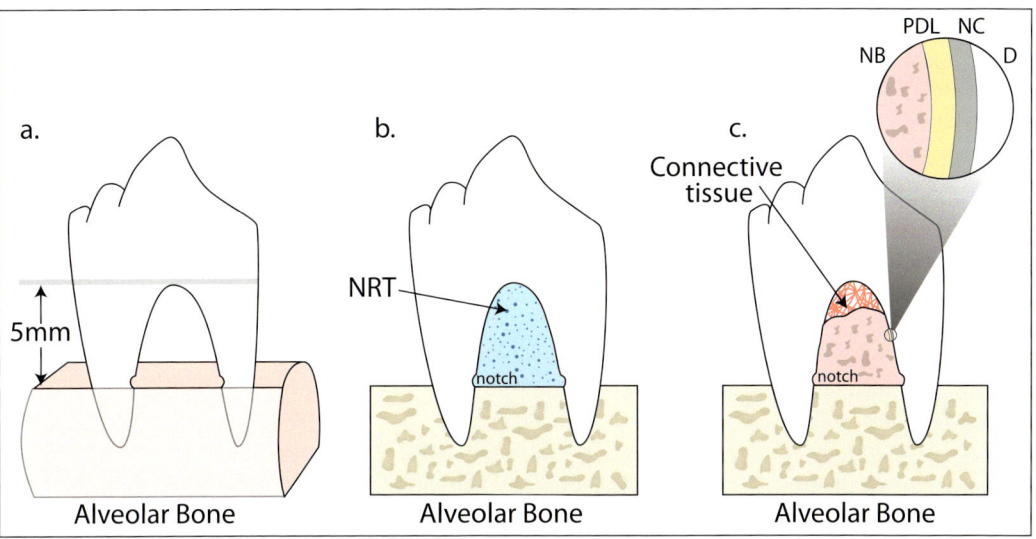

Fig 7-6 (a) Alveolar bone is removed around the third and the fourth premolars to create a horizontal defect of height 4 to 5 mm from reduced bone to the fornix of the furcation. Notches on the internal root surfaces are created at the level of the reduced bone. (b) The furcation lesion is filled with the regenerative agent or construct and the soft tissues are coronally advanced to cover the defect. Tissue samples are harvested at 4, 8, and 12 weeks after surgery. (c) Formation of new PDL, new cementum (NC), and new bone (NB) is evaluated in the furcation region. D, dentin. Reproduced from Pellegrini et al. (2009), with permission from SAGE Publications.

- For the canine intrabony regeneration model, an intraoral approach should be used. After sulcular incisions and mucoperiosteal flap elevations, alveolar bone is removed from around the teeth to make a circumferential defect using chisels and burs with saline irrigation.
- Supra-alveolar critical-size periodontal defects are produced by resection of buccal and lingual bone around the premolars.
- Resection can be restricted to the interdental area, which measures ~4 mm in height and 3 mm in width (Araujo et al., 1998; Araujo et al., 1999; Chen et al., 2006), or extended to create a horizontal circumferential defect up to 5 mm below the fornix of furcation (Fig 7-6 and Fig 7-7) (Wikesjö and Nilveus, 1991; Wikesjö et al., 2003c). Some protocols elect to extract the first mandibular premolar followed by amputation of the first molar level with the crest of the surgically reduced alveolar bone (Wikesjö et al., 1994)
- After resection, bone and cementum are removed, and notches are created to mark the lowest point of exposed roots in order distinguish between the old and new bone levels during evaluation (Fig 7-6). Reducing the crowns of teeth allows submerged repositioning of the flap, although this approach is not recommended since it does not mimic the normal wound environment.
- In the acute defect model, lesions are immediately treated with test agents. In the chronic defect model, the root surface is exposed to the oral environment in order to minimize spontaneous tissue regeneration (Wikesjö et al., 1994). Regenerative surgery can be performed after 1 to 6 months (Wikesjö et al., 1994; Morris et al., 2008) of

Osteology Guidelines for Oral and Maxillofacial Regeneration

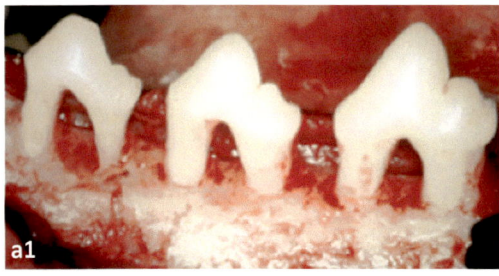
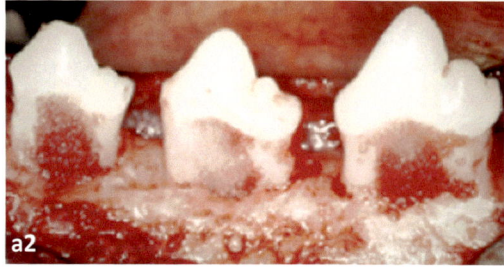
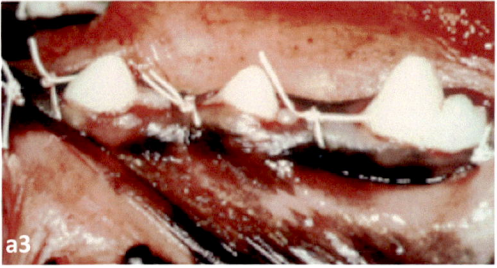

Fig 7-7 Full thickness flaps are designed to allow complete access to the surgical area. (**a: 1–3**) Supra-alveolar critical-size periodontal defects are produced by resection of buccal and lingual bone surrounding the premolars. Resection can be restricted to the interdental area or extended to create a horizontal circumferential defect below the furcation. Once the defects and notches are defined, the experimental factor or construct is delivered and secured into the defect. The flap is advanced and closure is achieved coronally by a simple interrupted suturing technique.
(**b: 1–4**) Histologically, evidence of no or limited regeneration can be obtained by identifying the surgically created notch (white arrows) and the adjacent periodontal structures. (**c: 1–4**) Successful periodontal regeneration can be clearly identified by the presence of new cementum formation (black arrows), new attachment of PDL fibers, as well as the presence of the alveolar bone. Repeoduced from Giannobile *et al*. (1998), with permission from the American Academy of Periodontology.

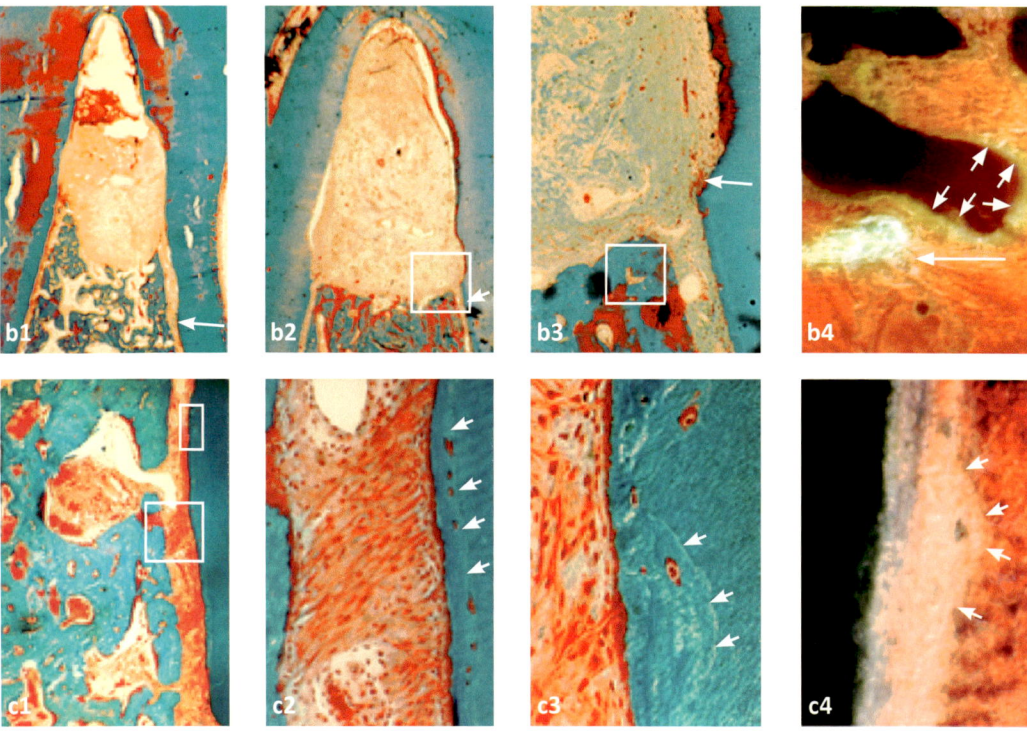

healing in combination with scaling and root planing via open flap surgery. Regenerative molecules are then applied around the defect area and flaps are closed.

7.4.5 Preparation

This is similar to the natural disease model (see Section 7.3.6 for more detail).

7.4.6 Anesthesia

Prior to anesthesia, dogs more than 10 weeks of age should be fasted for at least 6 hours, with the exception of water. They should be sedated using a combination of BAG as a presedative, approximately 30 to 60 minutes prior to propofol administration for induction.

Canine anesthetics. BAG (intravenous combination of 0.01 to 0.02 mg/kg buprenorphine, 0.03 to 0.05 mg/kg acepromazine, and 0.01 mg/kg glycopyrrolate) can be used as a sedative, 3 to 6 mg/kg of propofol (intravenously) can be given for anesthetic induction/intubation, and 1% to 2% isoflurane (inhalation) can be used to maintain general anesthesia during surgery. Atropine may be utilized as needed during canine surgery for the treatment of bradycardia while the animal is under general anesthesia. Local pain may be relieved by administering 1 to 2 mg/kg bupivacaine. Anesthesia depth can be monitored by loss of blink reflexes, jaw tone (tense = inadequate anesthesia), heart rate, and respiratory rate (60–80 beats per minute, 10–12 breaths per minute with anesthesia).

The canine will then be intubated and maintained under general anesthesia with isoflurane delivered through a volume-regulated aspirator (Giannobile *et al.*, 1998). Intravenous fluids, such as Ringer's solution (10 mL/kg/h), should be administered during surgery. If blood loss does occur during surgery, three times the estimated volume of blood loss should be administered via intravenous fluids.

Local infiltration anesthesia, for example lidocaine hydrochloride with epinephrine, is helpful to limit bleeding at and near to the surgical site. All animals should be provided with an external heat source, preferably a recirculating water blanket, to prevent hypothermia during the entire anesthesia and recovery period.

7.4.7 Postoperative Care, Including Analgesics and Wound Management

Postoperative Pain and Infection Control

Animals should be monitored until alert and active, and adequate homeostasis is achieved. While the animal is semiconscious it should be monitored every 15 minutes, and then monitored every hour until fully conscious. Once conscious, the animal must be monitored twice daily until fully recovered from the surgical procedure. Recovery should be carried out in a quiet, temperature-controlled, designated recovery area separate from the normal cage. Carprofen every 12 to 24 hours and/or buprenorphine every 8 to 12 hours can be administered for postsurgical pain relief (canine analgesics: 2 to 4.4 mg/kg carprofen [subcutaneous] and/or 0.01 to 0.02 mg/kg buprenorphine [subcutaneous] can be used for postoperative pain relief). Antibiotics, such as penicillin G benzathine (50,000 U/kg) should be administered subcutaneously on the day of surgery and every 5 days for up to 2 weeks.

Oral Hygiene Maintenance

For hygiene control, the treatment sites are to be cleaned with 0.1–0.2% chlorhexidine gel for 3 weeks following surgery. After the 3-week period, the dogs undergo supragingival debridement and prophylaxis every 2 weeks. Every effort should be made to maintain optimal oral hygiene for each animal. Acepromazine (0.03–0.25 mg/kg intramuscularly, intravenously, or subcutaneously) may be used as a tranquilizer prior to oral hygiene measures, if necessary.

Diet and Miscellaneous Remarks
The animals should be given a soft chow diet for up to 2 weeks following all surgical procedures to minimize trauma to the periodontium, until dry chow can be tolerated. The sutures must be removed between 10 and 14 days post surgery, under anesthesia if necessary. Surgical records should be kept in the animal housing area for 3 to 7 days following anesthesia and/or surgery.

7.4.8 Endpoint Measurements
At study endpoints animals can be sacrificed, and tissues harvested for analysis. Experimental endpoints are determined based on previous studies, published literature, and/or may be based on the biologic material properties themselves. If the molecule of interest acts early in the healing process, endpoints should be selected accordingly in order to capture important healing events involving the compound of interest. Euthanasia methods, such as barbiturate overdose, should be selected according to institutional guidelines. A second method should be employed to confirm animal death prior to tissue collection. Harvested samples should be immediately fixed to prevent degradation or damage occurring to the tissues. For canine jaw bone harvesting, a coping saw can be used to cut hard tissue. Each tooth segment can be sectioned by using a diamond saw.

The defect healing outcome is best evaluated histologically and the surgically created notches serve as guidance to assess the potential regenerative outcomes (Fig 7-7). Histomorphometric endpoint analyses quantify the following parameters (Wikesjö *et al.*, 2003a; Murano *et al.*, 2006):
- The length of the regenerated cementum
- Alveolar bone height
- PDL
- Junctional epithelium.

7.4.9 Statistical Analysis Plan
Sections 7.2.9 and 7.3.10 contain relevant information regarding proper power analysis and statistical analysis related to the use of this preclinical model. (See Chapter 4 for more details.)

7.4.10 Materials, Consumables, Equipment
- Initial incision: Surgical blade (#11, 15), periosteal elevator (Pritchard).
- Defect creation: Bur (¼, 4 round bur), low-speed and high-speed handpiece with engine and chisel.
- Surgical retractors, periodontal probe, 17/23 dental explorer.
- Small, sharp, hand instrument such as Gracey curette.
- Wound closure: Needle holder (Crile-Wood), suture material (resorbable), scissors (LaGrange double curved), and metal staples.
- Anesthesia; will vary with animal model.
- Sterile, sanitizable, surgical area with proper ventilation.
- External heat source(s).
- Hot-bead instrument sterilizer.
- Sterile, clean cages for post-surgery animal recovery.
- Staple remover.
- Tissue harvesting: Scissors, round disk and low speed engine for tissue harvesting.
- Upright optical microscope with imaging analysis apparatus.
- Micro-CT for additional three-dimensional analysis.

7.5 Surgically Created Periodontal Defects in Nonhuman Primates

7.5.1 Animal Model (Specific Animal Species)
Nonhuman primates possess anatomic and biologic features that closely resemble those of humans. These characteristics make the model valuable to evaluate the safety and efficacy of candidate factors or constructs for oral and periodontal regenerative therapies. However, the expense and demanding maintenance as well as regulatory requirements limit the use of nonhuman primates on a

broad scale. Different strains of nonhuman primates have been involved in biomedical research including macaque, baboon, squirrel monkey, cynomolgus macaque, and chimpanzee.

> **Box 7-4 Aim(s) of the Animal Model**
> Surgically created periodontal lesions in nonhuman primates have been used to test the effects of biologics such as growth factors and barrier membranes on periodontal regeneration.

7.5.2 Advantages/Disadvantages of the Presented Model

Advantages:
- Defects are rapidly created
- Standardized anatomic characteristics
- Similar morphology to human class II and III furcation defects.

Disadvantages:
- Fail to reproduce the microbiological and inflammatory condition
- Represents more an acute defect model
- Lesions are immediately treated with candidate factor or construct before wound closure
- Some spontaneous healing.

7.5.3 Timing

Histomorphometric endpoint analyses are generally performed within 5 months by measuring the length and/or area of new attachment, cementum, and bone. By 1 month, thin epithelium lines the coronal portion of the root surface and new cementum extends to the original cementum layer. Collagen fibers appear disorganized in the coronal area, while in the apical area collagen fibers are oriented parallel to the root surface and insert in the newly formed cementum (Sander and Karring, 1995). Periodontal regeneration progresses until about 5 months when new bone with a mature periodontium is found (Karatzas et al., 1999; Sculean et al., 2000b; Donos et al., 2003; Zhang et al., 2004). Chronic periodontal defects do not regenerate spontaneously, allowing for a greater observation window of the regenerative response to candidate factors or constructs. Moreover, chronic defects closely resemble the human situation, with respect to the microbial flora and the inflammatory reaction (Caton et al., 1994; Karatzas et al., 1999). Surgically created periodontal defects have been used to study the impact of guided bone regeneration and the application of biologics including enamel matrix proteins, BMP-2, FGF-2, TGF-β3 and PDGF (Sculean et al., 1997; Sculean et al., 2000b; Ripamonti et al., 2001; Takayama et al., 2001; Donos et al., 2003; Teare et al., 2008).

7.5.4 Surgical Procedures

A variety of defect configurations have been surgically created including palatal dehiscence (Laurell et al., 2006), intrabony (Sculean et al., 1997; Sculean et al., 2002), class II–III furcation (Ripamonti et al., 2001; Hovey et al., 2006), and fenestration lesions (Sculean et al., 2000a; Sculean et al., 2001). Fenestration defects heal spontaneously due to the residual periodontal tissues whereby mesenchymal progenitor cells can easily repopulate the defect. Thus, the fenestration model is not considered optimal to study the effects of candidate factors or constructs on periodontal regeneration (Caton et al., 1994; Sculean et al., 2000a). For the acute model, mucoperiosteal flaps are raised and bone defects, including the PDL and the cementum, are created. The reconstructive therapy can be performed immediately after creation of the defect (Ripamonti et al., 2001); however, to reduce spontaneous regeneration, the lesions are filled with space-filling mechanical devices (Ramfjord, 1951; Ellegaard et al., 1973; Ellegaard et al., 1974; Wirthlin and Hancock, 1982). Mechanical devices are metal strips, orthodontic wires, and bands or cotton floss ligatures that are positioned in the defects for 1 to 3 months, and are capable of provoking a chronic inflammation. At re-entry, the mechanical devices are removed and the lesions are debrided of granulation tissue, plaque, and calculus. After the root surface is scaled, candidate factors or constructs can be positioned into the defects (Takayama et al., 2001; Graziani et al., 2005; Laurell et al., 2006).

7.5.5 Preparation

Animals require an acclimation period of approximately 4 days to 1 week after arrival in a new housing facility. The surgical area should be easily sanitizable, and undergo careful preparation to ensure the aseptic surgical technique is carried out according to government and institutional guidelines. Ideally, the surgical area can be located within the housing facilities, but should be separated from human occupancy areas, therefore limiting stress and potential health hazards to the animals. Glutaraldehyde and sodium hypochlorite-based disinfectants can be used to clean and disinfect the surgery area, although some may not be effective at eliminating all contaminants.

Animals and instruments must also be prepared in a way to limit or prevent contamination and ensure success of the survival surgery. Surgeons should undergo appropriate preparation in a room separate from the operating areas, including, but not limited to surgical staff, wearing sterile gloves, gowns, caps, shoe covers, and masks for each animal's surgical procedures.

The presurgical oral hygiene phase is especially necessary for canine and nonhuman primates to obtain a healing response following surgery by ensuring biofilm removal, and to begin with healthy periodontal tissues. Scaling and root planing procedures should be performed in an area separate from the surgical operating room to prevent contamination, and can be carried out approximately 10 days prior to surgery.

7.5.6 Anesthesia

Nonhuman primates should be sedated using an intramuscular approach by ketamine injection (10 mg/kg) and subcutaneous injection of atropine (0.05 mg/kg), followed by halothane anesthesia to effect. Local pain, as with the canine models, can be relieved by administering 1 to 2 mg/kg bupivacaine. Anesthesia depth can be monitored by loss of blink reflexes, jaw tone (tense = inadequate anesthesia), heart rate, and respiratory rate (60 to 80 beats per minute, 10 to 12 breaths per minute with anesthesia).

Similar to dogs, nonhuman primates can be intubated, and maintained under general anesthesia with isoflurane delivered through a volume-regulated aspirator (Giannobile et al., 1998). Intravenous fluids, such as Ringer's solution (10 mL/kg/h), should be administered during surgery. If blood loss does occur during surgery, three times the estimated volume of blood loss should be administered via intravenous fluids.

Local infiltration anesthesia, for example lidocaine hydrochloride with epinephrine, is helpful to limit bleeding at and near to the surgical site. All animals should be provided an external heat source, preferably a recirculating water blanket, to prevent hypothermia during the entire anesthesia and recovery period.

7.5.7 Postoperative Care, Including Analgesics and Wound Management

Postoperative Pain and Infection Control
As for the intrabony or furacation periodontal regeneration model (see Section 7.4.7).

Oral Hygiene Maintenance
See Section 7.4.7 for details.

Diet and Miscellaneous Remarks
See Section 7.4.7 for details.

7.5.8 Endpoint Measurements

The histologic hard and soft tissue measurements often used include the following indices (Giannobile et al., 1994):
- Height of new crestal bone
- Area of coronal new bone
- Length of new attachment
- Complete new attachment apparatus
- Percentage of defect fill
- Percentage of new attachment
- Rate of ankylosis.

7.5.9 Statistical Analysis Plan

Sections 7.2.9 and 7.3.10 provide relevant information regarding proper power analysis and statistical analysis related to the use of this preclinical model. (See Chapter 4 for more details.)

7.5.10 Materials, Consumables, Equipment

- Visualizing microscope.
- Initial incision: Surgical blade (#11, 15), periosteal elevator (Pritchard).
- Defect creation: Bur (¼, 4 round bur), low-speed and high-speed handpiece with engine and chisel.
- Surgical retractors, periodontal probe, 17/23 dental explorer.
- Small, sharp, hand instrument such as Gracey curette.
- Wound closure: Needle holder (Crile-Wood), suture material (resorbable), scissors (LaGrange double curved).
- Anesthesia; will vary with animal model.
- Sterile, sanitizable, surgical area with proper ventilation.
- External heat source(s).
- Hot-bead instrument sterilizer.
- Sterile, clean cages for post-surgery animal recovery.
- Tissue harvesting: Scissors, round disk and Stryker saw.
- Optical microscope with imaging analysis apparatus.
- Micro-CT for additional three-dimensional analysis.

7.6 Ligature-induced Periodontal Lesions in the Nonhuman Primate

7.6.1 Animal Model (Specific Animal Species)

Nonhuman primates possess both primary and permanent dentitions highly similar to humans. These animals also form microbial plaque and calculus in the periodontium, however, they rarely exhibit spontaneous progression of gingival inflammation to periodontal disease (Schou et al., 1993). Various approaches have been designed to predictably induce periodontal defects (Kornman et al., 1981; Brecx et al., 1985). Thus, given the great similarities with relation to tooth size, anatomy, and healing characteristics, nonhuman primates make for an excellent model system for the evaluation of novel agents and constructs for periodontal regeneration.

> **Box 7-5 Aim(s) of the Animal Model**
> Nonhuman primate ligature-induced periodontal lesions have been used to evaluate the efficacy of biologics and guided tissue regeneration barriers (Giannobile et al., 1994; Giannobile et al., 1996)

7.6.2 Advantages/Disadvantages of the Presented Model

Advantages:
- Microbiological features similar to humans
- Morphological features similar to humans
- Minimal spontaneous repair
- Reasonable consistency in defect severity.

Disadvantages:
- Defects are restricted to the interproximal region
- Maintenance is expensive
- Establishment of the lesion requires significant time (Kornman et al., 1981; Caton et al., 1994).

7.6.3 Timing

The ligature-induced periodontal lesions in the nonhuman primate require at least 6 months to capture the clinical onset of the lesions. After 3 months, about 50% alveolar bone loss can be noted radiographically (Kostopoulos and Karring, 2004). Bone loss shows an angular pattern when the ligature is positioned around a single tooth, and has a horizontal pattern when ligatures are positioned around multiple teeth (Schou et al., 1993). The microflora is taxonomically comparable with that detected in human periodontitis (Brecx et al., 1985), with a shift of subgingival flora from Gram-positive cocci and rods to Gram-negative rods, and finally to Gram-negative anaerobes that are associated with disease progression (Kornman et al., 1981).

7.6.4 Surgical Procedures

- Periodontal lesions are induced by orthodontic elastic ligatures or silk sutures placed around the candidate teeth for 3 to 6 months. Both devices cause an ulceration of the junctional epithelium, the exposure to the oral environment, and plaque accumulation, together culminating in the initiation of periodontal disease.
- Additional inoculation of the devices with *Porphyromonas gingivalis* can accelerate disease progression (Holt et al., 1988).
- Bone loss shows an angular pattern when the ligature is positioned around a single tooth, and has a horizontal pattern when ligatures are positioned around multiple teeth.

7.6.5 Preparation

In ligature-induced periodontitis, the 4-0 silk or other material is placed and should be evaluated daily and replaced if it becomes loose. The animals are kept on a soft diet to promote plaque accumulation. The general recommendations followed are the same as with the surgically created defect model in nonhuman primates.

7.6.6 Anesthesia

See Section 7.5.6 for details.

7.6.7 Postoperative Care, Including Analgesics and Wound Management

The use of analgesics and wound management are similar to the surgically created defect model in nonhuman primates. The animals are able to continue with soft diet for 2 weeks postoperatively. Oral hygiene measures are similar to those recommended for the canine models.

7.6.8 Endpoint Measurements

After conventional periodontal surgery, spontaneous healing of ligature-induced lesions is characterized by formation of long junctional epithelium extending to the most apical level of the root. Thus, intervals suggested for the histomorphometric analysis are 1, 3, and 6 months (Giannobile et al., 1994). Main endpoints are the area/length of regenerated bone, cementum, and PDL. Even after 12 weeks, the main endpoint remains limited regeneration (Rutherford et al., 1992; Giannobile et al., 1994; Giannobile et al., 1996).

The histomorphometric analysis is aimed particularly at the evaluation of the following parameters (Giannobile et al., 1994):
- Area/length of regenerated bone, cementum and PDL
- Osseous defect fill
- Downgrowth of the junctional epithelium
- Root resorption
- Ankylosis.

7.6.9 Statistical Analysis Plan

Sections 7.2.9 and 7.3.10 provide relevant information regarding proper power analysis and statistical analysis related to the use of this preclinical model. (See Chapter 4 for more details.)

7.6.10 Materials, Consumables, Equipment
- Visualizing microscope.
- Initial incision: Surgical blade (#11, 15), periosteal elevator (Pritchard).
- Defect creation: Bur (¼, 4 round bur), low-speed and high-speed handpiece with engine and chisel.
- Surgical retractors, periodontal probe, 17/23 dental explorer.
- Small, sharp, hand instrument such as Gracey curette.
- Wound closure: Needle holder (Crile-Wood), suture material (resorbable), scissors (LaGrange double curved).
- Anesthesia; will vary with animal model.
- Sterile, sanitizable, surgical area with proper ventilation.
- External heat source(s).
- Hot-bead instrument sterilizer.
- Sterile, clean cages for post-surgical animal recovery.
- Tissue harvesting: Scissors, round disk and Stryker saw.
- Optical microscope with imaging analysis apparatus equipped with high-resolution CCD sensor.
- Micro-CT for additional three-dimensional analysis.

7.7 Conclusions and Future Directions

Preclinical animal models remain a critical component in the development and discovery of new approaches that will enhance our current regenerative approaches. *In vivo* models provide distinct advantages in the understanding of the complex molecular, cellular, and tissue reactions that occur in response to regenerative molecules or scaffolds to periodontal defects. Despite the limitations with preclinical models for human disease, *in vitro* investigations for the simulation of natural disease in humans remain inadequate prior to human trials for FDA or EMEA regulatory agency consideration. The increased investigation of biologics and devices for periodontal application requires a thorough examination of when and how the appropriate endpoints can be evaluated prior to entry into the human clinical trial arena. With continued innovations in noninvasive biomedical imaging, the need for extensive preclinical testing will decrease.

Advancements are still needed for the better exploitation of preclinical animal models for the evaluation of new regenerative alternatives prior to human testing. These include obvious differences in host–microbial interactions, defect morphology, and the implications of long-term (on the order of decades of disease progression in some cases with humans) disease development (Graves *et al.*, 2008). Furthermore, the size scale of periodontal lesions found in humans versus animals makes assessment of tissue neogenesis, oxygen, and nutrient diffusion through prototype scaffold matrices, especially in large defects, challenging (Cancedda *et al.*, 2007). As the clinical practice arena embraces personalized medicine, host susceptibility and identification of those patients who best respond to regenerative therapies may aid in the improvement of safety and effectiveness.

Acknowledgments

The authors appreciate Chris Jung and Chan Ho Park for assisting with the preparation of the figures. We also acknowledge the contribution of Drs Reinhard Gruber, Po-Chun Chang, Gaia Pellegrini, Qiming Jin, Jim Sugai, Andrei Taut, and Yong-Jo Seol in our animal studies. This work was supported by NIH Grant DE13397 and 1K23DE019872.

References

1. Araujo MG, Berglundh T, Lindhe J (1997). On the dynamics of periodontal tissue formation in degree III furcation defects. An experimental study in dogs. *J Clin Periodontol* 24:738–746.
2. Araujo MG, Berglundh T, Lindhe J (1998). GTR treatment of degree III furcation defects with 2 different resorbable barriers. An experimental study in dogs. *J Clin Periodontol* 25:253–259.
3. Araujo MG, Berglundh T, Albrekstsson T, Lindhe J (1999). Bone formation in furcation defects. An experimental study in the dog. *J Clin Periodontol* 26:643–652.
4. Attström R, Graf-de Beer M, Schroeder HE (1975). Clinical and histologic characteristics of normal gingiva in dogs. *J Periodontal Res* 10:115–127.
5. Belting CM, Schour I, Weinmann JP, Shepro MJ (1953). Age changes in the periodontal tissues of the rat molar. *J Dent Res* 32:332–353.
6. Benatti BB, Neto JB, Casati MZ, Sallum EA, Sallum AW, Nociti FH Jr (2006). Periodontal healing may be affected by aging: a histologic study in rats. *J Periodontal Res* 41:329–333.
7. Bonewald LF, Johnson ML (2008). Osteocytes, mechanosensing and Wnt signaling. *Bone* 42:606–615.
8. Brecx MC, Nalbandian J, Ooya K, Kornman KS, Robertson PB (1985). Morphological studies on periodontal disease in the cynomolgus monkey. II. Light microscopic observations on ligature-induced periodontitis. *J Periodontal Res* 20:165–175.
9. Burger EH, Klein-Nulend J, van der Plas A, Nijweide PJ (1995). Function of osteocytes in bone: their role in mechanotransduction. *J Nutr* 125(Suppl 7): 2020S–2023S.
10. Cancedda R, Giannoni P, Mastrogiacomo M (2007). A tissue engineering approach to bone repair in large animal models and in clinical practice. *Biomaterials* 28:4240–4250.
11. Caton J, Mota L, Gandini L, Laskaris B (1994). Non-human primate models for testing the efficacy and safety of periodontal regeneration procedures. *J Periodontol* 65:1143–1150.
12. Chen FM, Zhao YM, Wu H, Deng ZH, Wang QT, Zhou W et al. (2006). Enhancement of periodontal tissue regeneration by locally controlled delivery of insulin-like growth factor-I from dextran-co-gelatin microspheres. *J Control Release* 114:209–222.
13. Donos N, Sculean A, Glavind L, Reich E, Karring T (2003). Wound healing of degree III furcation involvements following guided tissue regeneration and/or Emdogain. A histologic study. *J Clin Periodontol* 30:1061–1068.
14. Duncan RL, Turner CH (1995). Mechanotransduction and the functional response of bone to mechanical strain. *Calcif Tissue Int* 57:344–358.
15. Ellegaard B, Karring T, Listgarten M, Löe H (1973). New attachment after treatment of interradicular lesions. *J Periodontol* 44:209–217.
16. Ellegaard B, Karring T, Davies R, Löe H (1974). New attachment after treatment of intrabony defects in monkeys. *J Periodontol* 45:368–377.
17. Frost H (1964). The laws of bone structure. Springfield, IL: Charles C. Thomas.
18. Giannobile WV, Finkelman RD, Lynch SE (1994). Comparison of canine and non-human primate animal models for periodontal regenerative therapy: results following a single administration of PDGF/IGF-I. *J Periodontol* 65:1158–1168.
19. Giannobile WV, Hernandez RA, Finkelman RD, Ryan S, Kiritsy CP, D'Andrea M et al. (1996). Comparative effects of platelet-derived growth factor-BB and insulin-like growth factor-I, individually and in combination, on periodontal regeneration in *Macaca fascicularis*. *J Periodontal Res* 31:301–312.
20. Giannobile WV, Ryan S, Shih MS, Su DL, Kaplan PL, Chan TC (1998). Recombinant human osteogenic protein-1 (OP-1) stimulates periodontal wound healing in class III furcation defects. *J Periodontol* 69:129–137.
21. Graves DT, Fine D, Teng YT, Van Dyke TE, Hajishengallis G (2008). The use of rodent models to investigate host-bacteria interactions related to periodontal diseases. *J Clin Periodontol* 35:89–105.
22. Graziani F, Laurell L, Tonetti M, Gottlow J, Berglundh T (2005). Periodontal wound healing following GTR therapy of dehiscence-type defects in the monkey: short-, medium- and long-term healing. *J Clin Periodontol* 32:905–914.
23. Hollinger JO, Kleinschmidt JC (1990). The critical size defect as an experimental model to test bone repair materials. *J Craniofac Surg* 1:60–68.
24. Holt SC, Ebersole J, Felton J, Brunsvold M, Kornman KS (1988). Implantation of *Bacteroides gingivalis* in non-human primates initiates progression of periodontitis. *Science* 239:55–57.
25. Hovey LR, Jones AA, McGuire M, Mellonig JT, Schoolfield J, Cochran DL (2006). Application of periodontal tissue engineering using enamel matrix derivative and a human fibroblast-derived dermal substitute to stimulate periodontal wound healing in Class III furcation defects. *J Periodontol* 77:790–799.
26. Huang KK, Shen C, Chiang CY, Hsieh YD, Fu E (2005). Effects of bone morphogenetic protein-6 on periodontal wound healing in a fenestration defect of rats. *J Periodontal Res* 40:1–10.
27. Jin QM, Anusaksathien O, Webb SA, Rutherford RB, Giannobile WV (2003). Gene therapy of bone morphogenetic protein for periodontal tissue engineering. *J Periodontol* 74:202–213.
28. Jin Q, Anusaksathien O, Webb SA, Printz MA, Giannobile WV (2004). Engineering of tooth-supporting structures by delivery of PDGF gene therapy vectors. *Mol Ther* 9:519–526.
29. Jin Q, Cirelli JA, Park CH, Sugai JV, Taba M Jr, Kostenuik PJ et al. (2007). RANKL inhibition through osteoprotegerin blocks bone loss in experimental periodontitis. *J Periodontol* 78:1300–1308.
30. Karatzas S, Zavras A, Greenspan D, Amar S (1999). Histologic observations of periodontal wound healing after treatment with PerioGlas in nonhuman primates. *Int J Periodontics Restorative Dent* 19:489–499.

References

31. King GN, Hughes FJ (1999). Effects of occlusal loading on ankylosis, bone, and cementum formation during bone morphogenetic protein-2-stimulated periodontal regeneration in vivo. *J Periodontol* 70:1125–1135.
32. King GN, Hughes FJ (2001). Bone morphogenetic protein-2 stimulates cell recruitment and cementogenesis during early wound healing. *J Clin Periodontol* 28:465–475.
33. King GN, King N, Cruchley AT, Wozney JM, Hughes FJ (1997). Recombinant human bone morphogenetic protein-2 promotes wound healing in rat periodontal fenestration defects. *J Dent Res* 76:1460–1470.
34. Klausen B (1991). Microbiological and immunological aspects of experimental periodontal disease in rats: a review article. *J Periodontol* 62:59–73.
35. Kornman KS, Holt SC, Robertson PB (1981). The microbiology of ligature-induced periodontitis in the cynomolgus monkey. *J Periodontal Res* 16:363–371.
36. Kostopoulos L, Karring T (2004). Susceptibility of GTR-regenerated periodontal attachment to ligature-induced periodontitis. *J Clin Periodontol* 31:336–340.
37. Laurell L, Bose M, Graziani F, Tonetti M, Berglundh T (2006). The structure of periodontal tissues formed following guided tissue regeneration therapy of intra-bony defects in the monkey. *J Clin Periodontol* 33:596–603.
38. Lekic P, Sodek J, McCulloch CA (1996a). Relationship of cellular proliferation to expression of osteopontin and bone sialoprotein in regenerating rat periodontium. *Cell Tissue Res* 285:491–500.
39. Lekic P, Sodek J, McCulloch CA (1996b). Osteopontin and bone sialoprotein expression in regenerating rat periodontal ligament and alveolar bone. *Anat Rec* 244:50–58.
40. Lekovic V, Klokkevold PR, Kenney EB, Dimitrijelic B, Nedic M, Weinlaender M (1998). Histologic evaluation of guided tissue regeneration using 4 barrier membranes: a comparative furcation study in dogs. *J Periodontol* 69:54–61.
41. Lindhe J, Hamp SE, Löe H (1975). Plaque induced periodontal disease in beagle dogs. A 4-year clinical, roentgenographical and histometrical study. *J Periodontal Res* 10:243–255.
42. Long P, Liu F, Piesco NP, Kapur R, Agarwal S (2002). Signaling by mechanical strain involves transcriptional regulation of proinflammatory genes in human periodontal ligament cells in vitro. *Bone* 30:547–552.
43. Lynch SE, de Castilla GR, Williams RC, Kiritsy CP, Howell TH, Reddy MS et al. (1991). The effects of short-term application of a combination of platelet-derived and insulin-like growth factors on periodontal wound healing. *J Periodontol* 62:458–467.
44. Marotti G (2000). The osteocyte as a wiring transmission system. *J Musculoskelet Neuronal Interact* 1:133–136.
45. Marotti G, Palumbo C (2007). The mechanism of transduction of mechanical strains into biological signals at the bone cellular level. *Eur J Histochem* 51(Suppl 1):15–19.
46. Martuscelli G, Fiorellini JP, Crohin CC, Howell TH (2000). The effect of interleukin-11 on the progression of ligature-induced periodontal disease in the beagle dog. *J Periodontol* 71:573–578.
47. Matsuura M, Herr Y, Han KY, Lin WL, Genco RJ, Cho MI (1995). Immunohistochemical expression of extracellular matrix components of normal and healing periodontal tissues in the beagle dog. *J Periodontol* 66:579–593.
48. Melcher AH (1970). Repair of wounds in the periodontium of the rat. Influence of periodontal ligament on osteogenesis. *Arch Oral Biol* 15:1183–1204.
49. Morris MS, Lee Y, Lavin MT, Giannini PJ, Schmid MJ, Marx DB et al. (2008). Injectable simvastatin in periodontal defects and alveolar ridges: pilot studies. *J Periodontol* 79:1465–1473.
50. Murano Y, Ota M, Katayama A, Sugito H, Shibukawa Y, Yamada S (2006). Periodontal regeneration following transplantation of proliferating tissue derived from periodontal ligament into class III furcation defects in dogs. *Biomed Res* 27:139–147.
51. Nociti FH Jr, Cesco De Toledo R, Machado MA, Stefani CM, Line SR, Goncalves RB (2001). Clinical and microbiological evaluation of ligature-induced peri-implantitis and periodontitis in dogs. *Clin Oral Implants Res* 12:295–300.
52. Page RC, Schroeder HE (1981). Spontaneous chronic periodontitis in adult dogs. A clinical and histopathological survey. *J Periodontol* 52:60–73.
53. Park CH, Abramson ZR, Taba M Jr, Jin Q, Chang J, Kreider JM et al. (2007). Three-dimensional micro-computed tomographic imaging of alveolar bone in experimental bone loss or repair. *J Periodontol* 78:273–281.
54. Park JB, Matsuura M, Han KY, Norderyd O, Lin WL, Genco RJ et al. (1995). Periodontal regeneration in class III furcation defects of beagle dogs using guided tissue regenerative therapy with platelet-derived growth factor. *J Periodontol* 66:462–477.
55. Pellegrini G, Seol YJ, Gruber R, Giannobile WV (2009). Pre-clinical models for oral and periodontal reconstructive therapies. *J Dent Res* 88:1065–1076.
56. Rajshankar D, McCulloch CA, Tenenbaum HC, Lekic PC (1998). Osteogenic inhibition by rat periodontal ligament cells: modulation of bone morphogenic protein-7 activity in vivo. *Cell Tissue Res* 294:475–483.
57. Ramfjord S (1951). Experimental periodontal reattachment in rhesus monkeys. *J Periodontol* 22:67–77.
58. Ripamonti U, Crooks J, Petit JC, Rueger DC (2001). Periodontal tissue regeneration by combined applications of recombinant human osteogenic protein-1 and bone morphogenetic protein-2. A pilot study in Chacma baboons (Papio ursinus). *Eur J Oral Sci* 109:241–248.
59. Roberts WE, Turley PK, Brezniak N, Fielder PJ (1987). Implants: Bone physiology and metabolism. *CDA J* 15:54–61.
60. Rogers JE, Li F, Coatney DD, Rossa C, Bronson P, Krieder JM et al. (2007). *Actinobacillus actinomycetemcomitans* lipopolysaccharide-mediated experimental bone loss model for aggressive periodontitis. *J Periodontol* 78:550–558.
61. Rutherford RB, Niekrash CE, Kennedy JE, Charette MF (1992). Platelet-derived and insulin-like growth factors stimulate regeneration of periodontal attachment in monkeys. *J Periodontal Res* 27(4 Pt 1):285–290.

62. Sander L, Karring T (1995). Healing of periodontal lesions in monkeys following the guided tissue regeneration procedure. A histological study. *J Clin Periodontol* 22:332–337.
63. Sato R, Yamamoto H, Kasai K, Yamauchi M (2002). Distribution pattern of versican, link protein and hyaluronic acid in the rat periodontal ligament during experimental tooth movement. *J Periodontal Res* 37:15–22.
64. Schectman LR, Ammons WF, Simpson DM, Page RC (1972). Host tissue response in chronic periodontal disease. 2. Histologic features of the normal periodontium, and histologic and ultrastructural manifestations of disease in the marmoset. *J Periodontal Res* 7:195–212.
65. Schou S, Holmstrup P, Kornman KS (1993). Non-human primates used in studies of periodontal disease pathogenesis: a review of the literature. *J Periodontol* 64:497–508.
66. Sculean A, Karring T, Theilade J, Lioubavina N (1997). The regenerative potential of oxytalan fibers. An experimental study in the monkey. *J Clin Periodontol* 24:932–936.
67. Sculean A, Donos N, Brecx M, Karring T, Reich E (2000a). Healing of fenestration-type defects following treatment with guided tissue regeneration or enamel matrix proteins. An experimental study in monkeys. *Clin Oral Investig* 4:50–56.
68. Sculean A, Donos N, Brecx M, Reich E, Karring T (2000b). Treatment of intrabony defects with guided tissue regeneration and enamel-matrix-proteins. An experimental study in monkeys. *J Clin Periodontol* 27:466–472.
69. Sculean A, Berakdar M, Pahl S, Windisch P, Brecx M, Reich E et al. (2001). Patterns of cytokeratin expression in monkey and human periodontium following regenerative and conventional periodontal surgery. *J Periodontal Res* 36:260–268.
70. Sculean A, Junker R, Donos N, Berakdar M, Brecx M, Dunker N (2002). Immunohistochemical evaluation of matrix molecules associated with wound healing following regenerative periodontal treatment in monkeys. *Clin Oral Investig* 6:175–182.
71. Shirakata Y, Yoshimoto T, Goto H, Yonamine Y, Kadomatsu H, Miyamoto M et al. (2007). Favorable periodontal healing of 1-wall infrabony defects after application of calcium phosphate cement wall alone or in combination with enamel matrix derivative: a pilot study with canine mandibles. *J Periodontol* 78:889–898.
72. Sorensen RG, Wikesjö UM, Kinoshita A, Wozney JM (2004). Periodontal repair in dogs: evaluation of a bioresorbable calcium phosphate cement (Ceredex) as a carrier for rhBMP-2. *J Clin Periodontol* 31:796–804.
73. Syed SA, Svanberg M, Svanberg G (1981). The predominant cultivable dental plaque flora of beagle dogs with periodontitis. *J Clin Periodontol* 8:45–56.
74. Takayama S, Murakami S, Shimabukuro Y, Kitamura M, Okada H (2001). Periodontal regeneration by FGF-2 (bFGF) in primate models. *J Dent Res* 80:2075–2079.
75. Talwar R, Di Silvio L, Hughes FJ, King GN (2001). Effects of carrier release kinetics on bone morphogenetic protein-2-induced periodontal regeneration *in vivo*. *J Clin Periodontol* 28:340–347.
76. Teare JA, Ramoshebi LN, Ripamonti U (2008). Periodontal tissue regeneration by recombinant human transforming growth factor-beta 3 in *Papio ursinus*. *J Periodontal Res* 43:1–8.
77. Tsuji K, Uno K, Zhang GX, Tamura M (2004). Periodontal ligament cells under intermittent tensile stress regulate mRNA expression of osteoprotegerin and tissue inhibitor of matrix metalloprotease-1 and -2. *J Bone Miner Metab* 22:94–103.
78. Wikesjö UM, Nilveus R (1991). Periodontal repair in dogs. Healing patterns in large circumferential periodontal defects. *J Clin Periodontol* 18:49–59.
79. Wikesjö UM, Kean CJ, Zimmerman GJ (1994). Periodontal repair in dogs: supraalveolar defect models for evaluation of safety and efficacy of periodontal reconstructive therapy. *J Periodontol* 65:1151–1157.
80. Wikesjö UM, Lim WH, Thomson RC, Cook AD, Wozney JM, Hardwick WR (2003a). Periodontal repair in dogs: evaluation of a bioabsorbable space-providing macroporous membrane with recombinant human bone morphogenetic protein-2. *J Periodontol* 74:635–647.
81. Wikesjö UM, Lim WH, Thomson RC, Hardwick WR (2003b). Periodontal repair in dogs: gingival tissue occlusion, a critical requirement for GTR? *J Clin Periodontol* 30:655–664.
82. Wikesjö UM, Xiropaidis AV, Thomson RC, Cook AD, Selvig KA, Hardwick WR (2003c). Periodontal repair in dogs: space-providing ePTFE devices increase rhBMP-2/ACS-induced bone formation. *J Clin Periodontol* 30:715–725.
83. Wikesjö UM, Sorensen RG, Kinoshita A, Jian Li X, Wozney JM (2004). Periodontal repair in dogs: effect of recombinant human bone morphogenetic protein-12 (rhBMP-12) on regeneration of alveolar bone and periodontal attachment. *J Clin Periodontol* 31:662–670.
84. Wirthlin MR, Hancock EB (1982). Regeneration and repair after biologic treatment of root surfaces in monkeys. II. Proximal surfaces posterior teeth. *J Periodontol* 53:302–306.
85. Yang YQ, Li XT, Rabie AB, Fu MK, Zhang D (2006). Human periodontal ligament cells express osteoblastic phenotypes under intermittent force loading *in vitro*. *Front Biosci* 11:776–781.
86. Zhang X, Kohli M, Zhou Q, Graves DT, Amar S (2004). Short- and long-term effects of IL-1 and TNF antagonists on periodontal wound healing. *J Immunol* 173:3514–3523.
87. Zhao M, Jin Q, Berry JE, Nociti FH Jr, Giannobile WV, Somerman MJ (2004). Cementoblast delivery for periodontal tissue engineering. *J Periodontol* 75:154–161.

CHAPTER 8

Osseointegration of Implants

Christer Dahlin and Carina B. Johansson

8.1 General Overview – Evaluating Osseointegration

Osseointegration was coincidently discovered more than 40 years ago when Brånemark and colleagues were about to retrieve a titanium implant, which had been used for evaluating microcirculation in bone, and experienced a very firm bone anchorage of the screw, i.e., the implant was osseointegrated. Still, there are no "exact numbers" or "exact values" that *describe* the osseointegration phenomena (Brånemark et al., 1969). The term osseointegration was coined and for the first time defined in 1981 (Albrektsson et al., 1981). The original definition was based on observations at a light microscopic level, although it did not indicate what percentage of bone needed to be in contact with the implant in order to call it osseointegration. Over the years osseointegration has been redefined to span a range of criteria from the original light microscopic level to more precise engineering approaches (Steinemann, 1998) as well as the clinical observations; the latter one is probably of most relevance since it describes "clinical measures" (Zarb and Albrektsson, 1991). The definition of osseointegration in Dorland's Medical Dictionary today is as follows: "the formation of a direct interface between an orthopedic or dental implant and bone without intervening soft tissue" (Dorland's Medical Dictionary, 2007), which is quite similar to the original light microscopic level definition in 1981.

Nevertheless, from time to time, the question arises as to when is an implant osseointegrated and to what extent should it be integrated in order to call it osseointegrated? To the best of our knowledge this is still not known. Bone is a living and dynamic tissue being constantly remodeled. There are no exact measures and no exact requirements set up in terms of how much bone needs to be in contact with the implant in order to fulfill the criteria for osseointegration. The major focus today is on the implant surface morphology (including all surface parameters, i.e., roughness, chemistry, oxide type, oxide thickness, etc.) and we have no exact knowledge of which surface structural parameter, or the combination of parameters, is the most important one to exactly describe and guide osseointegration (Coelho et al., 2009; Dohan Ehrenfest et al., 2010). This is even more complicated today since the targets of research are not only at the micro cellular level but also at the nano-protein and gene expression levels. Hence for the latter levels of investigations of osseointegration we are only in the beginning stages, and more tools and techniques are emerging rapidly which may well lead to further redefinitions of osseointegration in the near future. The research around osseointegration is as fascinating now as in the early days!

The development of an optimal interface between bone tissue and an orthopedic or dental implants is an ongoing process. In order to determine whether a newly developed implant material conforms to the requirements of *biocompatbility*, *mechanical stability*, and *safety*, it must undergo rigorous testing both *in vitro* and *in vivo*. As per the state of the art in biomaterial research today, characterization of bone-contacting materials is initiated by means of *in vitro* testing. The advantages of such procedures include a rapid response with regard to toxicity and cytocompatbility. Other reasons for the increasing popularity of *in vitro* testing within the medical field are the principles of animal reduction. It is accepted that *in vitro* testing is used as a first stage for acute toxicity and cytocompatibility to avoid the unnecessary use of animals.

In order to evaluate dental (and orthopedic) implants, it is essential to have a range of animal models suitable for various analysis. The present chapter will describe suitable animal models for dental implant research on three different levels as well as discuss the very special circumstances that exist when performing histological analysis involving hard and soft tissue in combination with an implanted biomaterial.

8.2 The Rat Model

8.2.1 Aim

The use of rat models for studying implant interfaces is a controversial issue in the literature. Although the rat is one of the most commonly used species in medical research, it has not been extensively used for implant research mainly due to concerns regarding limitation in size and dissimilarities between rat and human bone (ISO [International Organization for Standardization] 10993–6, 1994; Pearce et al., 2007). At the Department of Biomaterials in Gothenburg, we are of a different opinion and see several advantages of using a rat model for screening of novel implant surfaces and detailed analysis of tissue dynamics. The use of microimplants in the rat offers unique opportunities to combine state of the art histology, biomechanical torsion tests and analysis of gene expression in the same animal model (Omar et al., 2009; 2010a,b). The rat model is also suitable for studying osseointegration in compromised bone situations, i.e., radiation damage (Nyberg et al., 2010). Last but not least, these types of study can also be reasonably affordable due to the relatively low cost of animal and housing.

8.2.2 Advantages/Disadvantages of the Rat Model

Advantages:
- Low cost animal and housing.
- Easy surgical access. Few complications.
- Sufficient number of animals in groups.
- Access to wide range of antibodies etc. for sophisticated analysis.
- Possibility to combine histology, biomechanical testing, and gene expression in same animal model.

Disadvantages:
- Limitation in size = customized implants
- Dissimilarities between rat and human bone in tissue dynamics.

8.2.3 Timing
Important time points from the project start up to the collection of specimens and data analysis (graphical): ordering of animals, quarantine surgery, collection of specimen and preparation of sections.
- 2 to 3 weeks usually for ordering of animals (with huge individual variations between countries).
- Quarantine 1 week.
- Surgery x days.
- Healing period 0–x weeks.
- Specimen collection and preparation of sections: 2 to 3 months.

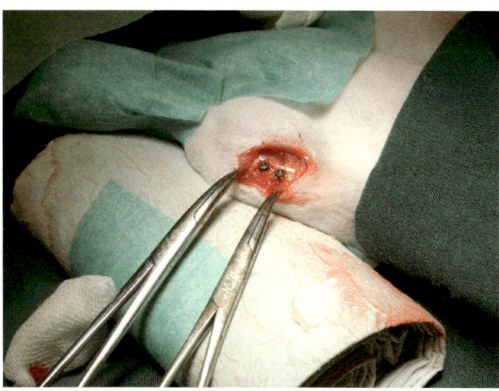

Fig 8-1 Installation of two microimplants in the rat tibia under clean conditions.

8.2.4 Surgical Procedure
After shaving and cleaning with chlorhexidine 5 mg/mL in 70% ethanol, the medial aspect of either the distal femoral epiphysis or tibial metaphysis is exposed via an anteromedial skin incision. This is followed by skin and periosteum reflection with blunt instruments (Fig 8-1). In the present model, specially manufactured implants 2 mm in diameter and 2.3 mm in length are used (Fig 8-2). The implant sites are prepared by using 1.4 and 1.8 mm spiral burs, respectively. All drilling is done under profuse irrigation with 0.9% NaCl. Implants are installed manually. The surgical wounds are closed in layers. The subcutaneous layer is closed with resorbable polyglactin sutures (5-0 Vicryl®, Ethicon, Johnson and Johnson, Brussels, Belgium).

8.2.5 Preparation – Anesthesia
Sprague-Dawley rats (200 to 250 g) are recommended for the model. The animals can be fed on standard laboratory diet with pellets and water *ad libitum*.

Anesthesia is performed using a Univentor 400 anesthesia unit (Univentor Ltd, Zejtun, Malta) under isoflurane (Isoba® Vet, Schering-Plough, Uxbridge, UK) ventilation. Anesthesia should be maintained by continous administration of isoflurane via a mask. Each rat receives an analgesic (Temgesic®, 0.03 mg/kg, Reckitt and Coleman, Hull, UK) subcutaneously prior to the implantation and daily postoperatively. Yet another method of rat anesthesia is to use a freshly prepared cocktail of fentanyl + midazolam (2 parts sterile water, 1 part fentanyl/fluanizone [Hypnorm® Vet, Saunderton, UK] and 1 part midazolam, 5mg/mL, Dormicum®, Roche, France). The cocktail is administered by intraperitoneal injections to each animal initially with dose of 2.7 mL/kg (Flecknell, 1996). Additional anesthesia is given when needed.

8.2.6 Detailed Methodology
See Section 8.5.

8.2.7 Postoperative Care
For pain relief, see above. After surgery, the animals are allowed free postoperative movement with food and water *ad libitum*.

Retrieval Procedure
Sacrifice by an intraperitoneal overdose of sodium pentobarbital (60 mg/mL; ATL Apoteket Production & Laboratories, Kungens Kurva, Sweden) under anesthesia with a 0.5 mL mixture of pentobarbital (60 mg/mL), sodium chloride, and diazepam (1:1:2).

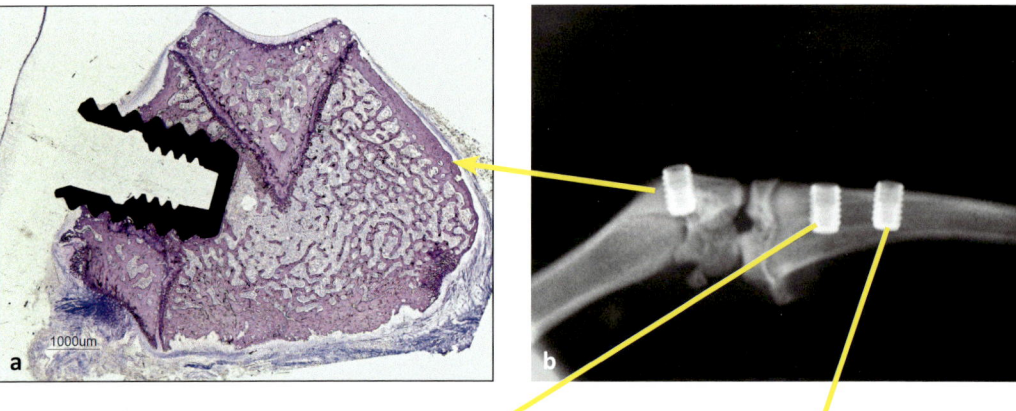
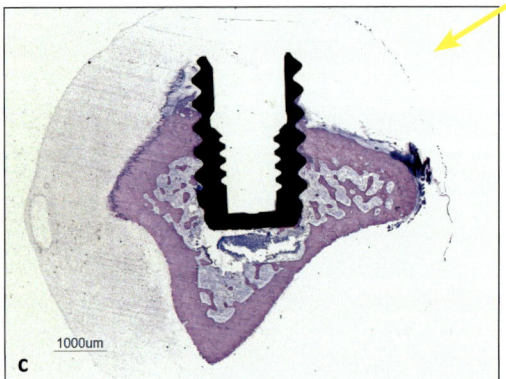
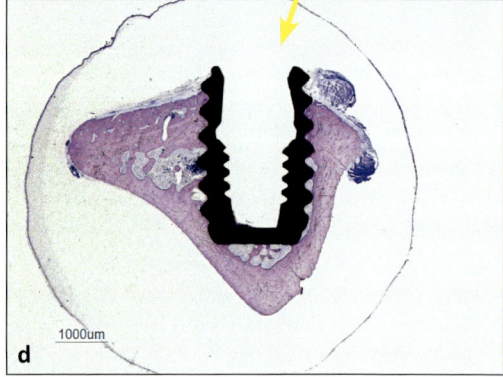

Fig 8-2 Radiographic image and histologic sections of the implant insertion sites in rat bone; one implant placed in the femur condyle region and two implants in the tibia region. The implant diameter is 2.0 mm. The proximal implant (c) has been removal torque tested prior to histological sectioning.

Healing Periods
This model is suitable for early analysis as well as more long-term studies. In brief, this means that healing dynamics can be studied from day 1. Solid osseointegration can be expected even around 4 weeks postoperatively.

8.2.8 Endpoint Measurements
See Section 8.5.

8.2.9 Statistical Analysis Plan
See Chapter 4.

8.2.10 Materials, Consumables, Equipment
See Section 8.5.

8.3 The Rabbit Model

8.3.1 Aim
The rabbit is one of the most commonly used animals for dental implant research. It is used in approximately 35% of all musculoskeletal research studies (Neyt et al., 1998). The rabbit attains skeletal maturity at around 6 to 8 months of age (Gilsanz et al., 1988). This can be studied by radiographs of the metaphysis (Fig 8-3).

The most commonly used experimental sites are the femoral diaphyseal bone and the tibial bone. The former is considered more ideal for studying bone dynamics and the interaction between surfaces and adjacent tissues. The

8.3 The Rabbit Model

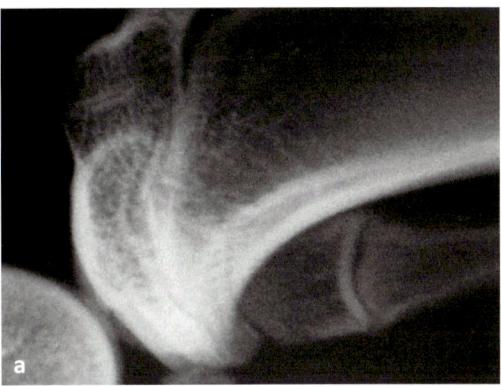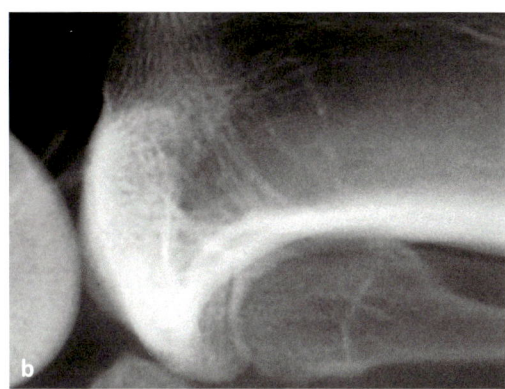

Fig 8-3 Radiographs of rabbit bone. (**a**) The rabbit is 7 months old. Note the open growth zones. (**b**) The rabbit is 10 months old with closed epiphyseal lines.

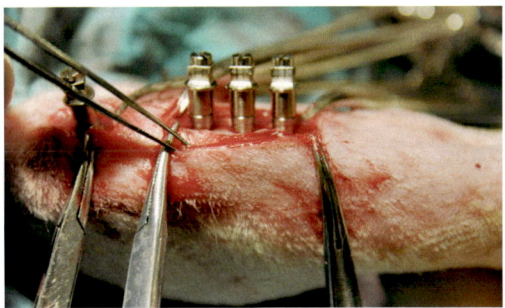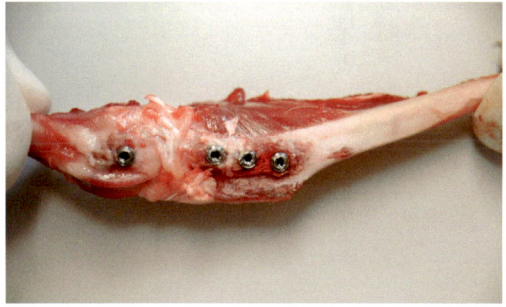

Fig 8-4 Installation of three implants in the rabbit tibia.

Fig 8-5 A specimen of a rabbit hindleg with one implant inserted in the femur condyle region and three implants placed in the tuberositas tibia region. The mean implant diameter is 3.7 mm. Illustration courtesy of Dr Young-Taeg Sul.

tibial bone is also suitable for some mechanical testing including torque removal tests and push-out tests. These methods will be described in more depth in Section 8.5. There are certain size limitations associated with the use of rabbit models. The international standard for the biologic evaluation of medical devices recommends a maximum of six implants (three test and three control implants) (ISO 10993–6, 1994). In order to avoid pathologic fractures of the test sites, the same ISO report suggests that cylindrical implants placed into the rabbit tibial and femoral diaphyseal bone should be no larger than 2 mm in diameter and 6 mm in length (Fig 8-4 and Fig 8-5). However, larger-sized implants such as a bone harvest chamber (BHC) can also succesfully be used. The BHC is an implant with a penetrating canal that permits bone ingrowth. The ingrown tissue may be harvested after removal of a titanium lid without disturbing the anchorage of the implant. This device is approximately 6 mm in dimension. Hence, only one device per site can be used (Albrektsson et al., 1981).

8.3.2 Advantages/Disadvantages of the Rabbit Model

The femoral and tibial bone of the rabbit has several advantages. The dimensions and the anatomy of the bone corresponds fairly well with the edentulous jaw in humans. It is easily accessible and seems to generate a minimum of morbidity for the animals.

Prior to surgery the animals should be kept in a purpose-designed room and be fed *ad libitum* with water, a standard laboratory animal diet, and carrots.

8.3.3 Timing
- Important time points from the project start up to the collection of specimens and data analysis (graphical):
- Ordering of animals 3 months in advance (huge variations in different countries)
- Quarantine approx 2 weeks
- Surgery, collection of specimen, x = weeks
- Preparation of sections 2 to 3 months

8.3.4 Surgical Procedure
After shaving and appropriate cleaning with, e.g., Panadyme®, the tibial or femoral bone is exposed via a skin incision followed by a careful subperiosteal incision. It is advisable to slightly overlap the skin–periosteal flap in order to secure an optimal primary closure. The periosteal flap and the skin should be closed in separate layers with slow resorbable sutures (4-0 or 5-0) (see Fig 8-8 and Fig 8-9 below).

8.3.5 Preparation – Anesthesia
- General anesthesia is given by an intramuscular injection of fluanison and fentanyl (Hypnorm®, Janssen Pharmaceutica, Brussels, Belgium) 0.2 mg/ kg body weight and intraperitoneal injection of diazepam (Stesolid®, Dumex, Copenhagen, Denmark) 1.5 mg/kg body weight.
- Additional Hypnorm® should be administered when needed.

Local Anesthesia
Local anesthesia should always be given at the surgical site. Both for hemostasis as well as postoperative pain prophylaxis (1 mL 2.0% lidocaine/epinephrine solution, Astra AB, Södertälje, Sweden).

8.3.6 Detailed Methodology
See Section 8.5.

8.3.7 Postoperative Care

Postoperative Antibiotics and Analgesics
The animals should be given antibiotics (Intenpenicillin 2,250,000 IU/5 mL 0.1 mL/kg body weight, LEO, Helsingborg, Sweden) for 3 days.

Temgesic® 0.05 mg/kg (Reckitt and Colman, NJ, USA) is given as single intramuscular injection for pain relief for 3 days.

8.3.8 Endpoint Measurements
See Section 8.5.

8.3.9 Statistical Analysis Plan
See Chapter 6.

8.3.11 Materials, Consumables, Equipment
See Section 8.5.

8.4 The Canine Model

8.4.1 Aim
The dog is one of the more frequently used large animal species for musculoskeletal and dental research. It has been found that there is most similarity in bone composition (ash weight, hydroxyproline, extractable proteins and insulin growth factor-1 content) between the dog and humans (Aerssens *et al.*, 1998). In terms of bone density the dog most closely represent the human situation (Pearce *et al.*, 2007). Depending on the size and the breed of dog, there may be some discrepancy in the size and shape of the canine bones. However, commercially dental implants can be utilized in particular in the mandible. It should be mentioned that there are increasing ethical issues relating to the use of dogs in medical research due to their status as companion animals. This model is ideally suited for studies on functional loading of implants.

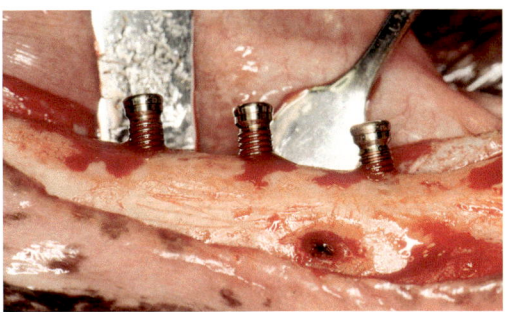

Fig 8-6 Placement of standard Brånemark Implants® in edentulous mandible in conjunction with bone augmentation study.

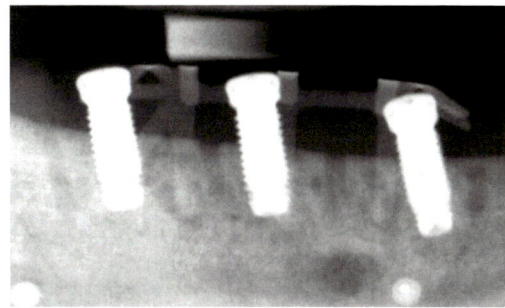

Fig 8-7 Radiographs demonstrating implants placed in mandibular bone of dog.

8.4.2 Advantages/Disadvantages of the Canine Model

Advantages:
- Bone density and quality most closely resemble humans
- Standard size implants
- Study of functional load.

Disadvantages:
- Expensive (including housing)
- Ethical concerns.

8.4.3 Timing
Important time points from the project start up to the collection of specimens and data analysis (graphical):
- Ordering (3 months)
- Quarantine (3 weeks)
- Surgery (day 0)
- Collection of specimen (2 months to × months)
- Processing (3 to 4 months)

8.4.4 Surgical Procedures – Baseline Surgery
Since an edentulous space is required for implant installation, so-called baseline surgery has to be performed, which includes bilateral surgical extractions of all the four mandibular premolars and the first molar. A healing period of 3 to 4 months is usually recommended prior to the placement of oral implants.

Implant Selection
According to ISO recommendations, cylindrical implants with a 4 mm diameter and up to 12 mm in length (Fig 8-6, Fig 8-7, Fig 8-8, and Fig 8-9) should be used. The breed of animal used in the study must of course be considered when choosing the exact implant dimensions. It is extremely important that control implants are included in the study design. These implants should preferably be of a material already in clinical use (ISO 10993–6, 1994).

The chosen implant design will determine the experimental techniques used to evaluate the material. Common mechanical testing used on tissues harvested from *in vivo* studies include torque removal tests, and pull-out and push-out tests. These tests are used to evaluate the strength of the bone–implant surface contact. A high force encountered is considered indirect evidence of a solid osseointegration. Regarding the histologic analysis, see below.

8.4.5 Preparation
The following description is based on a sequence related to implant placement in the mandible of canines.

Adult mongrel dogs, with a body weight of a minimum of 20 kg, are usually recommended. In compliance with guidelines for the care and use of laboratory animals the animals should be vaccinated, receiving anti-vermin drugs, and

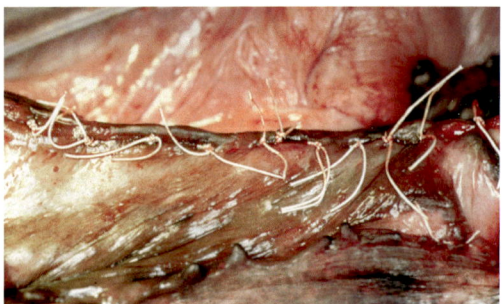

Fig 8-8 Tension-free suturing following surgery in edentulous mandible of dogs. Note the multiple single sutures in combination with horizontal mattress sutures. Nonresorbable Teflon 4-0 suture has been used.

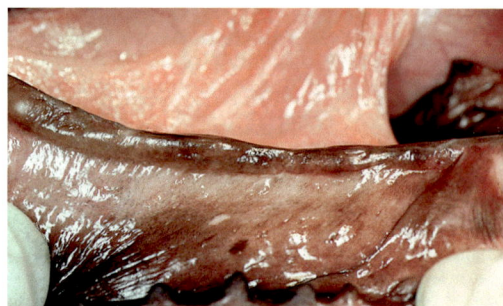

Fig 8-9 Uneventful healing after suture removal (10 days) in the mandible of dogs.

put into quarantine for clinical observation prior to the experiment.

Anesthesia
Local variations with regards to access to drugs etc. will apply in different countries. However, the following protocol is well established within this type of study:
- Pre-anesthesia with xilazine (Ronpum®, 20 mg/kg intramuscularly and Ketamine 1 g (Dopalen® 0.8 g/kg intramuscularly).
- Anaesthetized with thionembutal 1 g (Tiopental®, 20 mg/kg intravenously).

The animal should be kept on intravenous infusion of saline during surgery.

Analgesic
Anti-inflammatory/analgesic drug postoperatively (Banamine®).

Antibiotics
Postsurgical infection control includes 1.0 mg dexamethasone the day following surgery, Amoxicillin 500 to 750 mg BID or Pentabiotic® for 10 days.

8.4.6 Detailed Methodology
See Section 8.5.

8.4.7 Postoperative Care
Chlorhexidine (0.2%) rinse should be done twice a week during the duration of the study.

The sutures are removed when adequate healing is observed, usually around 7 to 10 days postoperatively.

The dogs are maintained on a soft diet for the duration of the study.

8.4.8 Endpoint Measurements
See Section 8.5.

8.4.9 Statistical Analysis Plan
See Chapter 6.

8.4.10 Materials, Consumables, Equipment
See Section 8.5.

8.5 Evaluating Osseointegration

8.5.1 Aim
What is osseointegration, how can we evaluate and measure it and how it is measured today – these are some questions that will be elaborated on in this section. Below we present some of our in-house materials and methods related to the techniques used for preparing samples as well as final tools and techniques used for evaluation of osseointegration. We start with a

8.5 Evaluating Osseointegration

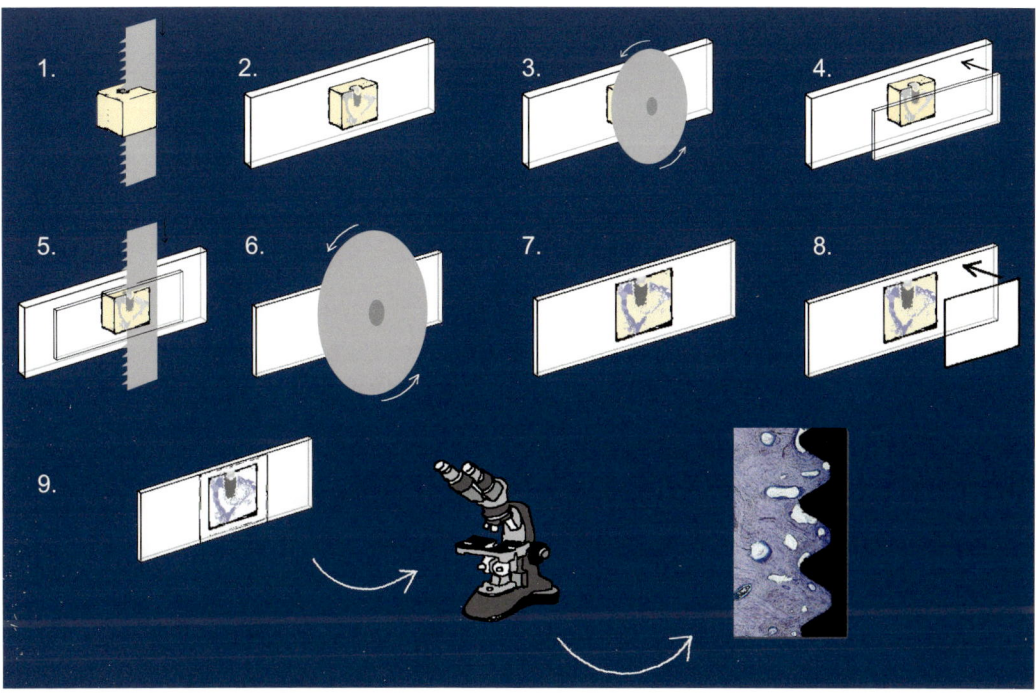

Fig 8-10 The preparation of cut and ground sections is illustrated here. **(1)** The resin-embedded implant is divided in the long axis of the implant. **(2)** The sample block is attached onto a supporting glass. **(3)** The surface of the divided implant is ground parallel on wet grinding paper in water-cooled grinding equipment. **(4)** A Plexiglas™ of known thickness is glued onto the plan sample. **(5)** A section of thickness of about 200 µm is prepared. **(6)** The thick section is further ground to a thickness of about 15 µm. **(7)** The section is histologically stained. **(8)** After drying, the samples are cover-slipped. **(9)** Qualitative inspection under the light microscope.

brief explanation of the preparation of cut and ground sections used for light microscopy. The methods presented are related to nondecalcified bone tissue with implants *in situ*. Almost all steps in the handling and treatment of samples will render some artifacts. This includes everything from fixation artifacts to evaluation artifacts. Human-made and technical artifacts are rather easy to identify but technical unexpected and unaccounted artifacts can arise and thus clear and standardized protocols should be used.

Our routine quantification techniques of tissue reactions to biomaterials will be explained. Biomechanical tests will briefly be mentioned in the end of the section since these are techniques that are frequently used in research studies. Some other novel methods are also presented.

8.5.2 Undecalcified Cut and Ground Sections With the Biomaterial *In Situ*

The concept of preparing undecalcified cut and ground sections was already implemented by one of the authors (CBJ) in 1983 when collaboration was started with Professor Karl Donath, oral pathologist at the Department of Pathology, University of Hamburg, Germany (Donath and Breuner, 1982; Donath, 1985) (Fig 8-10). Throughout the years the laboratories have used the so-called Donath technique involving the machine part related to the Exakt cutting and grinding system (Exakt Apparatebau, Norderstedt, Germany). All changes made by Professor Donath in collaboration with the author have been implemented and this is an ongoing issue. Despite being a well-known technique, it must be regarded as a "rough" technique and it does not allow serial sectioning; however, it is considered the state of the art technique when using biomaterials *in situ*. As with all special instruments and techniques it requires specially trained technicians. One major drawback of the equipment is that it is time consuming and costly. Having said this, one positive aspect is that samples, e.g., small cochlea wall implants up to human knee and hip samples, can be prepared using the very same equipment. Note that all steps during the tissue handling both before and during cutting and grinding should be performed strictly observing appropriate laboratory safety conditions. This involves avoidance of skin contact with the solutions and usage of lab coats and gloves as well as working in a hood during some of the steps.

8.5.3 Preparation of Samples for Undecalcified Sections

Fixation of Samples
In research animal studies it is quite common to apply perfusion fixation with, e.g., glutaraldehyde. This is strongly recommended if samples are going to be evaluated at the electron microscopic level. However, for routine morphology of retrieved human and animal samples it is common to immerse samples in fixative. Four percent neutral buffered formaldehyde is a suitable solution for fixation via immersion. However, for proper fixation it is important to trim and decrease the sample size as much as possible. Moreover, it is important to use a generous amount of fixative including stirring and vacuum treatment.

When the samples are fully fixed it is recommended to store them in 70% ethanol. Storage in formaldehyde solution for a long time renders artifacts such as difficulties in the staining ability. If enzyme- and immunohistochemical methods are the target then it is a must to use a fixative that will preserve the proteins. (Johansson *et al.*, 1999; Röser *et al.*, 2000). In order to succeed with such samples it is recommended to follow the protocol strictly, i.e., freshly made solutions with exact pH adjustment right before usage and exact timing of the steps involved in the methodology. The initial fixative steps are the most important and crucial ones for a positive result. Recently we have used a commercially available fixative containing zinc and formalin (4% zinc formaldehyde [Zn-F], Mallinckrodt Baker B.V., Holland). The rat bones were immersed for a few days in the Zn-F fixative followed by routine dehydration. Some specimens were decalcified using EDTA with PVP (ethylenediaminetetraacetic acid disodium salt dehydrate with polyvinylpyrrolidone), which is a mild decalcification solution that preserves proteins. The latter samples were embedded in paraffin followed by routine sectioning. Such sections were tested with von Willbrand factor (factor VIII) rendering positive results of bone marrow cells (megacariocytes) (Nyberg *et al.*, 2010).

Dehydration
All samples must be fully dehydrated before being embedded in supporting material. Among dehydration solutions, ethanol is the most commonly used one. After appropriate fixation time the routine immerse-fixed samples are rinsed in tap water. Dehydration starts in 70% ethanol followed by 80%, 96%, and absolute ethanol. It is recommended to change each solution at least twice during the dehydration process. Hence, this depends on the sample size as well as the amount of solution used. The exact dehydration time depends on the sample size, the number of samples and the size of the jar. The latter means that a generous amount of solution must be used.

Preinfiltration and Infiltration

The first step in sample treatment with resin solution involves a dilution of the pure resin. Usually we use three dilutions and each step is conducted under stirring and vacuum conditions. Following this, we use two batches of pure resin before the samples are embedded in pure resin. The routine resin in the laboratories is the Technovit 7200 VLC (Kulzer, Germany). However, for enzyme- and immunohistochemical samples one must use a resin that can be dissolved and for such we use Technovit 9100 NEW (Kulzer).

Embedding

Some extra planning in this last embedding step will save time when preparing the final cut and ground sections. This means that the preferred cutting direction should be known beforehand so that the samples can be embedded "smart". It is advisable to let the sample have a few extra days of "surface drying" before handling and cutting and grinding starts.

Sawing

The embedded sample is divided for example in the long axis of the implant in the bandsaw. Note that all samples in the same study must be sectioned in the same "anatomical manner" in order to avoid comparisons of apples to pears. The histomorphometric outcome is dependent on section direction (Johansson and Morberg, 1995a). Implants retrieved with a trephine must be marked so that all samples will be divided in the same manner.

1. The sample surface is ground parallel, and the thickness (1) of this is registered, before a supporting Plexiglas of known thickness (2) is mounted on the sample.
2. Measure the sandwich, i.e., the mounted sample with the Plexiglas (3). Knowing (1) and (2) and deducting this from (3) will result in the glue thickness between the sample and the Plexiglas. This is important to know since the glue thickness varies both between sample sizes and between batches (older glue is less viscous and results in a thicker glue compared to new).
3. A section of approximately 150 to 200 µm is prepared in the bandsaw. According to own experience, preparation of sections around 100 µm with an implant *in situ* is not recommended since this more often results in implant detachment. However, if no implant is *in situ* one may well prepare thinner sections and by using a thinner sawing-band the actual loss of material is reduced.

Grinding

Following this the grinding starts by using wet grinding papers of rough (800) to fine grains (1200). Due to the so-called water-planing effect, resulting in "shadow effects" in the interface (which will be visualized in the microscope as an interfacial artifact) it is advisable to avoid using too much weight during grinding. Moreover, too smooth grinding papers will also cause similar artifacts and should therefore be avoided. A sample thickness of 10 to 15 µm is optimal for histomorphometry. And it must be noted that the thicker the section the greater is the overestimation of the bony contact (Johansson and Morberg, 1995b). However, if enzyme and immunohistochemical studies are conducted one must prepare sections below 10 µm. Such sections are not prepared on Plexiglas but on precoated glass slides. This is due to the fact that the sections must be de-plastified before commencement of the subsequent "immune-protocol" (Johansson et al., 1999; Röser et al., 2000).

Staining

Almost all histologic stainings (with some modifications) can be used on cut and ground sections. It is recommended to use a routine staining that differentiates between various bone, i.e., old- and new bone as well as soft tissue. Our in-house routine staining technique is referred to as the toluidine blue mixed with pyronin G (Johansson, 1991). Bone stains in various purple grades (old bone light purple and new bone dark purple). The cement lines in the bone are sharply demarcated being darker stained. Osteoid is stained blue-grey and osteoblasts are most often clearly observed on osteoid. The trapped osteoblasts in the osteoid, i.e., the osteocytes, are clearly visible in its various stages. Osteoclasts are also recognized and sometimes the ruffled boarders are clearly distinguished. Muscle and other soft tissue stains blue. One can clearly discriminate between various cell types such as macrophages, multinucleated giant cells, plasma cells and other inflammatory cells. Mast cells are also clearly depicted using this staining protocol. Note that it is very important that the sections are not too thick because cellular details cannot be observed on thick sections. This is probably a reason why several scientific papers are lacking information regarding the cellular findings on cut and ground sections. In fact, it is quite common to find scientific papers where thick sections (from 50 μm up to a few 100 μm) have been used for evaluating osseointegration as well as other features (Ohashi et al., 2000; Becker et al., 2006; Cordaro et al., 2008; Iwaniec et al., 2008). Such studies are methodologically inappropriate since the thicker the sample the greater is the overestimation of the bone-to-implant contact. We have shown that, cut and ground, a section of a thickness above 30 μm up to 100 μm renders overestimations of at least 30% (Johansson and Morberg, 1995a).

8.5.4 Histomorphometry

"The quantitative measurement and characterization of microscopic images using a computer; manual or automated digital image analysis typically involves measurements and comparisons of selected geometric areas, perimeters, length angle or orientation, form factors, center or gravity coordinates, as well as image enhancement." (www.mondofacto.com/facts/dictionary?histomorphometry)

The image analysis tools and techniques are an issue that is sometimes frustrating. This is due to the lack of consensus in what and how to perform measurements. How to perform measurements: manually, automatically, or semi-automatically? It is our opinion that one cannot rely on automatic programs. A trained and experienced eye is required to judge whether something is an artifact or not. Moreover in order to understand the biologic processes we must rely not only on figures and data. The qualitative description is a must but unfortunately it seems that it has less priority in the analysis part. The methods and equipments used for histomorphometrical quantifications vary among laboratories and it is difficult to compare in-house data with out-house results and from one study to another. However, in our laboratories we emphasize that the same equipment and the same person perform all measurements in the same study. Our in-house routine quantifications are described below.

8.5.5 Assessing the Bone Quality

Bone-to-implant Contact
The undecalcified cut and ground sections are histologically stained with toluidine blue mixed in pyronin G prior to observations under the light microscope. This is our in-house standard and rule (Fig 8-11).

The bone-to-implant contact measurement requires a trained person to judge the interface. Learning time and practice involves measurements performed by an experienced person and the nonexperienced person together. Discussions and test measurements are conducted and individual as well as cross-comparisons are performed. The laboratories have internal criteria set up for judging whether or not an artifact is of relevance for the measurement, and all analysis and judgments follow the internal standards. Such artifacts are, for example, related to shrinking and staining errors.

The laboratories started with PC-based histomorphometric analyses about 25 years ago. The first PhD project reported using this tool was in 1991 (Johansson, 1991). The original semiautomatic Microvid program coupled to a PC and a Leitz Aristoplan light microscope is still in use (Leitz Wetzlar, Germany). In fact most of the PhD theses from the laboratories related to histomorphometric comparisons have used this program (i.e., Wennerberg et al., 1996; Ivanoff et al., 2001). We find it very useful, not only as a research and training tool, but also since the researchers can study the section with various magnifications and judge the interface in very high magnifications before performing the actual measurements on the preselected magnification. The advantage with this system is that one conducts histomorphometric analysis directly in the microscope. This means that all measurements are performed directly with the eyepiece of the microscope. Unfortunately this piece of equipment is no longer available on the market.

The enlargement used in the majority of histomorphometric studies involves one region of interest (ROI) at a time. For screw-shaped implants, our in-house rule is that one implant thread at a time is in focus. The implants curvature is outlined followed by marking nonbone lengths. The program automatically depicts the bone length measured as well as bone and nonbony contacts. The percentage of bone-to-implant contact is also shown. The laboratories are equipped with other image analysis tools but they will not be discussed here since they do not render any additional information related to this issue. To give one example of what has been observed in terms of the osseointegration process when measured as bone-to-implant contact, a unique clinical material related to 275 retrieved Brånemark implants was published by Bolind et al. (2005). Selected samples, both unloaded and loaded with various times of follow-up, were investigated along various regions of the implant, i.e., four different areas/regions were selected in

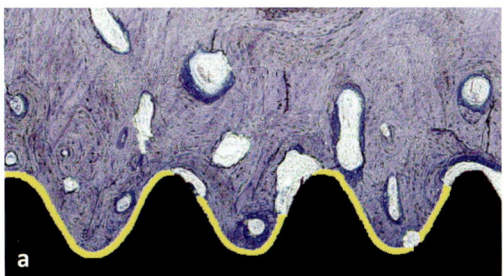
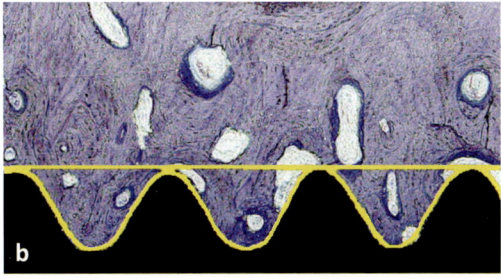
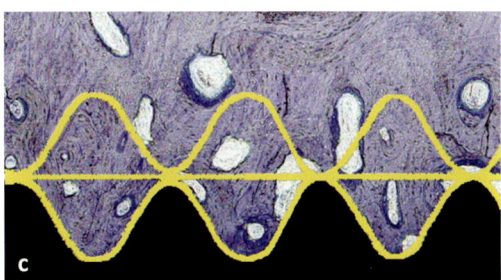

Fig 8-11 (a) Bone-to-implant contact (BIC) is outlined in the interface region. (b) Bone area (BA) measurements are performed in the inner threads. (c) The area of the inside threads is out-folded depicting the mirror image (MI) area. (These figures illustrate a toluidine blue stained section with subsequent quantitative histomorphometric methods that are used routinely. Note that all measurements are performed with only one thread visible in the eyepiece of the microscope.)

each ROI along the surface. A different bone remodeling pattern could be observed and thus the osseointegration varied both with time of insertion as well as within the implant geometry (Fig 8-12). Hence, the specific quality of the bone tissue could not be commented on and to the best of our knowledge this is seldom reported in scientific papers.

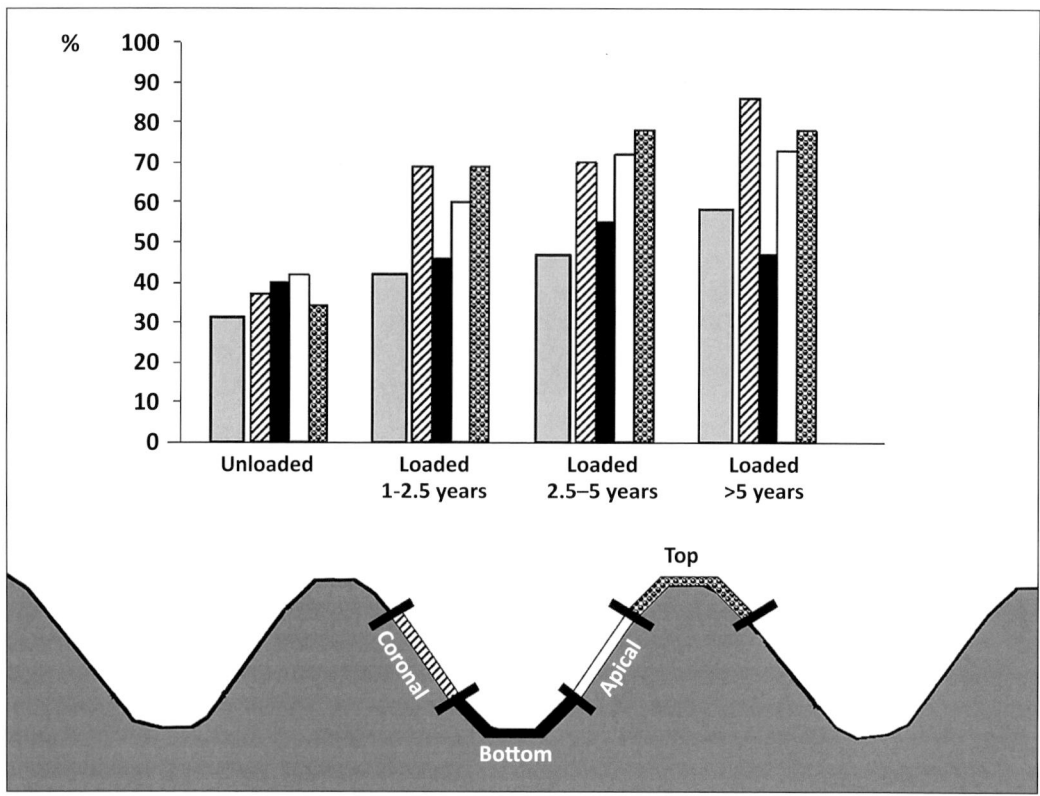

Fig 8-12 This figure illustrates bone-to-implant contact (BIC) measurements performed on retrieved human samples after being either unloaded or loaded with various times of follow-up. The first gray bar to the left in each group demonstrates the mean BIC of the entire implant. As can be seen the longer the loading time the greater is the BIC. The four bars to the right represent mean values of BIC when performed in selected regions, i.e., the coronal, bottom, apical, and top regions of the implant surface. The unloaded implants demonstrated the lowest BIC in the thread peaks (top) while with increasing time of loading the greatest BIC values varied along the four regions. After a loading time of more than 5 years the greatest BIC values were observed in the bottom part of the implant surface. Note the left side of the enlarged implant is facing the upper, coronal part of the implant while the right side depicts the apical region of the implant.

Bone Area
Another in-house method used is to quantify the bone area in a thread region or any preselected ROI (Fig 8-11). While the former bone-to-implant contact measurements may be more related to osseointegration per se, the area measurements reflect the remodeling activity in the threaded region as a whole. The quality of bone can vary quite substantially in a ROI. For example in rabbit cortical bone the remodeling pattern in the old cortical region is different compared with the newly formed bone in the threads in the marrow cavity. With increasing time of follow-up it is more difficult to depict new versus old bone. This is not so much elaborated on in the presentation of results and to the best of our knowledge, it is common to present data as bone area, i.e., old and newly formed bone.

One example of comparing newly formed and old bone inside threads was presented in combination with *in vivo* fluorescent labeling of bone

(Carlsson et al., 2009). The occurrence of fluorescence was in agreement with the amount of newly formed bone; however, the amount and type of fluorochrome (alizarin complexon and calcein) varied between test and control implants. Such data cannot be obtained based on newly formed bone alone when compared to the toluidine blue stained section.

Mirror Image Bone Area
Yet another in-house standard measurement is related to the mirror images. Here one outlines the inner area and folds it out, reflecting a mirror area (Johansson, 1991) (Fig 8-11). This type of measurement may be of importance for studying various bone remodeling activities and reasons; if various biomaterials are used, one may expect differences in the inner area compared with the mirror images (Johansson et al., 1998). Naturally this depends on the follow-up time as well. Hypothetically one may expect a greater bone area inside the threads if a more "tissue friendly material" has been used. A ratio of 1:1 between the inside area to mirror image may depict similar tissue reactions or time-dependent healing. However, if there is a 1:2 ratio between in and out this may indicate that there are material disturbances or the healing time is too short. A 2:1 ratio between in and out on the other hand may indicate that the implant surface condition is very prone to attract bone tissue. Having said this, there are times when the bone-to-implant contact is very high although the bone areas in the inner threads are low.

This may reflect chemical reactions and attachments, demonstrating that the bone-to-implant contact does not have to be "all over" but the contact points that are between bone and implant are "strong enough" (Ellingsen et al., 2004). These types of results and observations need to be further elaborated on. Nowadays one may not have to have high bone-to-implant contact but the contacts that are there may involve much stronger forces (and forces difficult to measure with the tools and techniques available as of today) compared with earlier times when the implant chemistry was not in focus. Quite similar quantitative interfacial analysis of bone inside and outside the inner threads (mirror image) has been conducted by Jansen (2003), who refers to these area measurements as "bone density". True or not, this is an effort from other biomaterials research groups to investigate the bone tissue formation occurring around the implant in various regions, and thus not only focusing on the interface. Whether or not we will find area measurements of significant value for the osseointegration process remains unknown for the time being but at least we are reporting data that can help and increase the understanding of the complex process of osseointegration.

Bone-to-Implant Contact and Bone Volume Measurement on 3D Material
Micro-computed tomography (CT) techniques are emerging in the field of biomaterials research when studying integration of medical devices in bone tissue. To the best of our knowledge and with our own experience there is no such technique or resolution available with the ordinary micro-CT equipment. The interface is most often occupied by an artifact-layer of various thickness (beam-hardening) resulting in the impossibility of judging osseointegration (Barrett and Keat, 2004). We have performed CT tests at the Synchrotron Radiation facility (SR micro-CT) at the Institute for Materials Research, GKSS Research Centre Geesthacht, Hamburg, Germany (www.desy.de). This technique yields more accurate tomographic reconstructions due to the parallel beam acquisition and higher resolution compared to standard micro-CT and avoids the beam-hardening effect. The aim of our SR micro-CT studies varies. For example, the results from the two-dimensional histologic sections are compared to the three-dimensional material. The method for finding the two-dimensional slice in the three-dimensional material (image registra-

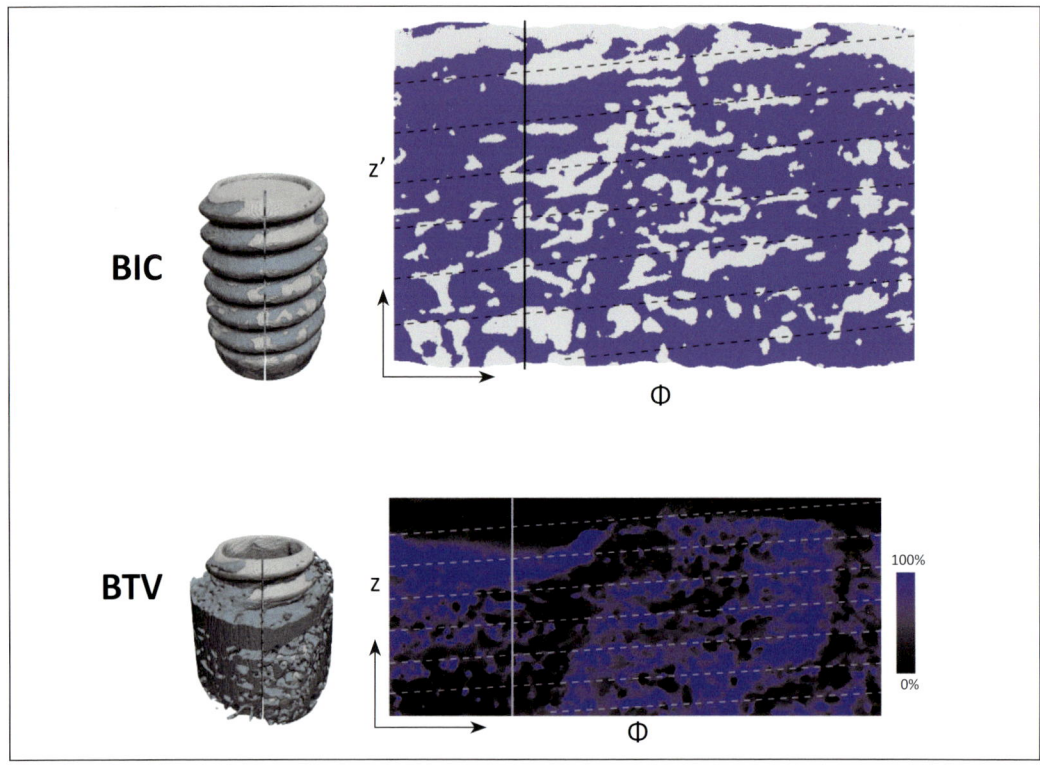

Fig 8-13 Computer tomography pictures are often shown as three-dimensional (3D) illustrations only. The material to these figures is originally rendered from SR micro-CT (Synchrotron Radiation micro-tomography). The upper part of the figures illustrates the entire bone implant contact (left) unfolded to a 2D-image (right). Black dashed lines show the approximate location of the peaks of the threads. The vertical line indicates the corresponding angles in the two images. The lower part of the figure illustrates the entire bone implant volume (left) unfolded to a 2D-image (right). This lower part illustrates the bone tissue volumes. White dashed lines show the peaks of the threads. The vertical line indicates the corresponding angles in the two images. Illustrations courtesy of Mr Hamid Sarve.

tion) is a challenge. This has been reported by Sarve et al. (2009). One of our recent papers describes a novel method related to bone tissue registration around implants. The bone-to-implant contact, bone area, and mirror image were extracted from the three-dimensional material and the results could be followed simultaneously in a helix structure (Fig 8-11) (Sarve et al., 2010). Yet another novel method is to "unfold" the tissue both as bone-to-implant and bone tissue volumes (Fig 8-13) (Sarve et al., 2010). Whether this will impact how to evaluate osseointegration is not fully understood. However, for research purposes and eventually to perform studies related to, for example, loading conditions, we foresee increased usage of equipment such as SR micro-CT. The drawback is the limited time available in the facilities and their location.

8.5.6 Biomechanical Tests for Evaluating Osseointegration

Removal Torque Tests (RTQ)
Removal torque tests as well as other destructive biomechanical tests such as push- and pull-

out tests cannot be performed in the clinical situation but in preclinical animal studies they are rapid tests revealing the actual osseointegration strength. The results depict the shear strength in a three-dimensional manner of the force needed to loosen an implant from its bone bed. Such destructive biomechanical tests of implant integration in research animals are performed with a variety of equipment. These range from manual hand-held Tonichi devices (Johansson and Albrektsson, 1987; Sennerby et al., 1992) to user-friendly and one-of-a-kind electronic products, where the in-house 1992 products is still in use (Detektor, Göteborg, Sweden). Several commercially available and larger equipment such as the Instron equipment are also frequently used for biomechanical tests (Brånemark, 1996; Buser et al., 1998). However, such equipment is not easily movable and tissue needs to be retrieved and transported to the test facilities, which may render artifacts. In fact it is rather common that the tissue is immersed in fixative on transportation to the test facility, and this will affect the results and the obtained data (Johansson CB, personal communication, 2009). Recently we have implemented and tested new user-friendly removal torque equipment (Johansson et al., 2010). The major advantages are the size of the instrument including the possibility of monitoring the release torque over a selected time span. The equipment has recently been verified for its accuracy and the results were as expected both when performed *ex vivo* on materials of different hardness as well as *in vivo* tests of C.p. Ti and TiAlV implants in rabbit bone.

Shear Strength Tests
The 3D removal torque tests roughly reflect the shear strength. The removal torque results are presented in Ncm. These results can be converted to shear strength in N/mm^2. For this purpose one has to leave the torque tested implant in the bone bed. The bone block with the implant *in situ* is retrieved, treated routinely and processed to a cut and ground section. The section is stained and evaluated under the light microscope. Estimation of the bone length close to the implant is performed, and by applying a geometrical formula, the shear strength data can be calculated (Derezende and Johansson, 1993; Stenport and Johansson, 2008; Johansson et al., 2010). For more information regarding shear strength calculations see Derezende and Johansson (1993), Stenport and Johansson (2009), and Johansson et al. (2010).

Combination of Biomechanical Tests
Yet another evaluation of osseointegration is to combine biomechanical tests, i.e., removal torque and pull-away tests. This was recently performed with a novel medical device component in rabbit bone (Sul et al., 2010). With this device it is possible to measure the removal torque/shear strength on screws and the bone bonding force between a disk-shaped implant and bone. The device also renders the possibility to investigate the qualitative and quantitative bone tissue reactions (bone-to-implant contact, bone area, mirror image) to implants since one of the two screws attaching the device to the bone is not RTQ tested but retrieved with surrounding bone and treated to cut and ground sections. For more information about this device see Sul et al. (2010).

Resonance Frequency Tests
The nondestructive resonance frequency analyses (RFA) test is nowadays mostly performed clinically and relates to the "implant stability as a function of the stiffness" (Meredith et al., 1996). The test is referred to as "a bending test of the implant–bone complex where a transducer applies an extremely small bending force" (Sennerby and Meredith, 2008). However, performing RFA tests in research animals is not a simple task and for more details related to this see Sennerby et al. (2005). In a study by Sul et al. (2010), the RFA measurements were performed on six groups of implants, with various topographies

and surface chemical properties, at the time of installation in rabbit bone and 6 weeks after. Significant differences were observed for bone measurements performed both in a longitudinal and in a perpendicular manner, comparing baseline to 6 weeks (Sul et al., 2010). Various RFA studies were reviewed by Quesada-García et al. (2009) who reported "The studies reviewed demonstrate the usefulness of RFA as a non-invasive method to assess implant stability. Further research is required to determine whether this system is also capable of measuring the degree of dental implant osseointegration".

References

1. Aerssens J, Boonen S, Joly J, Dequeker J (1997). Variations in trabecular bone composition with anatomical site and age: potential implications for bone quality assessment. *J Endocrinol* 155:411–421.
2. Albrektsson T, Brånemark PI, Hansson HA, Lindström J (1981). Osseointegrated titanium implants. *Acta Orthop Scand* 52:155–179.
3. Barrett JF, Keat N (2004). Artifacts in CT: Recognition and avoidance. *RadioGraphics* 24:1679–1691.
4. Becker J, Kirsch A, Schwarz F, Chatzinikolaidou M, Rothamel D, Lekovic V et al. (2006). Bone apposition to titanium implants biocoated with recombinant human bone morphogenetic protein-2 (rhBMP-2). A pilot study in dogs. *Clin Oral Invest* 10:217–224.
5. Bolind P, Johansson CB, Balshi T, Langer B, Albrektsson T (2005). A study of 275 retrieved Brånemark oral implants. *Int J Periodontics Restorative Dent* 25:425–437.
6. Brånemark PI, Breiner U, Lindström J, Adell R, Hansson BO, Ohlsson P (1969). Intraosseous anchorage of dental prostheses. I. Experimental studies. *Scand J Plast Reconstr Surg* 3:81.
7. Brånemark R (1996). A biomechanical study of osseointegration *in-vivo* measurements in rat, rabbit, dog and men. PhD Thesis. University of Göteborg, Göteborg, Sweden.
8. Buser D, Nydegger T, Hirt H, Cochran D, Nolte LP (1998). Removal torque of titanium implants in the maxilla of miniature pigs. *Int J Oral Maxillofac Implants* 13:611–619.
9. Carlsson C, Holmgren-Peterson K, Jönsson J, Johansson P, Albrektsson A, Hoffman M et al. (2009). Comparing light- and fluorescence microscopic data: A pilot study of titanium- and magnesium oxide implant integration in rabbit bone. Online. *TITANIUM Int Sci J Dent Implants Biomater* 1:61–70.
10. Coelho PG, Granjeiro JM, Romanos GE, Suzuki M, Silva NRF, Cardaropoli G et al. (2009). Basic research methods and current trends of dental implant surfaces. *J Biomed Res Part B: Appl Biomater* 88:579–596.
11. Cordaro L, Bosshardt DD, Palattella P, Rao W, Serion G, Chiapasco M (2008). Maxillary sinus grafting with Bio-oss or Straumann bone ceramic: histomorphometric results from a randomized controlled multicenter clinical trial. *Clin Oral Implants Res* 19:796–803.
12. Derezende MLR, Johansson CB (1993). Quantitative bone tissue response to commercially pure titanium implants. *J Mater Sci Mater Med* 4(3):233–239.
13. Dohan Ehrenfest DM, Coelho PG, Kang B-S, Sul Y-T, Albrektsson T (2010). Classification of osseointegrated implant surfaces: materials, chemistry and topography. *Trends Biotechnol* 28:198–206.
14. Donath K (1985). The diagnostic value of the new method for the study of undecalcified bones and teeth with attached soft tissue (Säge-Schliff (sawing and grinding) technique). *Pathol Res Pract* 179:631–633.
15. Donath K, Breuner G (1982). A method for the study of undecalcified bones and teeth with attached soft tissues. The Säge-Schliff (sawing and grinding) technique. *J Oral Pathol* 11:318–326.
16. Dorland´s Medical Dictionary (2007). Edinburgh: Elsevier.
17. Ellingsen JE, Johansson CB, Wennerberg A, Holmen A (2004). Improved retention and bone-to implant contact with fluoride-modified titanium implants. *Int J Oral Maxillofac Implants* 19:659–666.
18. Flecknell P (1996). Laboratory animal anaesthesia, 2nd ed. Maryland Heights: Academic Press, Elsevier.
19. Gilsanz V, Roe TF, Gibbens DT, Schulz EE, Carlson ME, Gonzalez O, Boechat MI (1988). Effects of sex steroids on peak bone density of growing rabbits. *Am J Physiol* 255: E416-E421.
20. ISO 10993-6 (1994). Biological evaluation of medical devices. Part 6. Tests for local effects after implantation. Geneva: International Organization for Standardization, pp 1–11.
21. Ivanoff CJ, Hallgren C, Widmark G, Sennerby L, Wennerberg A (2001). Histologic evaluation of the bone integration of TiO_2 blasted and turned titanium microimplants in humans. *Clin Oral Implants Res* 12:128–134.
22. Iwaniec UT, Wronski TJ Turner RT (2008). Histological analysis of bone. In: Alcohol: Methods and protocols 325, methods in molecular biology. Nagy LE, editor. No. 447. Toronto, New Jersey: Humana Press.
23. Jansen JA (2003). Histological analysis of bone-implant interface. In: Handbook of histology methods for bone and cartilage. An YH, Martin KL, editors. Toronto, New Jersey: Humana Press, pp 353–360.
24. Johansson C, Albrektsson T (1987). Integration of screw implants in the rabbit. A 1-year follow-up of removal torque of Ti implants. *Int J Oral Maxillofac Implants* 2:69–75.
25. Johansson CB (1991). On tissue reactions to metal implants. PhD Thesis. Gothenburg, Sweden: Department of Handicap Research, Biomaterials, University of Gothenburg.
26. Johansson CB, Morberg P (1995a). Importance of ground section thickness for reliable histomorphometrical results. *Biomaterials* 2:91–95.

References

27. Johansson CB, Morberg P (1995b). Cutting directions of bone with biomaterials in situ does influence the outcome of the histomorphometrical quantification. *Biomaterials* 13:1037–1039.
28. Johansson CB, Han CH, Wennerberg A, Albrektsson T (1998). A quantitative comparison of commercially pure (c.p.) titanium and Titanium-6Aluminum-4Vanadium (Ti6Al4V) implants in rabbit bone. *J Oral Maxillofac Implants* 13:315–321.
29. Johansson CB, Röser K, Bolind P, Donath K, Albrektsson T (1999). Bone-tissue formation and integration of titanium implants: an evaluation with newly developed enzyme and immunohistochemical techniques. *Clin Implant Dent Relat Res* 1:33–40.
30. Johansson CB, Jimbo R, Stefenson P (2010). *Ex vivo* and *in vivo* biomechanical test of implant attachment to various materials. Introduction of a new user-friendly removal torque equipment. *Clin Implant Dent Relat Res*. 17 July .[Epub ahead of print].
31. Meredith N, Alleyne D, Cawley P (1996). Quantitative determination of the stability of the implant interface using resonance frequency analysis. *Clin Oral Implants Res* 7:261–267.
32. Neyt JG, Buckwalter JA, Carrol NC (1988). Use of animal models in musculoskeletal research. *Iowa Orthop J* 18: 118–123.
33. Nyberg J, Hertzman S, Svensson B, Johansson C, Granström G, Johansson CB (2010). Single-dose irradiation followed by implant insertion in rat bone. An investigative study to find a critical level for osseointegration. *J Osseointegration* 2:93–101.
34. Ohashi H, Kobayashi A, Kadoya Y, Yamano Y, Oonishi H, Iwaki H (2000). Effect of particles and interface conditions on fibrous tissue interposition between bone and implant. A particle challenge model in rabbit. *J Mater Sci Mater Med* 11:255–259.
35. Omar O, Lennerås M, Svensson S, Suska F, Emanuelsson L, Hall J *et al*. (2010a). Integrin and chemokine receptor gene expression in implant-adherent cells during early osseointegration. *J Mater Sci Mater Med* 21:969–980.
36. Omar O, Svensson S, Zoric N, Lennerås M, Suska F, Wigren S *et al*. (2010b). In vivo gene expression in response to anodically oxidized versus machined titanium implants. *J Biomed Mater Res A* 92:1552–1566.
37. Omar O, Suska F, Lennerås M, Zoric N, Svensson S, Hall J *et al*. (2009). The influence of bone type on the gene expression in normal bone and at the bone-implant interface: experiment in animal model. *Clin Implant Dent Relat Res*. May 7 [Epub ahead of print].
38. Pearce AI, Richards RG, Milz S, Schneider E, Pearce SG (2007). Animal models for implant biomaterial research in bone: A review. European Cells and Materials 13:1–10.
39. Quesada-García MP, Prados-Sánchez E, Olmedo-Gaya MV, Muñoz-Soto E, González-Rodríguez MP, Vallecillo-Capilla M (2009). Measurement of dental implant stability by resonance frequency analysis: a review of the literature. *Medicina Oral Patología Oral Cirugía Bucal* 14:e538–e546.
40. Röser K, Johansson CB, Donath K, Albrektsson T (2000). A new approach to demonstrate cellular activity in bone formation adjacent to implants. *J Biomed Mater Res* 51:280–291.
41. Sarve H, Lindblad J, Johansson CB (2009). Quantification of bone remodeling in SRuCT images of implants. *Lect Notes Comput Sci* 5575:770–779.
42. Sarve H, Lindblad J, Johansson CB, Borgefors G (2010). Methods for visualization of bone tissue in the proximity of implants. In: Computer vision and graphics. Bolc L, Tadeusiewicz R, Chmielewski LJ, editors. Proc. ICCVG.
43. Sennerby L, Meredith N (2008). Implant stability measurements using resonance frequency analysis: biological and biomechanical aspects and clinical implications. *Periodontology 2000* 47:51–65.
44. Sennerby L, Thomsen P, Ericson LE (1992). A morphometric and biomechanic comparison of titanium implants inserted in rabbit cortical and cancellous bone. *Int J Oral Maxillofac Implants* 7:62–71.
45. Sennerby L, Dasmah A, Larsson B, Iverhed M (2005). Bone tissue responses to surface-modified zirconia implants: A histomorphometric and removal torque study in the rabbit. *Clin Implant Dent Relat Res* 7 (Suppl 1):S13–20.
46. Steinemann SG (1998). Titanium: the material of choice? *Periodontology 2000* 17:7–21.
47. Stenport VF, Johansson CB (2008). Evaluation of the tissue integration to pure titanium and titanium alloy implants. *Clin Implant Dent Relat Res* 10:191–199.
48. Sul YT, Johansson CB, Albrektsson T (2010). A novel *in vivo* method for quantifying the interfacial biochemical bond strength of bone implants. *J R Soc Interface* 7:81–90.
49. Wennerberg A, Albrektsson T, Lausmaa J (1996). Torque and histomorphometric evaluation of c.p. titanium screws blasted with 25- and 75- microns-sized-particles of Al_2O_3. *J Biomed Mater Res* 30:251–260.
50. Zarb G, Albrektsson T (1991). Osseointegration – A requiem for the periodontal ligament? An Editorial. *Int J Periodontics Restorative Dent* 11:88–91.

CHAPTER 9

Ridge Preservation

Maurício G. Araújo, Cléverson O. Silva, and Juliana C. Mesti

9.1 General Overview and Decision Tree/Table

Ridge preservation is a clinical procedure aimed at preventing, diminishing, or avoiding dimensional alteration of the alveolar process following tooth extraction. Thus, preclinical experiments in the field of ridge preservation are carried out in order to test a clinical procedure, an implanted material (graft or dental implant) or even a drug, which may provide relevant data before the onset of clinical trials. In addition, preclinical studies on ridge preservation may also be designed after clinical trials have started to evaluate aspects that clinically may not be feasible, i.e., details of the wound's healing process.

Almost all preclinical studies on ridge preservation have been performed on the dog (Table 9-1 and Table 9-2). Therefore, first the canine model will be comprehensively described in this chapter and then some information will be provided about the rat and minipig models. As in human beings, the alveolar process in dogs is formed during the eruption of the teeth. Most species have 28 primary teeth and 42 permanent teeth. In general, the primary teeth begin to erupt at about 3 to 4 weeks of age and the permanent teeth begin to emerge at about 3 to 4 months of age. Around 6 months of age, the permanent teeth are fully erupted.

Dogs have a set of 20 teeth in the maxilla and 22 in the mandible (Fig 9-1). They are divided into four types as in humans: incisors (maxilla and mandible: six), canines (maxilla and mandible: two), premolars (maxilla and mandible: four) and molars (maxilla: four; mandible: six). The incisors, canines, and first premolars have a single root while the remaining premolars and molars are multi-rooted teeth. The roots of the incisors are straight and relatively short while the canines have long and curved roots. The premolars and molars have two roots that are parallel or slightly divergent (Fig 9-2). It is

Table 9-1 Summary of the ridge preservation studies in the dog model

Author	N	Species	Procedure (immediately after tooth extraction)	Methods	Healing interval	Postoperative care	Endpoint measurements
Araújo et al., 2005	5	Beagle	Implant	Histometric measurements	3 months	Soft-food diet; plaque control (3×/week); antibiotic (7 days)	Socket wall height
Araújo et al., 2006a	6	Beagle	Implant	Histometric measurements	1 and 3 months	Soft-food diet; plaque control (3×/week)	Socket wall height
Araújo et al., 2006b	7	Beagle	Implant	Histometric measurements	0, 1, and 3 months	Soft-food diet; plaque control (3×/week); antibiotic (7 days)	Socket wall height
Boix et al., 2006	3	Beagle	Biphasic calcium phosphate ceramic	Histomorphometric measurements	3 months	Soft-food diet; antibiotic (2 days)	Presence of mineralized tissue above and below socket walls Composition of newly formed tissue
Shi et al., 2007	5	Mongrel	Surgical-grade calcium sulfate + platelet-rich plasma	Histomorphometric measurements CT scans evaluation	3 months	Soft-food diet; antibiotic (5 days)	New bone formation activities Alveolar ridge height
Araújo et al., 2008	5	Mongrel	Deproteinized bovine bone mineral	Histomorphometric measurements	3 months	Soft-food diet; plaque control (3×/week)	Socket wall height Alveolar process area
Rothamel et al., 2008	10	Foxhound	Nanocrystalline hydroxyapatite paste	Histomorphometric measurements	3 and 6 months	Soft-food diet	Socket wall height and width Total bone width
Fickl et al., 2008a	5	Beagle	Deproteinized bovine bone mineral ± soft tissue graft	Tissue contour changes	0, 2, and 4 months	Plaque control (3×/week); antibiotic (7 days); anti-inflammatory (6 days); analgesic (2 days)	Volumetric measurements of casts with digital imaging system

Study	N	Animal	Material	Measurement	Time	Protocol	Outcomes
Fickl et al., 2008b	5	Beagle	Deproteinized bovine mineral ± soft tissue graft	Histometric measurements	4 months	Plaque control (3×/week); antibiotic (7 days); anti-inflammatory (6 days); analgesic (2 days)	Socket wall height; Alveolar ridge width
Araújo et al., 2009	5	Beagle	Deproteinized bovine bone mineral	Histomorpho-metric measurements	2 weeks	Plaque control (days 3, 7 and 10)	Composition of newly formed tissue
Araújo and Lindhe, 2009a	5	Beagle	Deproteinized bovine bone mineral	Histomorpho-metric measurements	6 months	Plaque control (3×/week)	Socket wall height; Alveolar process area; Composition of newly formed tissue
Araújo and Lindhe, 2009b	5	Beagle	With or without flap elevation	Histomorpho-metric measurements	6 months	Plaque control (3×/week)	Socket wall height; Alveolar process area
Fickl et al., 2009a	5	Beagle	Deproteinized bovine bone mineral ± buccal connective tissue graft	Tissue contour changes	2 weeks and 4 months	Soft-food diet; plaque control (3×/week); antibiotic (13 days); anti-inflammatory (13 days); analgesic (2 days)	Volumetric measurements of casts with digital imaging system
Fickl et al., 2009b	5	Beagle	Deproteinized bovine bone mineral ± buccal connective tissue graft	Histometric measurements	4 months	Soft-food diet; plaque control (3×/week); antibiotic (13 days); anti-inflammatory (13 days); analgesic (2 days)	Socket wall height; Alveolar ridge width
Araújo et al., 2010a	5	Beagle	Deproteinized bovine bone mineral	Histomorpho-metric measurements	1 and 3 days, 1, 2, and 4 weeks	Plaque control (3×/week)	Composition of newly formed tissue
Araújo et al., 2010b	5	Beagle	Beta-tricalcium phosphate	Histomorpho-metric measurements	1 and 3 days, 1, 2, and 4 weeks	Plaque control (3×/week)	Composition of newly formed tissue

Table 9-2 Summary of the ridge preservation studies in the rat and minipig models. BMP, bone morphogenic protein.

Author	Animal	N	Procedure (immediately after tooth extraction)	Methods	Healing interval	Postoperative care	Endpoint measurements
Hahn et al., 1988	Rats	24	Hydroxyapatite collagen	Xeroradiographic and histologic measurements	1 day and 2, 4, 8, and 12 weeks	Soft-food diet	Alveolar ridge height Composition of newly formed tissue
Matin et al., 2001	Rats	60	Recombinant human BMP-2	Scanning electron microscopy, histomorphometric measurements, and immunohistochemical analysis	3, 5, 7, 14, 21, 28, 56, and 84 days	Commercial rat food	Alveolar ridge height Composition of newly formed tissue, alkaline phosphatase activity, 5-bromodeoxyuridine localization
Oltramari et al., 2007	Minipigs	6	Association of bovine bone, collagen, bBMP, and hydroxyapatite	Radiographic measurements	3 months	Commercial pig food	Bone height and density
Aguirre et al., 2010	Rats	90	Subcutaneous alendronate	Histomorphometry	10, 21, 35, and 70 days	Not informed	Bone volume, bone height, bone cells, blood vessels
Jee et al., 2010	Rats	20	Subcutaneous alendronate	Tomography	2, 4, and 6 weeks	Not informed	Alveolar bone radiographic densities and dimensions

important to note that the tooth size varies according to the size of the animal. Thus, a 30 kg Labrador is expected to have significantly larger teeth than a 10 kg Beagle. A larger dog has also the propensity to alveolar processes with wider bony walls than a smaller dog.

9.2 The Dog Model

9.2.1 Aim of the Dog Model

As the name indicates, ridge preservation is about preserving the alveolar process and a full description of the tissue to be preserved is mandatory. The alveolar process may be defined as the bone tissue that surrounds a fully erupted tooth. It is limited coronally by the bone margins of the socket walls and apically by an imaginary line at the bottom of the socket in a perpendicular direction to the long axis of the root. Beyond this line is the basal bone of the mandible or the maxilla (Fig 9-1).

The choice of the experimental site should answer the specific question (aim) of the study. If the aim of the study is to evaluate the outcome of a ridge preservation technique, it is logical to choose alveolar sockets that exhibit a thin buccal wall because they are expected to undergo marked dimensional alterations. In addition, such sites may relate better to the anterior dentition of the maxilla in humans where the ridge preservation technique may be more frequently used. On the other hand, if the aim of the study is to evaluate the inflammatory tissue reaction to a bone graft, the thickness of the

9.2 The Dog Model

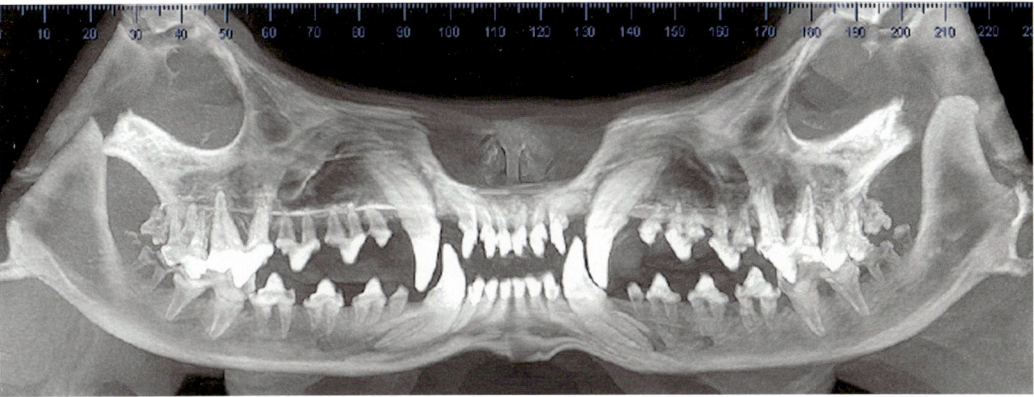

Fig 9-1 Panoramic tomographic radiograph of the dog maxilla and mandible.

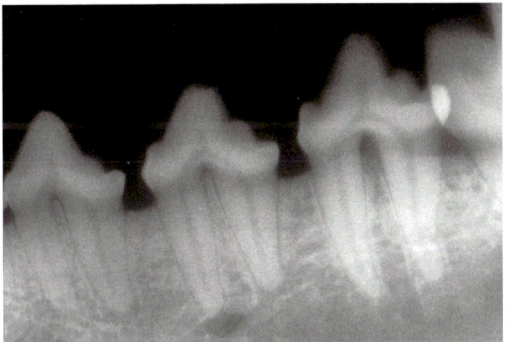

Fig 9-2 Periapical radiograph of the fourth, third, and second mandibular premolars.

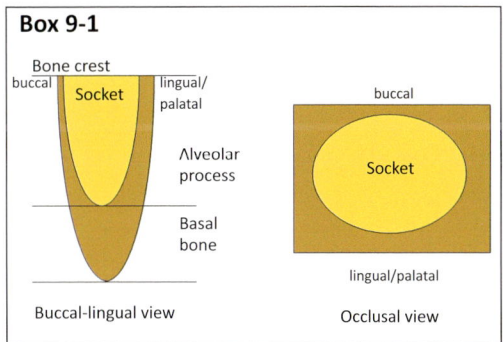

Fig 9-3 Schematic drawing illustrating the buccolingual and occlusal view of the alveolar process. Note that the alveolar socket may be described as a self-containing defect in which the buccal wall is frequently thinner than its lingual counterpart.

bone wall is not critical and the experimental site can be located in alveolar sockets with different anatomic characteristics.

9.2.2 Advantages/Disadvantages of the Presented Model

Advantages:
- The alveolar socket has a very similar shape to that of humans.
- The healing process of the extraction socket is obviously the same as humans and has already been extensively described (Cardaropoli *et al.*, 2003; Araújo and Lindhe, 2005; Trombelli *et al.*, 2008).
- Some dog species such as the Beagle can be kept under a plaque control regimen where teeth can be brushed by the animal caretaker with relative ease.
- Finally, the roots of the teeth that are usually used for the experiments on ridge preservation, the premolars and molars, can be easily removed without much effort or danger of fracturing the socket walls.

Table 9-3 Study chronogram

Activities to be carried out	Period (from baseline; months)					
	1–3	4	5–9	10–13	14–16	17–20
Animal selection and preparation	×					
Extraction and experimental graft procedure		×				
Wound healing			×			
Animal sacrifice, biopsy retrieval and onset of the histologic processing				×		
Data analyses					×	
Manuscript production						×

Disadvantages:
The disadvantages of the dog model are related to the size of the wound and to the speed of the modeling and remodeling phase of the healing. The size of a premolar alveolar socket in a Beagle dog is significantly smaller than the corresponding socket in humans. It is expected, therefore, in this case for the socket healing in the dog to be faster than in humans. In addition, it must be acknowledged that the remodeling process in dogs is much quicker than in humans, by three to five times (National Research Council, 1980). Consequently, even if two alveolar sockets, one in a dog and the other in a human, exhibit the same size, the wound process as a whole will take a longer time in humans. In summary, socket healing is similar in dogs and humans but the time interval in which it takes place is different. The faster wound healing process in the dog allows completion of studies in a shorter amount of time than in humans.

An important potential disadvantage in the dog model is the wide variations of dog species. Care should be taken when comparing the outcome of the experimental procedures performed in animals that are physically different, as with large Foxhound and small Beagle. The remodeling and modeling phase of the wound may be the same but the whole healing process may take longer or produce a different outcome due to size differences.

9.2.3 Timing

Once the research project has been finalized and approved by the local ethical committee, it is time to organize the various phases of the project in terms of timing. Such division should occur in accordance to the corresponding methodology and the time required for carrying out each one of the phases. A table should be made clearly displaying this information. The time intervals may be divided into days, weeks, months, or even years.

As an example, the research chronogram utilized by Araújo and Lindhe (2009a) is shown in Table 9-3. The aim of their study was to evaluate the use of a biomaterial as a graft material to preserve the alveolar ridge. Six months of healing was allowed for the grafted sockets.

9.2.4 Surgical Procedures

Proper knowledge of the basics of surgical technique is fundamental to avoid unnecessary damage to the tissues. An inappropriate surgical technique may jeopardize the healing and hide the real effect of the evaluated procedure. In all experiments on ridge preservation, tooth extraction is performed. In dogs, extraction should be performed with an exact technique in order to avoid fracture of the roots and socket walls, as well as contamination of the wound. Before the extraction, root scaling should be done to prevent any fragments of dislodged calculus or plaque to penetrate the alveolar socket or the graft material (Fig 9-4).

Extraction of a premolar distal root is described below. Before the onset of the surgery (Fig 9-5a), the crown is ground to its cervical third to expose the pulp chamber (Fig 9-5b). The mesial pulp is extirpated and the canal is instrumented with the use of endodontic files (Fig 9-5c). The canal is then rinsed with sodium hypochlorite 1%. Subsequently, the canal is dried with paper points and filled with guttapercha and endodontic cement.

The extraction is initiated by a sulcus incision (Fig 9-5d). A periotome or fine Freer elevator is used to elevate the buccal and lingual/palatal flap to the level of the bone crest (Fig 9-5e). A high-speed fissure bur is then used to cut the crown in a buccolingual direction in order to separate the mesial and distal roots. Care should be taken with the fissure bur to avoid damage of the soft and hard tissues (Fig 9-5f). Indeed, the fissure bur should not be inserted too deep so as to touch the interradicular bone crest. A thin layer of the pulp chamber should remain; subsequently, a luxator will be used to break it and separate the roots. The luxators should be used in sequence from the thinnest to the thickest instrument in a horizontal direction in relation to the long axis of the tooth (Fig 9-6a). Gentle movement should be applied in such a way that it will pull out the distal root from the socket. Once the root presents a clear movement, forceps can be used. The beaks of the forceps should be located at the cementoenamel junction level and care should be taken to avoid damaging the bone crest (Fig 9-6c). The movement is circular and parallel to the base of the mandible. Jingling movement may cause root and bone fracture. The root is then removed and the entrance of the pulp chamber on the remaining mesial root is restored with composite. Cross or singles sutures are placed at the socket entrance and removed after 10 days. In order

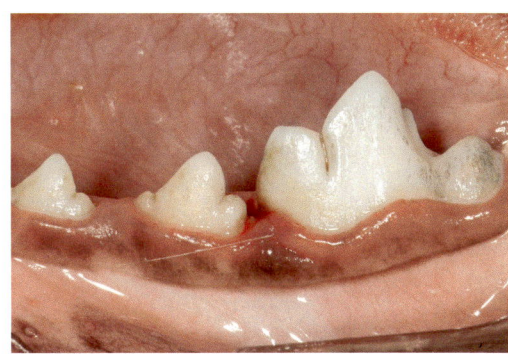

Fig 9-4 The mandibular premolar and molar region before root scaling.

to obtain primary wound closure, the soft tissues can be mobilized by elevating them beyond the level of the mucogingival junction and by incising the periosteum. If this approach is not enough for the desired wound closure, flap elevation including incision of the interproximal gingiva, followed by the procedures described above promote further release of the soft tissues. The same extraction procedure is performed, however, no root canal treatment is necessary when the entire multi-rooted tooth is to be removed.

The placement of a test material in the fresh extraction socket needs some consideration. The manufacturer's instructions should be followed. The following instructions refer to the use of a graft material. Before its use, the graft material should be moisturized with saline or blood for a few minutes (Fig 9-6b). The handling should also be done with care to avoid contamination with saliva etc. Before the grafting procedure takes place, rinsing of the socket and checking for the presence of any contaminant is necessary. Ideally, the graft should occupy the entire volume of the socket; therefore the graft material should be of a size that easily reaches the bottom of the socket. A wise way to graft the socket is to use small portions of the graft material at a time. The graft is packed with a blunt instrument until it fills the entire socket

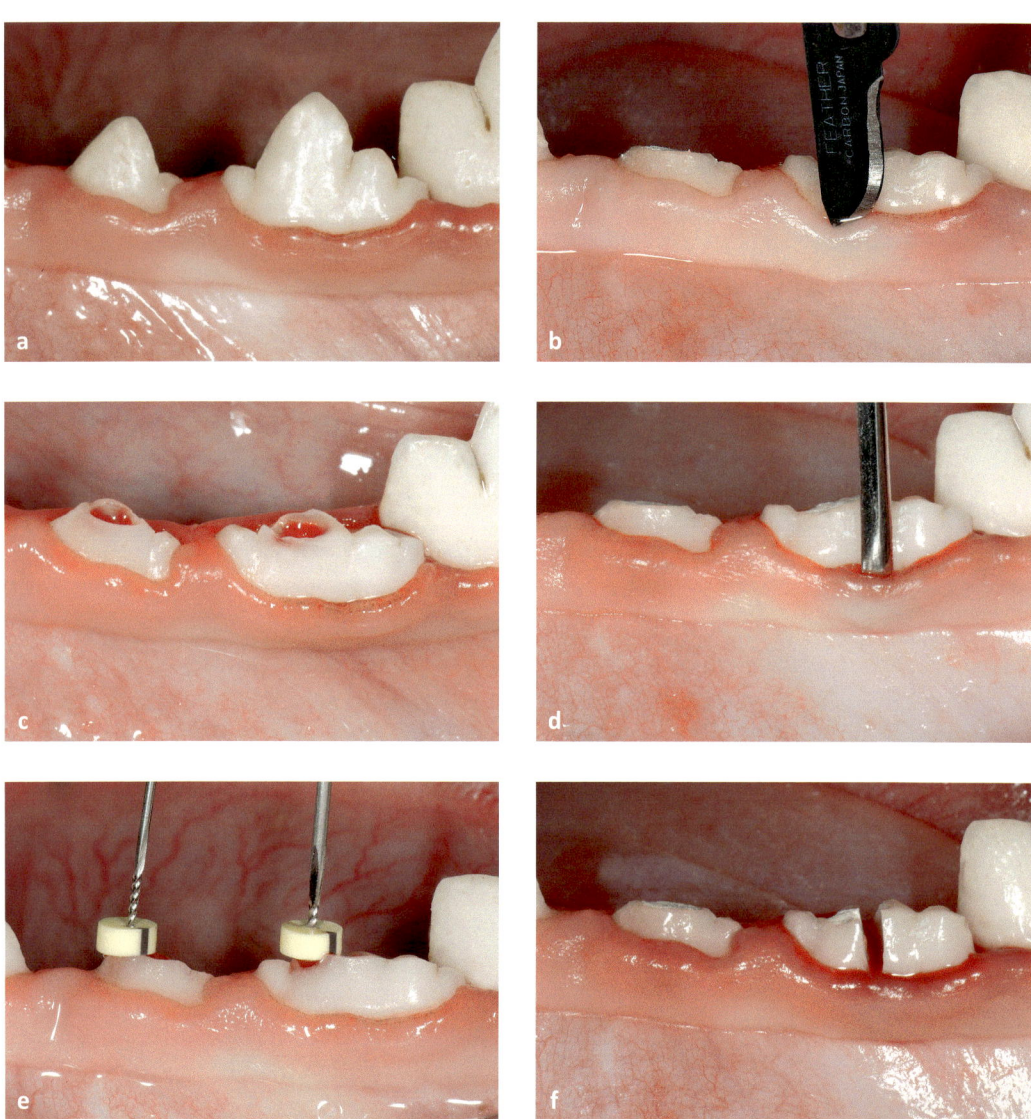

Fig 9-5 Clinical photographs illustrating various steps of the extraction and grafting of the fourth and third mandibular premolars (**a**). The crown is ground to the cervical third to expose the pulp chamber (**b**). The pulp is extirpated and the canals are instrumented with the use of endodontic files (**c**). Sulcus incision in the fourth mandibular premolar region (**d**). A periotome is use to elevate the buccal and lingual/palatal flap to the level of the bone crest (**e**). A cut is made between the mesial and distal roots of fourth mandibular premolar (**f**).

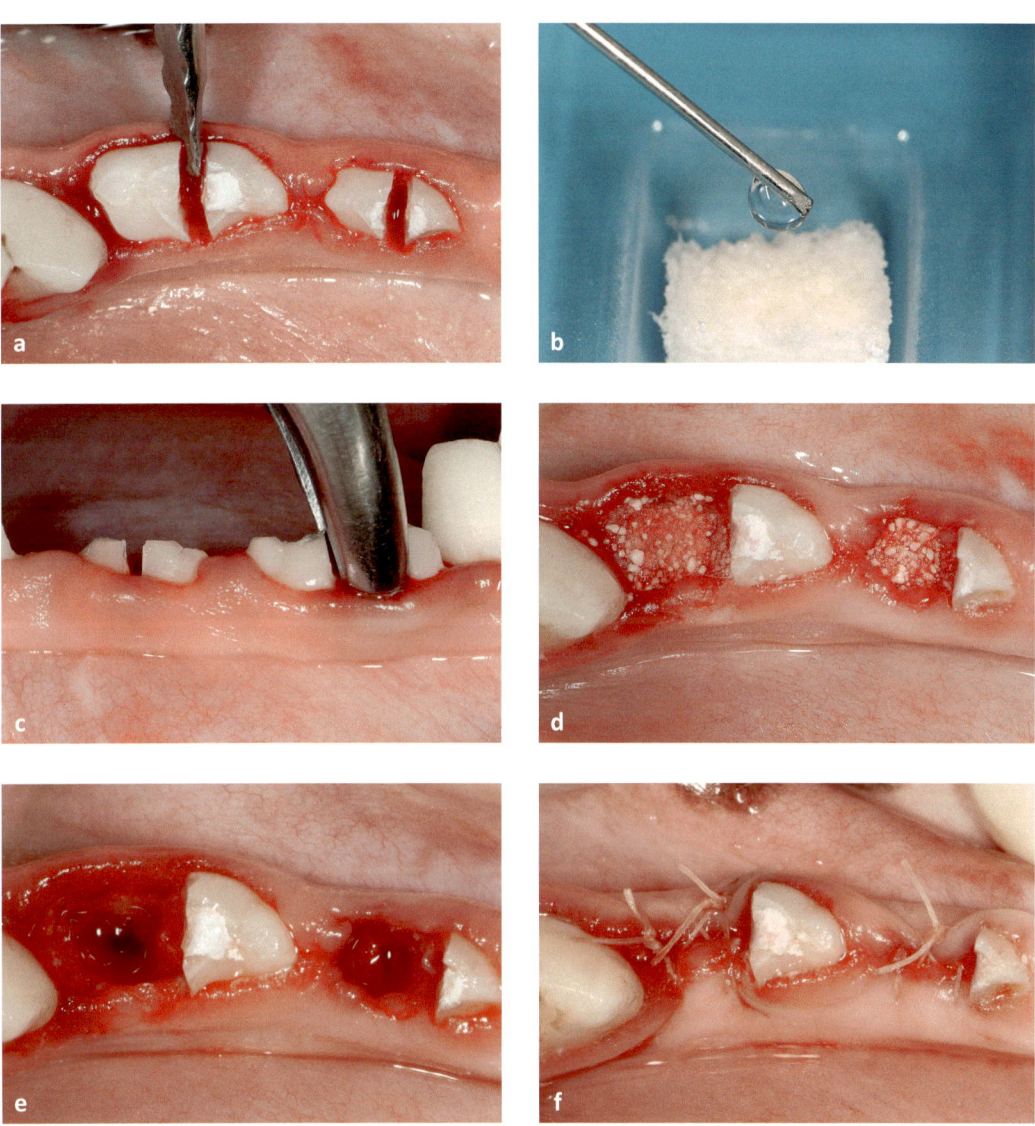

Fig 9-6 Clinical photographs illustrating various steps of the extraction and grafting of the fourth and third mandibular premolars. (**a**) A luxator is used to break and separate the mesial and distal roots of fourth mandibular premolar. The pulp chamber of the remaining mesial root is filled with composite. (**b**) The graft material is moisturized with saline. (**c**) The cementoenamel junction is grasped with the beaks of the forceps. (**d**) The socket of the distal root. (**e**) The graft material in place. (**f**) Sutured extraction sites.

(Fig 9-6e). Unless planned otherwise, the graft material should extend coronally to the level of the bone crest and primary wound closure is obtained as described previously (Fig 9-6f). If membranes, implants, or other products are used in the research project, the same basic care used for grafting should be followed.

9.2.5 Preparation

The dogs are selected for inclusion in the study after assessment of their general health, age, and weight. A certified veterinarian should examine the animals and be responsible for their systemic health during entire study. Animals that are approximately 1 year of age are preferable for the study because they are already adults but still young enough to allow uneventful tooth extraction. The weight depends on the surgical procedure planned; however, for easy maneuverability, it is reasonable to select animals that are 10 to 20 kg.

All teeth in the region to be included in the experimental surgical procedure should be cleaned and scaled 1 week before the procedure. For the procedure, the animal can be anesthetized with an intramuscular administration of ketamine hydrochloride (8 mg/kg) with xylazine (0.1 mg/kg). For the surgical procedure, the animal may be preanesthetized as described above and during surgery anesthesia may be maintained with intravenous administration of ketamine. The animals may also be anesthetized with the intravenous administration of propofol (3 mg/kg) combined with ketamine hydrochloride (2 mg/kg) and maintained with the inhaled anesthetic isoflurane. The advantages of the use of inhaled anesthetic are better control of the depth of anesthesia and quick postoperative recovery. The animals should receive lactated Ringer's solution during the entire procedure. Then careful decontamination of the mucosa and skin in the surgical area is carried out with chlorhexidine 0.12%, after which the experimental procedure may be initiated.

9.2.6 Detailed Methodology

The literature shows different materials being used to preserve the alveolar ridge after tooth extraction. Bone substitutes (Boix et al., 2006; Shi et al., 2007; Araújo et al., 2008; Fickl et al., 2008a, 2008b; Rothamel et al., 2008; Araújo and Lindhe, 2009a; Araújo et al., 2009; Fickl et al., 2009a, 2009b; Araújo et al., 2010a, 2010b), implants (Araújo et al., 2005, 2006a, 2006b), and buccal overbuilding with soft tissue grafts (Fickl et al., 2009a, 2009b) have been used to avoid or compensate for bone plate resorption during the healing process; the success rate varies according to the study. Independently of the material used, the methods to achieve the desirable outcomes are very similar.

As mentioned before, the dog is the main animal used in the ridge preservation studies. The dog species used include the Beagle (Araújo et al., 2005, 2006a, 2006b; Boix et al., 2006; Araújo et al., 2008; Fickl et al., 2008a, 2008b; Araújo et al., 2009; Araújo and Lindhe, 2009a; Fickl et al., 2009a, 2009b; Araújo et al., 2010a, 2010b), the foxhound (Rothamel et al., 2008), and mongrel dogs (Shi et al., 2007). Usually, five to seven dogs are enough for an experiment. Care should be taken not to include animals of different sizes and species in the same study. Foxhounds are usually larger than Beagles and mongrel dogs may present different sizes.

In ridge preservation procedures, many regions in the dog's mouth may be used for the experiment. The mandible is the most used arch and the third and fourth premolars (P3 and P4) the most preferred teeth (Araújo et al., 2005, 2006b; Fickl et al., 2008a, 2008b; Araújo et al., 2009; Fickl et al., 2009a, 2009b; Araújo et al., 2010a); but, the second premolar and first molars are also used (Araújo et al., 2006a; Rothamel et al., 2008) and the maxilla is a possible option (Boix et al., 2006; Araújo et al., 2010a, 2010b). Control sites are frequently used in the ridge preservation studies. Some studies use a pristine site as control. The best example of such a site is the alveolar ridge that contains the mesial root of the involved tooth (Araújo et al., 2005, 2008, 2009). This approach allows comparison with a fully preserved ridge. Comparison with a contralateral untreated fresh extraction socket is also possible, however, this allows only a relative assessment of the ridge preservation procedure. If the aim of the study is to describe the healing process that occurs under the influence of a particular treatment, comparison with an untreated or pristine site may not be necessary. On the other hand, in this type of study, evaluation at different time points is mandatory (Araújo et al., 2010a, 2010b).

Variations in the methods occur due to differences in aims of studies on ridge preservation. Some studies have intended to show the effect on osseous resorption of: a flap (Araújo and Lindhe, 2009b) or lack of periodontal ligament (Cardaropoli et al., 2005), the size of hard tissue walls of the socket (Araújo et al., 2006a) or buccal overbuilding (Fickl et al., 2009a, 2009b). Other studies have assessed the placement of a biomaterial (Boix et al., 2006; Shi et al., 2007; Araújo et al., 2008; Fickl et al., 2008b, 2009b; Rothamel et al., 2008; Araújo et al., 2010b) or an implant (Araújo et al., 2005, 2006b) in fresh extraction sockets to verify if it is able to avoid or compensate for alveolar plate resorption during healing or bone changes in the vertical and horizontal dimensions (Fickl et al., 2008a, 2009a). Furthermore, some studies have looked at the inflammatory reaction caused by these biomaterials (Araújo and Lindhe, 2009a; Araújo et al., 2009, 2010a).

If the objective of the study is to verify whether a procedure (i.e., kind of flap, absence of periodontal ligament, size of walls, alveolar overbuilding, use of biomaterials) can prevent or reduce alveolar bone resorption, the alveolar ridge wall dimensions have to be analyzed after, at least, 2 to 3 months. For the analysis of a long-term effect, 6 months of healing is mandatory (Araújo and Lindhe, 2009a). Moreover, it is necessary to use a method of analysis that can effectively measure the bone shrinkage, such as volumetric measurements of the alveolar bone walls.

In addition, if the study aims to verify the entire ridge shrinkage (soft and hard tissue), analysis of the vertical and horizontal alterations of ridge dimensions can be done using casts or computed tomography (CT) scans taken before and after treatment. For evaluation of inflammatory reactions caused by the placement of different graft materials in fresh alveolar sockets, histologic description and histomorphometric measurements have to be done early, i.e., 1 and 3 days, and 1, 2, and 4 weeks into healing. In summary, all the studies mentioned above were performed in the same way: tooth extraction included or followed by an experimental procedure and healing allowed for a variety of time intervals. The reasoning behind the experiment is always the same: the possibility to alter socket healing so as to preserve the ridge volume.

9.2.7 Postoperative Care

Antibiotics may be prescribed after ridge preservation procedures in the dog. A protocol including the administration via systemic route of 1 g/day of amoxicillin for 5 days is an option. The use of cephalosporin, penicillin, spiramycin, and ampicillin in different dosages and length of time has also been described in the literature. In some cases antibiotic therapy may be replaced successfully with a careful local mechanical plaque control regimen for the entire duration of the study (gentle site cleaning three times a week with the use of a toothbrush and dentifrice containing chlorhexidine 0.12%). For postoperative pain control, 2 mL (1 mL/10 kg) of sodium dipyrone 50% 2 to 3 times/day for 2 to 3 days can be used.

During the first 12 hours after the surgical procedure, the dog should rest in a peaceful and clean place with water *ad libitum*. After that period and during the following 2 weeks, a soft diet should be offered in quantities according to the size of the dog. Subsequently, the dog is fed with conventional dog food for the rest of the study.

9.2.8 Endpoint Measurements

There are different ways to evaluate a ridge preservation procedure in regard to its effect on the dimensional alterations of the alveolar ridge following tooth extraction as well as on the wound healing associated with such change. It is possible to analyze the height and width of the bone walls, the volume of the alveolar process and alveolar ridge, the soft tissue reaction, etc. Below, some of these measurements are described. Most of these measurements involve the preparation of undecalcified, decalcified or deparaffinized histologic sections; examinations are performed with a microscope equipped with an image system. In general, undecalcified ground sections can be used when histologic assessments of tissue are related to distances between landmarks or when tissue volume needs to be determined. Decalcified sections embedded in paraffin or epon are used when assessment of cell type is required (morphometry), i.e., volume occupied by erythrocytes, neutrophilic leukocytes, mesenchymal cells. Deparaffinized sections are used for the identification of specific cell or cell products by the use of chemical or immuno-histochemical reactions.

The height and width of the socket walls can be evaluated as described by Araújo and Lindhe (2005). On the captured image of a buccolingual section of a healing socket, the height of the cortical walls is determine by drawing a line parallel to the long axis of the root in the center of the socket (C-C) to separate the buccal and lingual compartments. Subsequently, horizontal lines perpendicular to C-C are drawn to connect the most coronal portions of the buccal and lingual bone crests to C-C. The vertical distance between the buccal and lingual intersections with C-C is measured and expressed in millimeters. Also the width of the buccal and lingual bone walls is determined and expressed in millimeters at three different levels, 1, 3, and 5 mm apical to the buccal and lingual bone crest (Fig 9-7). The method described by Araújo and Lindhe (2005) has become a standard and has been used in different studies on alveolar ridge preservation (Cardaropoli et al., 2005; Fickl et al., 2008b, 2009b; Rothamel et al., 2008), with few modifications. Boix et al. (2006), using scanning electron microscopy (SEM), drew a vector tangent to the buccal and lingual bone crests and determined the surface above this vector occupied by bone and biomaterials or the empty space below the vector.

The ridge alteration following extraction and implant placement may be evaluated using different landmarks on the implant and on the socket walls (Araújo et al., 2005, 2006a, 2006b). Therefore, the shoulder of the implant, the marginal border of the treated implant surface, the margin of bone-to-implant contact on the lingual and buccal sides, the margin of peri-implant mucosa and the apical cells of barrier epithelium are identified. The distance between these landmarks is measured to determine any difference in relation to the control site. It is also possible to determine the width of the buccal and lingual walls at different levels below the implant shoulder by measuring the distance between the outer surface of the bone and the implant surface (Fig 9-8).

The volume of the alveolar process can be determined in a histologic buccolingual section by dividing the alveolar process into three different portions (apical, middle, and coronal); the cross-sectional area occupied by each portion is measured with a cursor and expressed in square millimeters (Araújo et al., 2008; Araújo and Lindhe, 2009b). The relative alterations in the size of the alveolar process that occurred following tooth extraction are estimated by subtracting the value obtained at the extraction site from the corresponding value at a pristine site (Fig 9-9). Tomography scans and scintigraphy can also be used to evaluate the volume

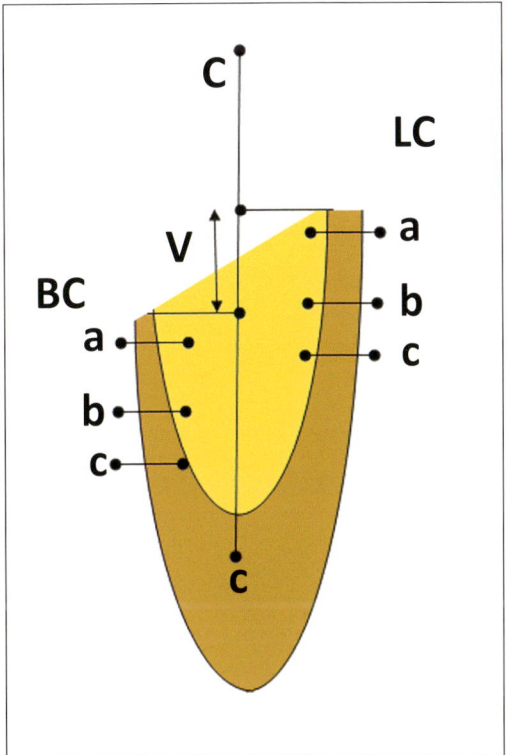

Fig 9-7 Schematic drawing illustrating the various landmarks used for histometric measurements; a = segment 1 mm; b = segment 3 mm; c = segment 5 mm apical to the buccal and lingual bone crest. BC, buccal crest of the tooth site; LC, lingual crest of the tooth site; C-C, long axis of the root; V, vertical distance between the buccal and lingual bone crests.

of the alveolar socket in different time intervals (Shi *et al.*, 2007).

If the aim of the study is to volumetrically assess alterations of the ridge contour (mucosa and bone volume), the methodology described by Fickl *et al.* (2008a, 2009a) may be used. Impressions of the jaws are taken before and after socket preservation surgery and master casts are made out of dental stone for each dog. The casts are optically scanned with a three-dimensional camera and the obtained digital images reflecting the different treatment time points are superimposed, and the images

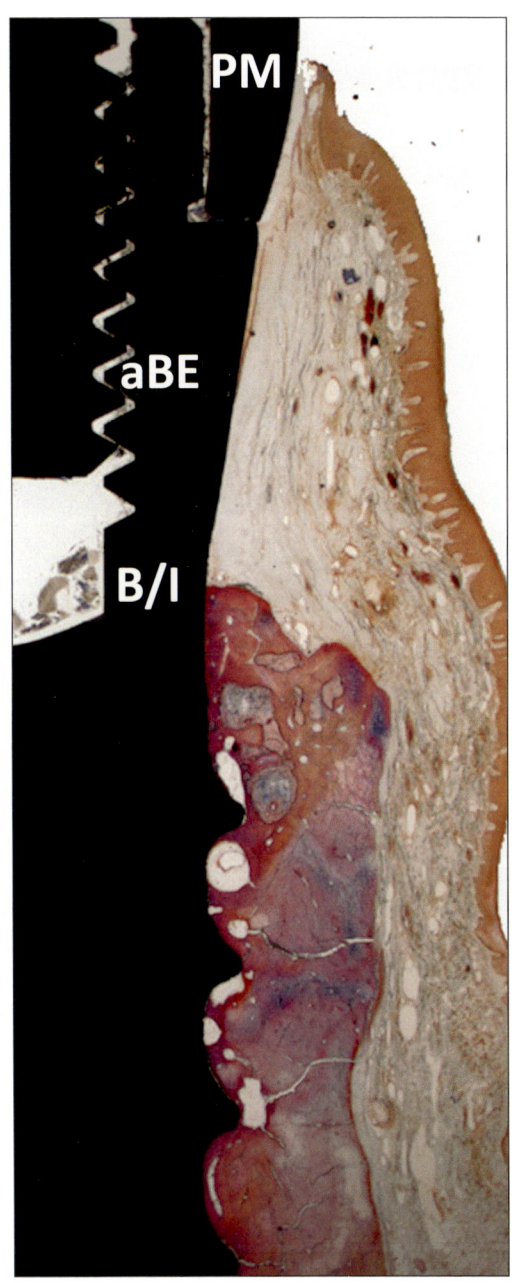

Fig 9-8 Buccolingual section describing different landmarks from which histometric measurements can be performed. aBE, apical portion of the barrier epithelium; B/I, marginal level of bone-to-implant contact; PM, peri-implant margin. Ladewig's fibrin staining; original magnification ×16.

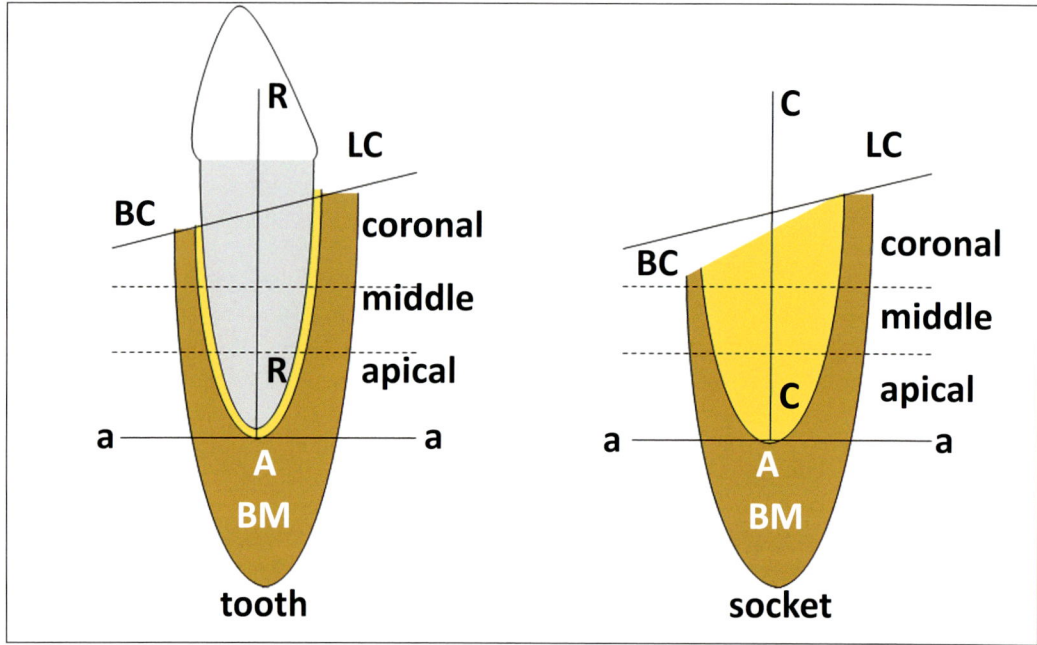

Fig 9-9 Schematic drawing (buccolingual view) illustrating the measurements made to determine the cross-sectional area of the apical, middle, and coronal thirds of the alveolar process. A, apex of the root; BC, buccal crest of the tooth site; LC, lingual crest of the tooth site; BM, base of mandible; a-a = line, perpendicular to R-R, that separates the alveolar process from the basal bone of the mandible.

matched in one common coordinate system. A defined area of interest is measured and the volume difference between the time points is calculated.

The relative volume occupied by different tissues as blood clot (mainly blood cells, network of fibrin), granulation tissue (highly vascularized tissue with an inflammatory cell infiltrate), provisional matrix (connective tissue including a multitude of mesenchymal cells embedded in a fibrous matrix), mineralized bone (woven bone, parallel fibered bone, and lamellar bone), bone marrow (intraosseous space mainly occupied by adipocytes), and graft materials in the alveolar socket can also be determined. For this aim, a point counting procedure on a lattice comprising 100 light points superimposed over the histologic image is used (Cardaropoli et al., 2003; Boix et al., 2006; Araújo et al., 2008, 2009; Araújo and Lindhe, 2009a).

This is a histologic technique based on a modification of the method described by Schroeder and Münzel-Pedrazzoli (1973). These measurements are frequently performed in locations representing the apical, middle, and coronal portions of the socket and buccolingual or mesiodistal sections may be used for this purpose.

Morphometric measurements of the relative volume occupied by mesenchymal cells, connective tissue fibers, vessels, mineralized bone, biomaterial granules, neutrophilic leukocytes, mononuclear leukocytes, and residual elements (e.g., erythrocytes, strands of fibrin, and undefined structures) can also be performed in decalcified paraffin embedded sections to evaluate the inflammatory reaction due to the presence of a biomaterial and the incorporation process of this biomaterial (Araújo et al., 2010a). Osteoclasts and osteoblasts may be identified, respectively, by their tartrate-resistant acid phosphatase (TRAP) and alkaline phosphatase activities. Furthermore, the expression of osteopontin during the socket healing process may be evaluated by immunohistochemical methods (Araújo et al., 2010b).

9.2.9 Statistical Analysis Plan

The correct indication of a statistical method is an important phase of the study preparation. Indeed, there are several statistical methods, each of them with a different characteristic. Below some basic guidelines for the use of statistical analyses are offered. For more detailed information, the reader is encouraged to refer to specific texts (Altman, 1990).

For statistical analysis, (i) mean values and standard deviation must be calculated for each animal, experimental group, and variable, (ii) the dog must be used as the statistical unit, and (iii) the level of significance established at 5% or 1%. Only descriptive analyses of the measurements can be done if there is great variability in data, the sample is too small or there is no need for group comparisons.

Before selecting the statistical test, some simple questions should be answered to guide the choice. First of all, you need to know how many groups will be compared. Will there be two groups or more? Second, the kind of data to be analyzed is important. Will the data be parametric (all values expressed in continuous measurements) or nonparametric (all data expressed as categorical)? Finally the relationship between groups must be identified. Will it be a dependent/paired (same group in different time point evaluation) or an independent/unpaired (comparison between different groups) relationship?

If two paired (dependent) groups are compared, differences for parametric data may be evaluated using paired t test and for nonparametric data, Wilcoxon and McNemar tests are possibilities. If two unpaired (independent) groups are compared, differences in parametric data may be evaluated using unpaired t test and for nonparametric data, the Mann-Whitney U test is the option.

For more than two paired (dependent) groups with parametric data, analysis may be performed using one-way analysis of variance (ANOVA), if data is nonparametric, the Friedman test is used. When more than two unpaired (independent) groups are involved and data is parametric, ANOVA is used, and for nonparametric data the choice is the Kruskal-Wallis test.

When three or more groups are compared, the results of the statistic test show only if there is a difference but do not show which groups are different from each other. Therefore, another statistical test must be applied, and this test is known as *post hoc analysis* and follows the same stages for its choice. For paired groups with parametric data, Fisher's test may be used for small samples, and for nonparametric data, the Friedman test can be used. For unpaired groups with parametric data, Tukey's test is usually used, and for nonparametric data, Kruskal-Wallis is the most common test.

9.2.10 Material, Consumables, Equipment

The instruments, materials and equipment necessary for ridge preservation experiments may be divided into surgical and laboratory. The former are common to any experiment that needs to produce histologic sections for tissue examination and will not be included in this text. The most important materials and instruments for the surgical part of the experiment are described below in the sequence that they should be used. A vast variety of surgical instruments and materials of different brands are available in terms of quality and cost. Personal choice has a role in selection of instruments and materials but this choice should not compromise the final results of the surgery. As in human surgery, the instruments should be kept in good shape and always used after proper sterilization.

Instruments
- Endodontic treatment, if needed: diamond burs, files and endodontic condensers.
- Soft tissue incision: 15 or 15C blades and handles.
- Root hemisection: carbide fissure burs.
- Soft tissue elevation: Freer elevator or similar.
- Tooth removal: luxators of different widths and forceps for roots.
- Insertion of grafts in the socket: socket curettes and condensers.
- Suture: Castro Viejo needle-holder and scissors.

Materials and Equipment
- Anesthesia and other medication: See Sections 9.2.5 and 9.2.7.
- Endodontic treatment: paper point, gutta-percha, and endodontic cement.
- Tested material.
- Suture: silk, Vicryl or polyfluorotetraethylene (PTFE) sutures 4-0 or 5-0.
- Surgical attire.
- For postoperative care: toothbrush and dentifrices.
- For pre- and postoperative care: ultrasonic device and tips.
- Anesthetic equipment for the use of inhaled anesthetic.

9.3 Rat and Minipig Models

The use of noncanine models for the study of ridge preservation procedures is very limited (Table 9-2). Here such models are briefly described. In the rat model, maxillary and mandibular molars have been used as experimental sites to evaluate, for example, the socket graft with hydroxyapatite-collagen implants (Hahn et al., 1988) and recombinant human bone morphogenetic protein-2 (Matin et al., 2001). The evaluation of the effect of ridge preservation procedures in the rat model can be done in terms of alveolar socket dimensions or tissue composition during healing as described for dogs (Hahn et al., 1988; Matin et al., 2001; Aguirre et al., 2010; Jee et al., 2010). There is only one paper on ridge preservation using the minipig model (Oltramari et al., 2007). In this study, a combination of bovine bone, collagen, bovine bone morphogenetic protein (bBMP), and hydroxyapatite was used as filler material in a ridge preservation procedure. The first permanent molar in the maxilla was used as the experimental site. Radiographic measurements were used to evaluate dimensional changes in the socket.

References

1. Aguirre JI, Altman MK, Vanegas SM, Franz SE, Bassit AC, Wronski TJ (2010). Effects of alendronate on bone healing after tooth extraction in rats. *Oral Dis* 16:674–685.
2. Altman DG (1990). Practical statistics for medical research. 1st ed. New York: Chapman & Hall/CRC.
3. Araújo MG, Lindhe J (2005). Dimensional ridge alterations following tooth extraction. An experimental study in the dog. *J Clin Periodontol* 32:212–218.
4. Araújo MG, Lindhe J (2009a). Ridge preservation with the use of bio-oss collagen: a 6-month study in the dog. *Clin Oral Implants Res* 20:433–440.
5. Araújo MG, Lindhe J (2009b). Ridge alterations following tooth extraction with and without flap elevation: and experimental study in the dog. *Clin Oral Implants Res* 20:545–549.
6. Araújo MG, Sukekava F, Wennström JL, Lindhe J (2005). Ridge alterations following implant placement in fresh extraction sockets: an experimental study in the dog. *J Clin Periodontol* 32:645–652.
7. Araújo MG, Wennström JL, Lindhe J (2006a). Modeling of the buccal and lingual bone walls of fresh extraction sites following implant installation. *Clin Oral Implants Res* 17:606–614.
8. Araújo MG, Sukekava F, Wennström JL, Lindhe J (2006b). Tissue modeling following implant placement in fresh extraction sockets. *Clin Oral Implants Res* 17:615–624.
9. Araújo M, Linder E, Wennström J, Lindhe J (2008). The influence of bio-oss collagen on healing of an extraction socket: an experimental study in the dog. *Int J Periodontics Restorative Dent* 28:123–135.
10. Araújo M, Linder E, Lindhe J (2009). Effect of a xenograft on early bone formation in extraction sockets: an experimental study in dog. *Clin Oral Implants Res* 20:1–6.
11. Araújo MG, Liljenberg B, Lindhe J (2010a). Dynamics of bio-oss collagen incorporation in fresh extraction wounds: an experimental study in the dog. *Clin Oral Implants Res* 21:55–64.

References

12. Araújo MG, Liljenberg B, Lindhe J (2010b). Beta-tricalcium phosphate in the early phase of socket healing: an experimental study in the dog. *Clin Oral Implants Res* 21:445–454.
13. Boix D, Weiss P, Gauthier O, Guicheux J, Bouler JM, Pilet P et al. (2006). Injectable bone substitute to preserve alveolar ridge resorption after tooth extraction: a study in dog. *J Mater Sci Mater Med* 17:1145–1152.
14. Cardaropoli G, Araújo M, Lindhe J (2003). Dynamics of bone tissue formation in tooth extraction sites. An experimental study in dogs. *J Clin Periodontol* 30:809–818.
15. Cardaropoli G, Araújo M, Hayacibara R, Sukekava F, Lindhe J (2005). Healing of extraction sockets and surgically produced – augmented and non-augmented – defects in the alveolar ridge. An experimental study in the dog. *J Clin Periodontol* 32:435–440.
16. Fickl S, Zuhr O, Wachtel H, Stappert CFJ, Stein JM, Hürzeler MB (2008a). Dimensional changes of the alveolar ridge contour after different socket preservation techniques. *J Clin Periodontol* 35:906–913.
17. Fickl S, Zuhr O, Wachtel H, Bolz W, Hürzeler MB (2008b). Hard tissue alterations after socket preservation: an experimental study in the beagle dog. *Clin Oral Implants Res* 19:1111–1118.
18. Fickl S, Schneider D, Zuhr O, Hinze M, Ender A, Jung RE et al. (2009a). Dimensional changes of the ridge contour after socket preservation and buccal overbuilding: an animal study. *J Clin Periodontol* 36:442–448.
19. Fickl S, Zuhr O, Wachtel H, Kebschull M, Hürzeler MB (2009b). Hard tissue alterations after socket preservation with additional buccal overbuilding: a study in the beagle dog. *J Clin Periodontol* 36:898–904.
20. Hahn E, Sonis S, Gallagher G, Atwood D (1988). Preservation of the alveolar ridge with hydroxyapatite-collagen implants in rats. *J Prosthet Dent* 60:729–734.
21. Jee JH, Lee W, Lee BD (2010). The influence of alendronate on the healing of extraction sockets of ovariectomized rats assessed by in vivo micro-computed tomography. *Oral Surg Oral Med Oral Pathol Oral Radiol Endod* 110:e44–e50.
22. Matin K, Nakamura H, Irie K, Ozawa H, Ejiri S (2001). Impact of recombinant human bone morphogenetic protein-2 on residual ridge resorption after tooth extraction: an experimental study in the rat. *Int J Oral Maxillofac Implants* 16:400–411.
23. National Research Council (1980). Committee on animal models for research on aging. Mammalian models for research on aging. 1st ed. Washington, DC: National Academy Press.
24. Oltramari PV, Navarro RdeL, Henriques JF, Taga R, Cestari TM, Janson G et al. (2007). Evaluation of bone height and bone density after tooth extraction: an experimental study in minipigs. *Oral Surg Oral Med Oral Pathol Oral Radiol Endod* 104:e9–e16.
25. Rothamel D, Schwarz F, Herten M, Engelhardt E, Donath K, Kuehn P et al. (2008). Dimensional ridge alterations following socket preservation using a nanocrystalline hydroxyapatite paste. A histomorphometrical study in dogs. *Int J Oral Maxillofac Surg* 37:741–747.
26. Schroeder HE, Münzel-Pedrazzoli S (1973). Correlated morphometric and biochemical analysis of gingival tissue. Morphometric model, tissue sampling and test of stereologic procedures. *J Microsc* 99:301–329.
27. Shi B, Zhou Y, Wang YN, Cheng XR (2007). Alveolar ridge preservation prior to implant placement with surgical-grade calcium sulfate and platelet-rich plasma: a pilot study in canine model. *Int J Oral Maxillofac Implants* 22:656–665.
28. Trombelli L, Farina R, Marzola A, Bozzi L, Liljenberg B, Lindhe J (2008). Modeling and remodeling of human extraction sockets. *J Clin Periodontol* 35:630–639.

CHAPTER 10

Horizontal Ridge Augmentation

Michael M. Bornstein, Dieter D. Bosshardt, Thomas von Arx, and Daniel Buser

10.1 General Overview

10.1.1 Background

Clinical or experimental studies analyzing outcomes of horizontal (lateral) ridge augmentation can be divided into two categories: first, studies on the surgical augmentation procedure itself, in which the principal outcome parameter is the possibility to place a dental implant in an ideal position for prosthodontic rehabilitation without the need for additional grafting; and studies evaluating implant survival or success in horizontally augmented alveolar ridges according to predefined criteria. Techniques for horizontal ridge augmentation can be divided according to the type of grafting material used to augment or cover the surgical site (block or particulate/autogenous versus bone-substitute material/combinations of grafting material) or the type of membrane (resorbable or nonresorbable/natural versus synthetic material). A recent systematic review of the literature including only those studies with at least 10 or more patients and a minimum follow-up period of 12 months after loading of the inserted implants analyzed the outcomes of bone augmentation procedures in localized defects in the alveolar ridge (Jensen and Terheyden, 2009). The authors concluded that the most predictable horizontal ridge augmentation procedure included an autogenous block graft alone or in combination with a particulate bone graft or bone-substitute material, with or without the concomitant use of a resorbable membrane. In another recent systematic review applying similar inclusion criteria, the authors evaluated clinical outcomes of guided bone regeneration (GBR) procedures to correct dehiscence or fenestration type defects associated with implant placement (Chiapasco and Zaniboni, 2009). The authors found that it was difficult to draw significant conclusions with regard to any grafting material or membrane barrier for the treatment of

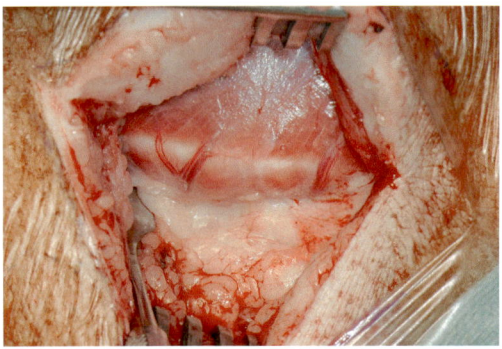 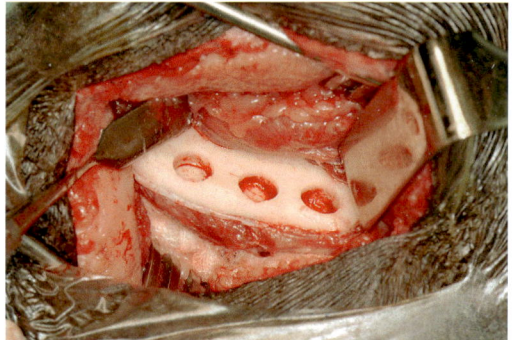

Fig 10-1 Through a subangular incision, the lateral portion of the mandibular body and ramus has been exposed to evaluate different grafting materials using minipigs.

Fig 10-2 Three standardized intraosseous defects (9 mm in diameter/4 mm in depth) prepared at the area of the mandibular angle using a trephine and copious saline irrigation.

dehiscence/fenestration defects. Problems encountered were the limited sample sizes, the wide variety of grafting materials and membranes applied, either alone or in combination, and a paucity of randomized clinical trials.

10.1.2 Animal Models

Regarding the limited knowledge of GBR procedures and outcomes as derived from human clinical trials, the use of appropriate animal models for translational research in bone tissue engineering and regenerative medicine appears crucial. When choosing a species of animal for a particular study model or a specific research question, several factors should be considered, including: costs of acquiring and caring for the animals, ease of housing and availability, acceptability to society, biologic characteristics analogous to humans, and tolerance to surgery. Further, the lifespan of the species chosen should be suitable for the duration of the study, and the size of the animal must be appropriate for the surgical technique to be evaluated (Schimandle and Boden, 1994). In addition, regarding the research field of *horizontal ridge augmentation*, there are specific clinically related issues that further guide the decision making for an appropriate animal model (von Arx et al., 2001a), including: surgical access to the area of augmentation (extraoral versus intraoral), type and size of bone defect (acute versus chronic, contained or transosseous), and defect localization (extraoral bone versus jawbone; ramus versus alveolar ridge). Taking into consideration all these factors, it is evident that within a specific field of research, no single animal model will be appropriate to study all purposes (Hazzard et al., 1992).

In general, preclinical translational testing is ideally performed in large and skeletally mature animals, rather than in rodents or rabbits. Mimicking the underlying bone biology of the human is one of the principal goals of selecting a given animal (Schimandle and Boden, 1994; Liebschner, 2004; Egermann et al., 2005). In rodents, the trabecular bone compartment is limited, even in metaphysic or long bones, and their skeleton continues to remodel throughout their lives at a faster rate than in humans. These are significant disadvantages when considering rodents as appropriate models of human bone biology. The dog, goat, sheep, and pig are the most utilized species when studying bone repair or bone regeneration (O'Loughlin et al., 2008). Although nonhuman primates (NHPs) such as Rhesus macaque (Hanisch et al., 2003) or baboons (Busenlechner et al., 2005; Miranda et al., 2005) have been used in experiments

Table 10-1 Overview of characteristics and key features of different animal species used for experimental research in the field of horizontal ridge augmentation

	Rat	Rabbit	Sheep	Pig	NHP	Dog
Different types (most common)	Norway rat (*Rattus norvegicus*), black rat (*Rattus rattus*), and albino strains	Californian, Florida White, and New Zealand White	Domestic sheep (*Ovis aries*)	Domestic pig (*Sus scrofa*)	Rhesus macaque (*Macaca mulatta*), baboon (*Papio anubis*)	Beagle, coonhound, mongrel
Adult weight	70–300 g	1.5–2.5 kg	>100 kg	50–350 kg	5–20 kg	<10 kg–>30 kg
Lifespan	4 years	9 years	10–12 years	10 years	20–40 years	15 years
Skeletal maturity	Continuous growth	1 year	1.5 years	1–1.5 years	5–7 years	1–1.5 years
Suitability/ applicability/ commonness	++	+	+	++	++	+++

+ = least suitable/common; ++ = moderately suitable/common; +++ = most suitable/common.
NHP, nonhuman primate.
Source: Pearce et al. (2007); Muschler et al. (2010).

analyzing the outcome of horizontal augmentation procedures of alveolar bone, the use of NHPs adds substantially to the cost of research and is associated with some cultural and ethical concerns (Muschler et al., 2010).

The dog is one of the more frequently used large animal species in orthopedic and dental research (Pearce et al., 2007). However, there are increasing ethical issues related to the use of dogs in medical research as well due to their status as companion animals. Sheep and goats have been used more frequently for orthopedic research in the last two decades, but for goats this was mostly limited to studies on cartilage, meniscal, and ligamentous repair (Pearce et al., 2007). Like sheep, goats are considered food-producing animals and thus also have the advantage of less critical public perception when used for research than companion animals such as dogs. Pigs are reported as the subject of choice for a variety of research topics including studies of fractures on cartilage and bone (Pearce et al., 2007) and studies assessing new dental implant surfaces (Buser et al., 1991, 2004) or bone grafting materials (Fig 10-1 and Fig 10-2; Buser et al., 1998; Jensen et al., 2006, 2009). Table 10-1 gives an overview of the animal species used for GBR research in the dental field.

Regarding the specific topic of lateral/horizontal ridge augmentation using different bone fillers with or without barrier membrane application and with or without simultaneous or staged implant insertion, different animal species have been utilized including rats (Kostopoulos and Karring, 1994; Donos et al., 2002), monkeys (Fonseca et al., 1983), sheep (Ylinen et al., 1991), and pigs (Buser et al., 1999; Mai et al., 2008; Bornstein et al., 2009). Some of these animal models do not represent the typical clinical situation encountered in patients with chronic and sometimes large bone defects on the buccal aspect of the alveolar ridge. Furthermore, there is a lack of literature reporting on failures or problems of specific experimental approaches evaluating horizontal ridge augmentation. One of the few studies to do so was published by Olsen and co-workers (2004), in which the authors reported complete failure of their experimental setup comparing block and particulated bone grafts for ridge augmentation in combination with immediate implant placement using an intraoral approach in minipigs.

In Olsen's study, standardized bone defects (10 mm × 10 mm × 30 mm) were prepared on each side of the mandible of eight minipigs. After a healing period of 3 months, the defects in four animals were augmented with iliac crest grafts as a block or particulated graft with simultaneous implant insertion. Clinical inspection was performed after 2 weeks, and complete exposure of grafts and implants was discovered. The surgical procedures were altered in the fifth animal, avoiding incision in the insertion area of the musculus depressor labii mandibularis and placing the graft closer to the first molar. But again, grafts and implants were exposed. Consequently, the study was discontinued and all eight animals were sacrificed. The authors mention that the reasons for exposure of grafts and implants could be due to inappropriate handling of the animals in the stable and/or problems with the surgical techniques causing decreased blood supply in the surgical site. The authors concluded that an intraoral surgical design as described above cannot be recommended.

Therefore, the following sections of this chapter will focus on the most widely used and best established animal species for GBR procedures, and especially horizontal ridge augmentation, in dental research, the dog. Treatment modalities for the canine model include acute (Schwarz et al., 2007) and chronic (von Arx et al., 2001b, 2002) types of defects with varying sizes and configurations, different bone fillers (autografts, allografts, xenografts, alloplasts, and combinations), and different membranes to cover the augmented sites (bioabsorbable versus nonresorbable) (Schwarz et al., 2008a).

10.2 The Canine Model for Experimental Research in the Field of Horizontal Ridge Augmentation

10.2.1 Aim of the Canine Model

The animal species chosen for an experimental study addressing a specific clinical question should ideally fulfill the following prerequisites:

- Performance of therapy in a way it will most probably be carried out in the clinical setting
- Choice of a location for therapy/surgery that will as closely as possibly match the location in a patient
- Use of clinical methods that are similar/identical to those in the clinic
- Use of an animal that is comparable with humans regarding metabolic and physiologic characteristics
- Use of materials (grafts/membranes/transplants, etc.) that are similar/identical to the future clinical products.

There is substantial literature demonstrating that the canine model is one of the preferred animals for research of bone regeneration regarding the rich background of experience, ease of housing, and accessibility (Muschler et al., 2010). Therefore, this chapter will focus on the canine model in a step-by-step description of the surgery to histomorphometric methods most often applied in the laboratory.

The different outcome parameters evaluated in experimental studies analyzing horizontal ridge augmentation procedures have already been mentioned in the first paragraph of Section 10.1.1: namely, studies in which the principal outcome parameter is the possibility to place a dental implant in an ideal position without the need for additional grafting; and studies that evaluate implant survival or success in horizontally augmented alveolar ridges. Furthermore, the different techniques for horizontal ridge augmentation can be

10.2 The Canine Model for Experimental Research in the Field of Horizontal Ridge Augmentation

Table 10-2 Potential variables for experimental studies evaluating horizontal ridge augmentation

Characteristics of the dog	Type of defect	Type of filler material	Type of barrier membrane	Implant insertion
Beagle dog (small) or mongrel dog (large)	Chronic type of horizontal ridge defect: Defect has to be prepared during extraction of teeth (initial surgery)	Negative control: no filler applied, represents physiologic regeneration/repair process	Negative control: no barrier membrane applied, represents physiologic regeneration/repair process	Outcome 1: Surgical augmentation procedure itself, in which the principal outcome parameter is the possibility to place a dental implant in an ideal position for prosthodontic rehabilitation
		Positive control: Usually autogenous bone in particulate or block form		
	Acute type of horizontal ridge defect: Defect is prepared during second stage surgery, e.g., simultaneously with augmentation procedure	Test sites: any modification of the situation mentioned above (allograft/xenograft/alloplast combinations in block or particulate form)	Positive control: Usually an ePTFE membrane	
			Test sites: Any modification of the situation mentioned above (non-resorbable/resorbable/combinations)	Outcome 2: Studies that evaluate implant survival or success according to predefined criteria in horizontally augmented alveolar ridges → dental implant placed during second stage surgery
Age: around 1 year				
Easy handling and manageability				
Intraoral approach				
Mandible > maxilla				
Extraction of teeth before horizontal ridge augmentation				
Macro- and microstructure of bone, and bone remodeling moderately similar to humans				
Bone composition most similar				

divided according to the grafting material used to augment or cover the surgical site (block or particulate/autogenous versus bone-substitute material/combinations of grafting materials) or the type of membrane (resorbable or nonresorbable/natural versus synthetic material).

Table 10-2 summarizes potential variables regarding the choice of dog species, the type of defect, type of filler material, and type of barrier membrane used for experimental horizontal ridge augmentation.

10.2.2 Advantages and Disadvantages of the Dog Model

The dog is one of the most frequently used large animal species for musculoskeletal and dental research. Regarding the macrostructure of bone, there may be some discrepancy in size and shape of canine bone in comparison with human bone, depending on the size and breed of the dog. This is an important aspect, as there is a wide variation between different dog species, and care should be taken when comparing the outcome of experimental procedures performed in animals that are physically different, as with large mongrel and small Beagle dogs. It is also interesting to note that despite similarities in organic composition, canine bone has a significantly higher mineral density than human bone (Wang et al., 1998). In terms of bone density, the dog and the pig most closely represent the human situation (Aerssens et al., 1998). In addition, it must be acknowledged that the remodeling process in dogs is much quicker than in humans, by approximately three to five times (Pearce et al., 2007; Reinwald and Burr, 2008). Consequently, even if two defects of the alveolar process regenerated with horizontal ridge augmentation procedures, one in a dog and the other in a human, exhibit the same size, the regeneration process as a whole will take longer for humans. Therefore, the regeneration process after horizontal ridge augmentation is similar in dogs and humans, but the time interval in which it takes place is different. On the other hand, the faster wound healing process in the dog model allows completion of experimental studies in a shorter time period than would be possible when performing a similar study with humans.

10.2.3 Timing of an Experimental Study Evaluating Horizontal Ridge Augmentation

Experimental studies evaluating horizontal ridge augmentation can be subdivided into four phases (Fig 10-3):

1. Planning phase – writing of the protocol, briefing of the coinvestigators including the veterinarian, submission of study plan to the local animal ethical committee for approval, inspection of the animal research facilities, and writing applications to various institutions and foundations for funding the study, if needed.
2. Surgical phase – extraction of teeth in the canine model described above, defect creation with/without simultaneous implant placement, augmentative procedures, healing phase, and sacrifice.
3. Histologic processing phase – for light microscopy, scanning electron microscopy (SEM), back-scattered SEM (BSEM), and transmission electron microscopy (TEM), descriptive morphology, histochemical and immunohistochemical methods, and histomorphometry with/without the help of specialized software.
4. Statistical analysis and manuscript draft preparation phase – depending on the number of animals included in the study, on the healing phases analyzed, and on the histologic techniques applied, the timeframe for an experimental study from the initial planning stages to the finalized manuscript may range from less than 1 to several years.

10.2.4 Surgical Procedures: General Thoughts

Experimental studies should only be initiated after approval has been granted by the responsible animal ethical committee. Writing a protocol for the committee should not only be regarded as a necessary bureaucratic step before beginning the study, but as a chance to critically assess the methods and outcome parameters chosen. Furthermore, this preparation period allows the scientist to talk to the veterinarian in charge about the study to choose adequate medication, diet, and follow-up visits, to inspect the housing facilities of the animals, and to check that after sacrifice, the necessary steps for the histologic processing

10.2 The Canine Model for Experimental Research in the Field of Horizontal Ridge Augmentation

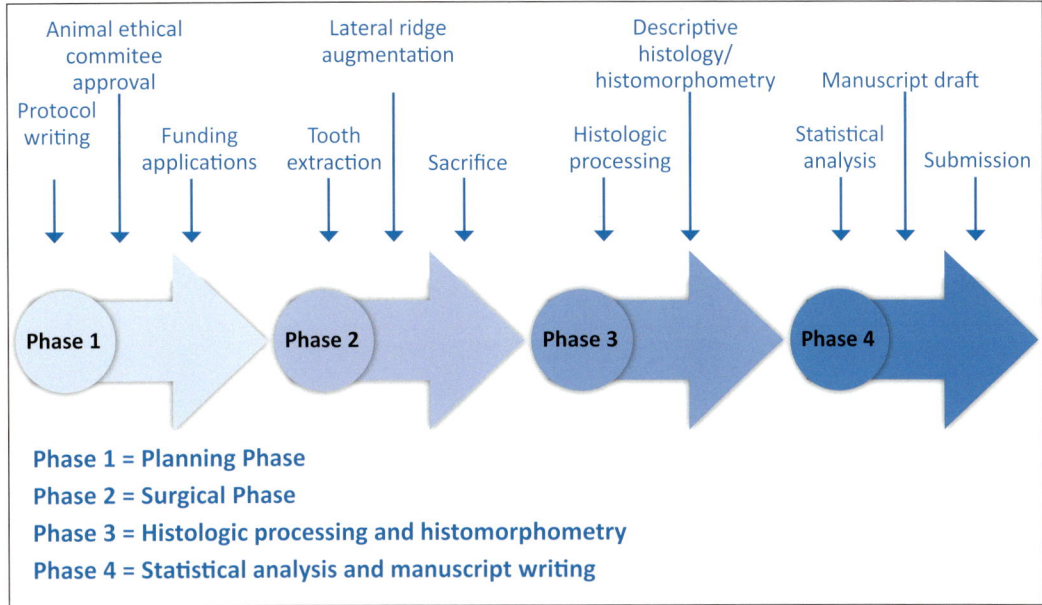

Fig 10-3 The four phases of an experimental project evaluating lateral/horizontal ridge augmentation in the canine model.

and analysis are clear to all involved investigators. Usually, all surgeries are performed under general anesthesia in an operating room under aseptic conditions. For horizontal ridge augmentation procedures in the dog model, usually two surgical procedures are necessary: (1) extraction of teeth (generally all premolars, and the first mandibular molar); and (2) horizontal ridge augmentation using one of the approaches specified in Table 10-2.

10.2.5 Preparation of the Animals

Dogs to be included in the study are selected in accordance to their general health, age, and weight. A certified veterinarian should examine the animals, and be responsible for their systemic health during the entire study. Animals that are approximately 1 year of age are preferred.

A typical setup for general anesthesia of a Beagle dog would be as follows (Bornstein et al., 2007): after intramuscular injection of atropine (0.05 mg/kg), anesthesia is induced by intramuscular administration of tiletamine-zolazepam (5 to 10 mg/kg), followed by a slow intravenous administration of sodium thiopental (10 to 15 mg/kg). Anesthesia is maintained with inhalation of an O_2/N_2O isoflurane (0.5% to 4%) mixture. Additionally, local anesthesia is achieved by buccal and lingual infiltration with 2% lidocaine combined with 1/100,000 epinephrine (adrenaline).

10.2.6 Detailed Surgical Methodology Including Sacrifice

Surgery 1 (tooth extraction)
This step prepares the alveolar crest for the experimental setup to be tested by removing the teeth in the area of interest. In general, sulcular incisions are made, with subsequent reflection of full mucoperiosteal flaps in the mandible from the canine to the second molar for better access and visualization of the teeth (Fig 10-4a). All premolars (PM1–PM4) and the first molar (M1) are then removed (Fig 10-4b). Prior to removal, all two-rooted teeth are sec-

Osteology Guidelines for Oral and Maxillofacial Regeneration

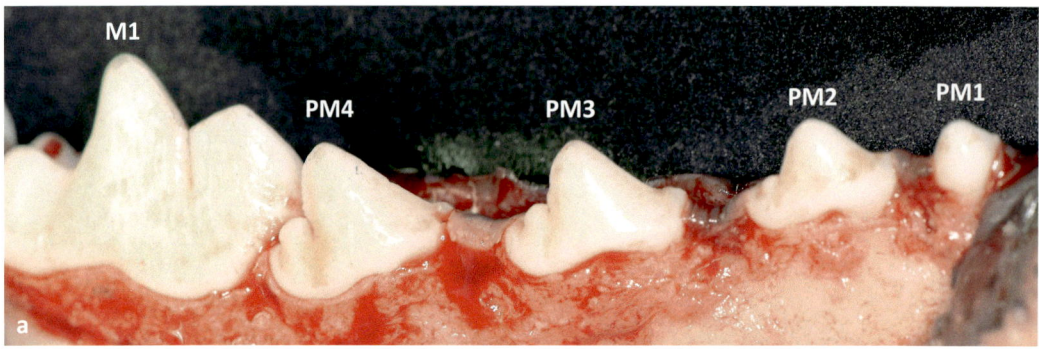

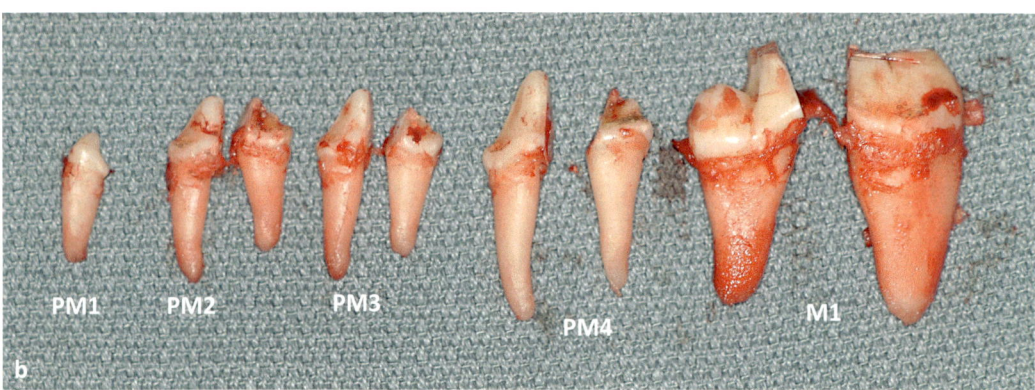

Fig 10-4 (**a**) Right mandible of a mongrel dog after preparation of lingual and buccal mucoperiosteal flaps from the first premolar (PM1) to the first molar (M1). Thus, access for extraction of the premolars (PM1 to PM4) and the first molar (M1) is simplified. (**b**) The extraction of the premolars (PM1 to PM4) and first molar (M1) should be done with great care not to fracture any root tips. Therefore, the two-rooted teeth (PM2, PM3, PM4, and M1) are sectioned using a separating disk before root extraction.

tioned with a separating disk, to ease root extraction. All drilling should be done under sterile saline irrigation. Finally, the flaps are closely approximated with interrupted sutures. Suture removal is generally done 1 to 2 weeks postoperatively. As modifications to this study design, defects of the alveolar ridge, ideally buccal defects, can be created at this stage (Figs 10-5a and 10-5b). This is always indicated when a chronic-type of defect is indicated for the study (von Arx et al., 2001a,b; Araújo et al., 2003; Schwarz et al., 2008b, 2009).

Surgery 2 (lateral/horizontal ridge augmentation)
Generally, the alveolar crests and/or defect sites are re-entered for lateral ridge augmentation 2 to 3 months after the first surgery (von Arx et al., 2001a,b, 2002; Araújo et al., 2003; Bornstein et al., 2007; Schwarz et al., 2008b, 2009). For the second intervention, midcrestal incisions are made from the canines to the second molars in the mandible, and full-thickness mucoperiosteal flaps are elevated on the buccal and lingual sides. As a variation of this procedure, especially if only two different time points will be evaluated, defects could be prepared only on one mandibular side for a specific time point (Bornstein et al., 2007). Using this

10.2 The Canine Model for Experimental Research in the Field of Horizontal Ridge Augmentation

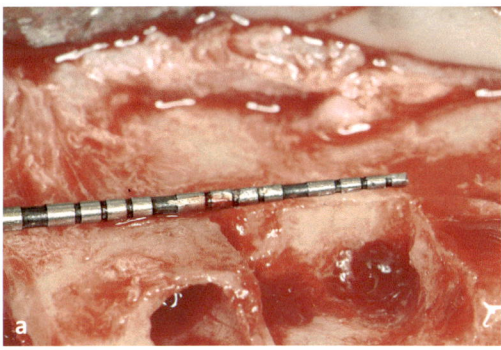
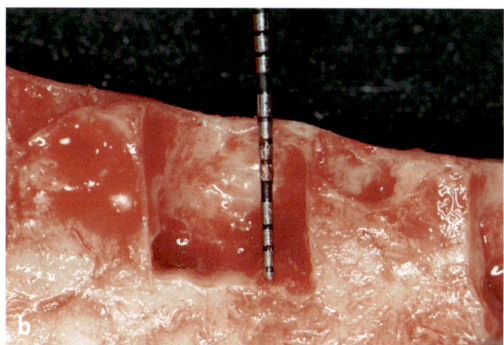

Fig 10-5 (a) After removal of the premolars and first molar in the right mandible of mongrel dogs, standardized defects on the buccal bone wall are created. For this experimental set-up, the mesiodistal width measures 9 mm (same canine mandible as in Fig 10-4a). (b) In the same canine mandible as in Fig 10-4a, the height from the crestal bone to the bottom of the defect measures 9 mm.

approach, each canine mandible comprises two different time points, and thus minimizes potential confounders (time or animal related). Nevertheless, randomization should be planned as regards location and different treatment options to be evaluated, when performing horizontal ridge augmentation procedures. If defects were not created during surgery 1 (= chronic-type defect), they are made at this stage in the edentulous alveolar mandibular area using rotary and hand instruments and chilled sterile saline irrigation (= acute-type defect). After defect creation in the alveolar ridge, horizontal ridge augmentation itself is performed. Many different variables exist for this procedure, ranging from autogenous bone blocks with varying sizes and configurations, particulate autografts, allografts, xenografts, alloplasts, and combinations thereof. Furthermore the defects can be covered without or with different membranes ranging from bioabsorbable to nonresorbable, and from collagen to synthetic polymers (Schwarz et al., 2008a; Fig 10-6). As a rule, the defects and augmented sites should ideally be measured with a periodontal probe. A further modification of this approach includes the simultaneous placement of dental implants, and the coverage/horizontal augmentation of any dehiscence

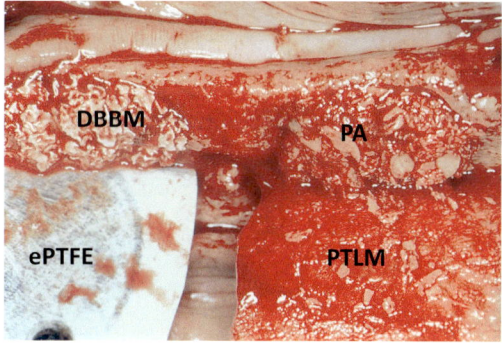

Fig 10-6 Two standardized lateral bone defects created in the mandible are augmented with bone graft material (PA, particulate autograft; DBBM, deproteinized bovine bone mineral) following stabilization of the membranes (bioresorbable prototype trilayer membrane [PTLM]; nonresorbable expanded polyfluorethylene [ePTFE]) at the lower buccal aspect with titanium screws.

defects (Fig 10-7). Before closure of the wound, the surgical site should be thoroughly irrigated with sterile saline to remove any residual debris. Following this, the wound margins are carefully approximated and closed with horizontal mattress and single interrupted sutures.

Sacrifice

Usually, dogs are sacrificed using an overdose of pentobarbital sodium 0.2 mL intravenously

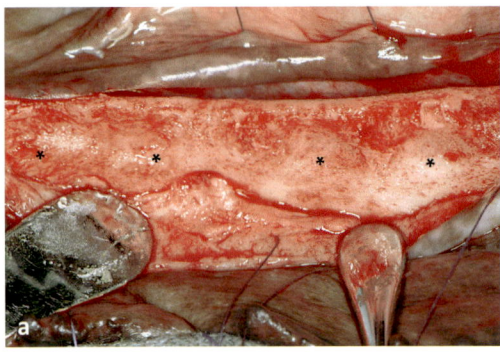
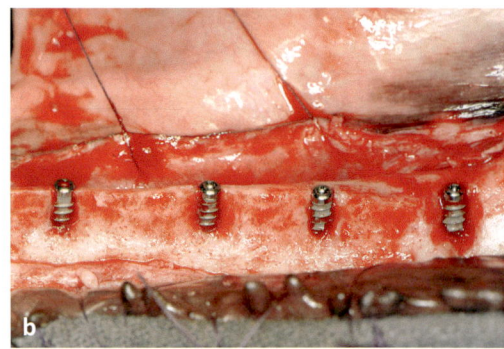
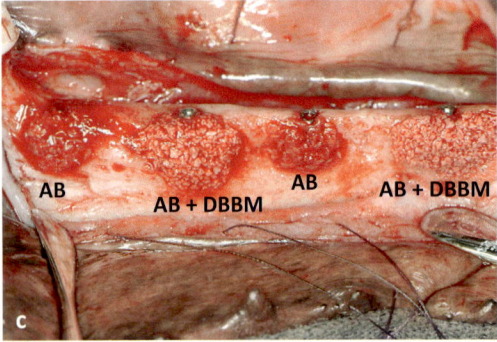
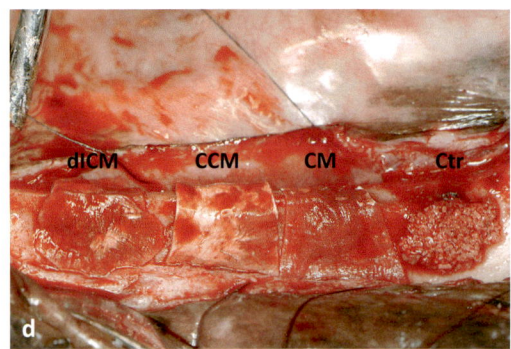

Fig 10-7 (**a**) Chronic-type defect 2 months after tooth extraction and creation of the defects (*) in the right canine mandible. (**b**) Insertion of four dental implants in the area of the chronic-type defects in the right canine mandible. All four implants exhibit pronounced buccal dehiscence defects. (**c**) The dehiscence defects are covered with either particulate autogenous bone grafts alone (AB) or in combination with particulate bovine bone mineral (AB + DBBM). (**d**) The grafted dehiscence defects are then covered with a commercially available non cross-linked collagen membrane (CM), a prototype cross-linked collagen membrane (CCM), and a double-layer of the non cross-linked collagen membrane (dlCM). Here, the control defect without membrane coverage (Ctr) is grafted with autogenous particulate bone in combination with particulate bovine bone mineral (AB + DBBM).

(65 mg/kg). There are also methods reporting perfusion with a fixative (formaldehyde-glutaraldehyde; Karnowsky, 1965), although the respective animals should be sedated before injection. Subsequently, the mandibles are resected en bloc, including the covering soft tissues, using an oscillating autopsy saw (Fig 10-8). The recovered specimens should be immediately immersed in a solution of formaldehyde (4%) combined with 1% calcium chloride prior to histologic preparation (alternative: neutral buffered 10% formalin solution).

10.2.7 Postoperative Care

After tooth extraction in the mandible (with or without simultaneous defect creation), animals normally receive an antimicrobial prophylaxis (for example: combination of spiramycin 750,000 IU and metronidazole 125 mg per day per os for at least 7 days), and an anti-inflammatory agent (for example: carprofen 50 mg per os and per day for three days). Additionally, animals receive a subcutaneous injection of an analgesic (for example: butorphanol). For suture removal under intravenous sedation, the following medications are used: atropine (0.05 mg/kg intramuscular) and tiletamine-zolazepam (5 mg/kg intra-

10.2 The Canine Model for Experimental Research in the Field of Horizontal Ridge Augmentation

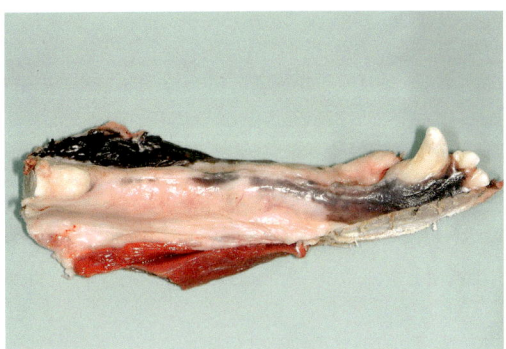

Fig 10-8 En-bloc-resected canine mandible, including the covering soft tissues, using an oscillating autopsy saw.

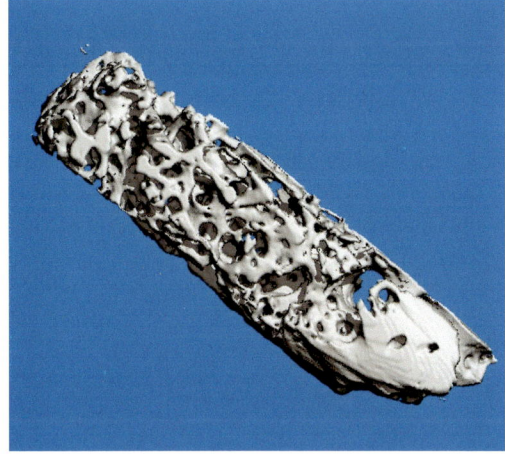

Fig 10-9 Micro-CT image of a central bone core retrieved during implant bed preparation.

muscular). A soft diet is generally maintained throughout the study, and the dogs should be regularly checked when in their cages to prevent them chewing on the bars or other bulky material with their operated mandibles.

10.2.8 Histologic Processing and Endpoint Measurements

Microscopic methods used to evaluate outcomes, efficacy, and quality of augmentative procedures in experimental studies include various techniques such as micro-computed tomography (micro-CT), light microscopy, scanning electron microscopy (SEM), backscattered electron microscopy (BSEM), transmission electron microscopy (TEM), confocal laser scanning microscopy (CLSM), and standard radiography, all of which provide excellent and useful information (Boyde et al., 1995).

Micro-CT
Following the fixation period, grafted regions of the retrieved specimens can be quantified via micro-CT analysis (Maréchal et al., 2005; Kon et al., 2009; Fig 10-9). Possible measurements include: total volume of newly formed bone (TBV; usually in cubic millimeters) and gain in bone height (BH). These measurements are based on standard two-dimensional image analysis that is further processed using stereologic methods (Saffarzadeh et al., 2009). TBV is acquired by the radiopaque voxels observed in the region of interest; the BH can be evaluated from the distance between the basal host (original) bone and the highest point of the regenerated bone.

Histologic Processing
Without applying the perfusion technique, the retrieved specimens are ready to be prepared for further histologic processing and analysis after a period of approximately 2 weeks. There are several procedures available for histologic processing, but one widely accepted method, and also the method favored by the authors of this chapter, is the histologic processing as described by Schenk and co-workers (1984). According to this procedure, the fixated block specimens are dehydrated and embedded in methylmethacrylate. The specimens are usually cut in a buccolingual direction in the regions of the defects. If dental implants are present, they should be cut parallel to their axis, resulting in two to three approximately 500 μm thick undecalcified sections per implant (with an implant

Osteology Guidelines for Oral and Maxillofacial Regeneration

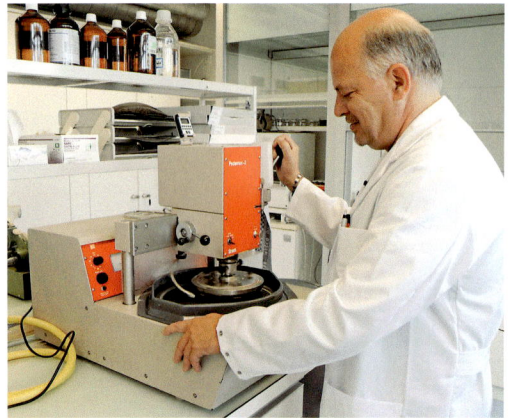

Fig 10-10 The ground sections are glued on a Plexiglas slab and ground to a final thickness of 80 to 100 μm.

diameter between 4 and 5 mm). Subsequently, the sections are glued to opaque Plexiglas slabs with acrylic cement, ground to a final thickness of approximately 80 μm (Fig 10-10), and stained superficially with toluidine blue alone or toluidine blue followed by basic fuchsin. Ideally, one should analyze as many coronal sections per defect as possible for descriptive histology and histomorphometry. However, implant diameter and technical issues such as tissue processing and cutting/grinding may reduce the number of sections available or suitable for analyses. If only one section is analyzed, it should comprise the most central coronal section.

Equipment for Histomorphometry

All measurements should be performed with a photomicroscope (color charge-coupled device camera mounted on a binocular light microscope) by an experienced examiner. Ideally, the observer should also be masked for the specific experimental condition(s). The digital images using different magnifications (between ×100 and ×200) can be evaluated using specific software programs. As an alternative, analysis can also be performed conventionally, for example by using a superimposed grid for point counting with standardized image magnifications. In fact,

observation directly in the microscope offers significant advantages including focusing during observation and distinction between different tissues or maturation stages in critical situations. Thus, conventional stereologic methods are often preferred over computer-based analyses.

Histomorphometric Measurements using Light Microscopy

There are numerous possible histomorphometric measurements, and the most common parameter to be measured is the calculation of a specific area (in square millimeters) of interest. As landmarks, the coronal extension of the bone crest adjacent to the defect area, and the bottom of the bone defect usually are defined (Fig 10-11). Using these landmarks, additional measurements include: the total area of the membrane-covered compartment, the proportion of the different tissues found in the regenerated area such as bone matrix/newly formed bone, soft tissue and residual graft/filler material (expressed for example as a percentage of the regenerated area; Bornstein *et al.*, 2007; Jensen *et al.*, 2009), the mineralized bone to osteoid ratio, the bone-to-filler contact (to assess osteoconduction), and the bone-to-implant contact, when dental implants were inserted. Bone-to-filler and bone-to-implant contacts can be analyzed directly under the microscope using a square grid (Buser *et al.*, 2004; Jensen *et al.*, 2009), or by calculating interface contact lengths between bone and implant–bone filler surface using a software package (Bornstein *et al.*, 2008). There are further selected light microscopy techniques to evaluate specific questions in experimental studies: the use of polarizing light microscopes (Fig 10-12; Saffarzadeh *et al.*, 2009), fluorescence microscopy using different labeling techniques/dyes to visualize and quantify bone formation (for example with calcein blue, xylenol orange, calcein, or alizarin complexone; Fig 10-13) that were injected at different stages of the experiment (Aida *et al.*, 2003; Katsaros *et*

10.2 The Canine Model for Experimental Research in the Field of Horizontal Ridge Augmentation

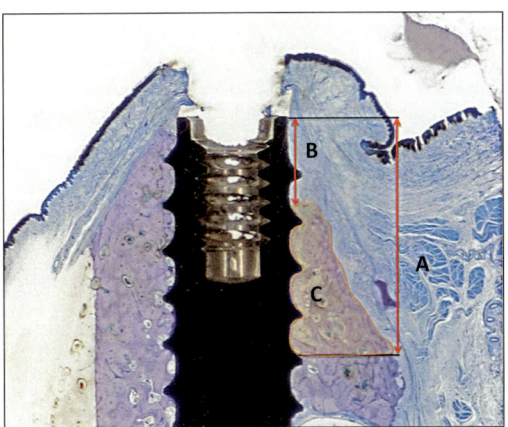

Fig 10-11 Histomorphometric measurement of a dental implant inserted in a canine mandible with a buccal dehiscence defect augmented with autogenous bone and covered with a cross-linked collagen membrane. A: distance from the bottom of the bone defect to the implant shoulder. B: distance from the first bone-to-implant contact to the implant shoulder. C: the total area of the membrane-covered regenerate.

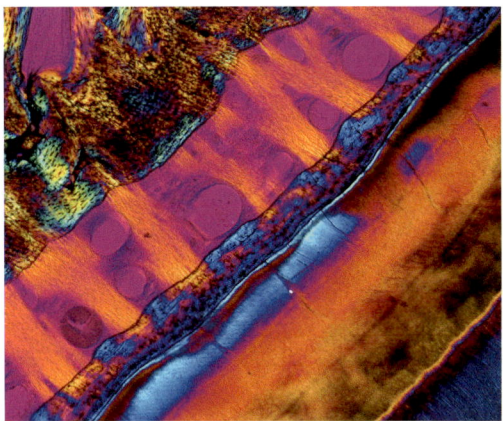

Fig 10-12 Ground section viewed under polarized light showing dentin, enamel, root cementum, periodontal ligament, and alveolar bone. This technique is particularly useful to illustrate the orientation of collagen fibers.

al., 2006), bright field microscopy (Hwang et al., 2000), and phase contrast (Dereka et al., 2006).

For descriptive purposes, osteoclast-like cells can be stained histochemically by evaluating the activity of tartrate-resistant acid phosphatase (TRAP) in multinucleated giant cells with azo staining using naphtol AS-TR phosphate coupled with fast red violet TR salt (Jensen et al., 2009; Fig 10-14). Additionally, immunohistochemical labeling of the specimens allows for an analysis of selected antigen reactivity. For example, osteocalcin, a non-collagenous protein, which is predominantly synthesized by osteoblasts, odontoblasts, and hypertrophic chondrocytes, can be visualized in the tissues indicating maturation of regenerated bone areas by highlighting osteoblastic differentiation (Schwarz et al., 2007, 2008a,b). Another example of immunohistochemical analysis is the use of monoclonal antibodies to transglutaminase II (TG) (Schwarz et al., 2008a, 2009). As the organization of the wound area by proliferating blood vessels is considered to be of crucial importance for the process of GBR, angiogenesis can be investigated by

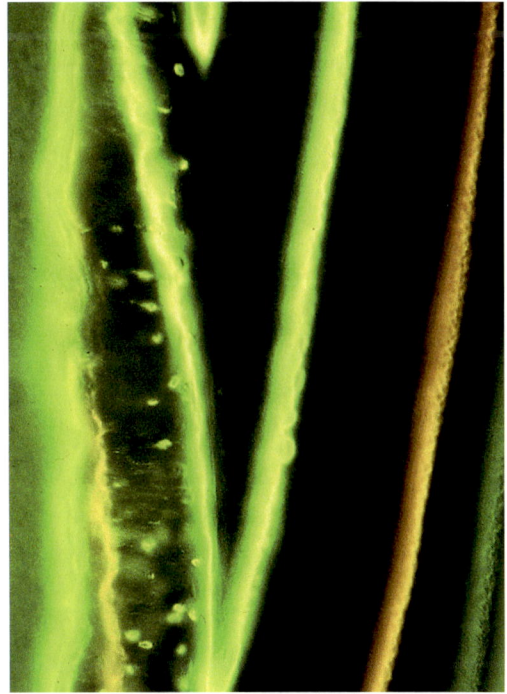

Fig 10-13 Fluorescent lines in cementum and dentin viewed in the fluorescence microscope. The animal received sequential injections of calcein (green lines) and xylenol orange (orange lines). The two fluorochromes bind to sites of ongoing mineralization and produce clear fluorescence lines.

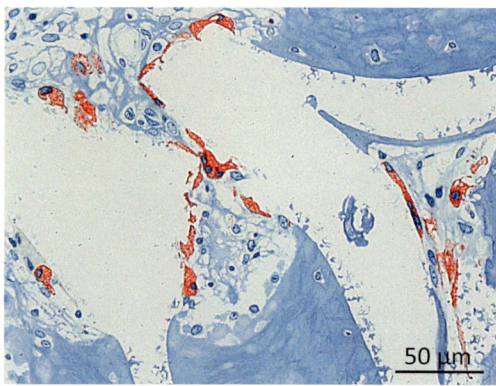

Fig 10-14 TRAP staining in a 1 μm thick section from a biopsy retrieved from a site augmented with a bone substitute material. The cytoplasm of TRAP-positive multinucleated cells, which are located at the biomaterial-soft tissue interface, stands out due to its dark red staining.

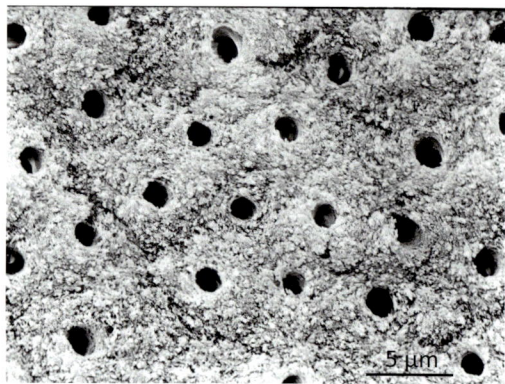

Fig 10-15 SEM view of the mineralized dentin after removal of the soft tissue of the dental pulp. Note the regularly arranged dentinal tubules.

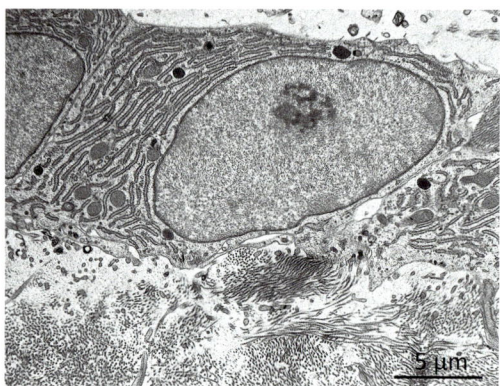

Fig 10-16 TEM illustrating a typical osteoblast adjacent to the osteoid matrix. Note the abundant rough endoplasmic reticulum in the cytoplasm.

labeling the tissues with antibodies to TG. Especially, the variations in transmembraneous angiogenesis between different types of barrier membranes can be studied using this technique (Schwarz et al. 2008a).

SEM/BSEM/TEM
SEM has been described in experimental studies after sputter-coating the fixated specimens with gold-palladium (de Kok *et al.*, 2003; Saffarzadeh *et al.*, 2009; Fig 10-15). With SEM imaging, bone filler particles with a low organic component and a relatively high atomic number of calcium and phosphate in hydroxyapatite crystals usually appear whitish-gray, whereas newly formed bone appears dark gray because of collagen, marrow, and fat components (Traini *et al.*, 2008).

BSEM offers considerable insight into the mineralized tissues at the graft–bone and/or implant–bone interface. BSEM is particularly useful in distinguishing one material from another, since the yield of the collected backscattered electrons increases monotonically with the specimen's atomic number (Boyde and Jones, 1983; Nanci *et al.*, 1990). A recent experimental study in the canine mandible used BSEM to analyze specimens in which bone was augmented both horizontally and vertically with a xenograft scaffold and recombinant human platelet-derived growth factor (rhPDGF-BB), with or without a resorbable collagen membrane (Rocchietta *et al.*, 2007).

For TEM, ultrathin sections (ideally less than 100 nm in thickness) are collected on copper grids, stained with lead citrate and uranyl acetate, and examined under the microscope

(Orsini et al., 2006; Fig 10-16). Using TEM, Orsini and coworkers were able to observe and differentiate the following features: regions rich in osteoid matrix and spaces between the collagen fibrils; areas in which there was a rich-interlaced framework of collagen fibrils that started to present circumscribed mineralization foci; regions of woven bone; and zones of well-organized mature bone. A disadvantage of TEM is its limitations when a metal implant is present in the biopsy material.

A technique that is a little less common, but still is worth noting here is contact microradiography. This technique is especially suitable for descriptive analyses due to the good contrast seen, for example, between metal implants and surrounding bone, for different stages of bony maturation/mineralization, or between native/older and newly regenerated bone (Sawai et al., 1996; Tung et al., 2006; Chikazu et al., 2007).

10.2.9 Thoughts on the Statistical Analysis

Researchers evaluating horizontal ridge augmentation procedures and outcomes invest great effort in terms of time and money to ensure that the experiment addresses an important question in a biologically valid and meaningful way. Nevertheless, often little thought is given to ensure that the experimental data will be collected and analyzed in such a way as to provide a valid answer to the research question that was framed with great care (Stratton and Neil, 2005). It is important to remember that inappropriate analyses and/or erroneous interpretations can invalidate the meaning and impact of the data collected. A thorough planning of an experimental study (phase 1, see 10.2.3 and Chapter 4) should therefore already include an evaluation of the statistical methods to be applied to ensure that the study is likely to yield conclusive results. Furthermore, given the expensive nature of in vivo experiments and the ethical concerns involved, careful planning is mandatory to ensure that animals are used efficiently (Hanfelt, 1997).

An analysis to identify the statistical significance should prove that the difference between groups did not happen by chance alone. It should be emphasized here that there is never 100% certainty that chance did not play a role in the data collected, but we can calculate the probability that chance alone was not the dominating factor in the results. That probability is called the P value (Baumgardner, 1997; Whitley and Ball, 2002a). Another important variable is the confidence interval that indicates the likely range of values for a certain effect in the population studied. Confidence intervals and P values are both strongly dependent on the size of the study sample, with larger samples generally resulting in narrower confidence intervals and smaller P values.

Sample sizes for experimental studies using a canine model should ideally be kept to a minimum and therefore, they should be rationally planned and not arbitrarily chosen. This makes calculation of an appropriate sample size important, and more and more animal ethical committees as well as grant-giving bodies are requiring adequate sample size calculations to be provided at the initial stage of the project (Whitley and Ball, 2002b). Factors that affect sample size calculations are: a cutoff for statistical significance based on a defined P value; the size of the effect to be detected, with a small effect requiring larger samples; the statistical power of the study, e.g. the probability of correctly identifying a difference between groups in the study sample when one genuinely exists. It should be kept in mind that sample size calculations, when performed at the initial stages of an experimental study (phase 1), are by large dependent on estimates of effect, power, and significance. Thus, a range of values should be initially provided in order to give several suitable sample sizes rather than a single number. To help researchers with this crucial step, several computer programs are available for adequate sample size calculation.

By being aware of the importance of accurate sample size calculation, researchers can avoid performing experimental studies that are too small to have adequate power to detect the hypothesized effect. In these studies, too few animals are included to demonstrate a statistically significant effect even when in reality a difference exists. This effect is often quoted as "absence of evidence is not evidence of absence" (Whitley and Ball, 2002b). On the other hand, well-designed studies that do not demonstrate a statistically significant treatment effect (so called *null studies*) are not less valid. These studies are clinically quite important, as they show that a particular procedure may not be indicated, preventing the implementation of potentially harmful procedures.

10.2.10 Materials, Consumables, and Equipment

The instruments, materials, and equipment necessary for horizontal ridge augmentation procedures may be divided into surgical and laboratorial. For the surgical instrumentarium, they should ideally represent instruments utilized in daily clinical practice. There are a vast variety of surgical instruments and materials of different brands, quality, and cost. Personal choice certainly has an important role in selecting instruments and materials, but this choice should not compromise the final results of the surgery. The instruments must be sterile, and the operating room and the animal should be covered with sterile drapes in the same manner as when performing surgery on a human being. To avoid contamination, all materials (bone filler, barrier membranes, or other) must be kept closed in their appropriate sterile packs until needed on the operating table. Ideally, sutures should be nonresorbable and preferably with low plaque retention. More details concerning specific instruments for the surgical part of the experiment or histologic processing and evaluation can be found in Sections 10.2.6 and 10.2.8, respectively.

References

1. Aerssens J, Boonen S, Lowet G, Dequeker J (1998). Interspecies differences in bone composition, density, and quality: potential implications for *in vivo* bone research. *Endocrinology* 139:663–670.
2. Aida T, Yoshioka I, Tominaga K, Fukuda J (2003). Effects of latency period in a rabbit mandibular distraction osteogenesis. *Int J Oral Maxillofac Surg* 32:54–62.
3. Araújo MG, Sonohara M, Hayacibara R, Cardaropoli G, Lindhe J (2003). Lateral ridge augmentation by the use of grafts comprised of autologous bone or a biomaterial. An experiment in the dog. *J Clin Peridontol* 29:1122–1131.
4. Baumgardner KR (1997). A review of key research design and statistical analysis issues. *Oral Surg Oral Med Oral Pathol Oral Radiol Endod* 84:550–556.
5. Bornstein MM, Bosshardt DD, Buser D (2007). Effect of two different bioresorbable collagen membranes on guided bone regeneration. A comparative histomorphometric study in the dog mandible. *J Periodontol* 78:1943–1953.
6. Bornstein MM, Valderrama P, Jones AA, Wilson TG, Seibl R, Cochran DL (2008). Bone apposition around two different sand-blasted and acid-etched titanium implant surfaces. A histomorphometric study in canine mandibles. *Clin Oral Implants Res* 19:233–241.
7. Bornstein MM, Heynen G, Bosshardt DD, Buser D (2009). Effect of two bioabsorbable barrier membranes on bone regeneration of standardized defects in calvarial bone. A comparative histomorphometric study in pigs. *J Periodontol* 80:1289–1299.
8. Boyde A, Jones SJ (1983). Backscattered electron imaging of dental tissues. *Anat Embryol (Berlin)* 168: 211–226.
9. Boyde A, Jones SJ, Aerssens J, Dequeker J (1995). Mineral density quantitation of the human cortical iliac crest by backscattered electron image analysis: Variations with age, sex, and degree of osteoarthritis. *Bone* 16:619–627.
10. Busenlechner D, Kantor M, Tangl S, Tepper G, Zechner W, Haas R *et al.* (2005). Alveolar ridge augmentation with a prototype trilayer membrane and various bone grafts: a histomorphometric study in baboons. *Clin Oral Implants Res* 16:220–227.
11. Buser D, Schenk RK, Steinemann S, Fiorellini J, Fox C, Stich H (1991). Influence of surface characteristics on bone integration of titanium implants. A histometric study in miniature pigs. *J Biomed Mater Res* 25: 889–902.
12. Buser D, Hoffmann B, Bernard JP, Lussi A, Mettler D, Schenk RK (1998). Evaluation of filling materials in membrane-protected bone defects. A comparative histomorphometric study in the mandible of miniature pigs. *Clin Oral Implants Res* 9:137–150.
13. Buser D, Nydegger T, Oxland T, Cochran DL, Schenk RK, Hirt HP *et al.* (1999). Interface shear strength of titanium implants with a sandblasted and acid-etched surface: a biomechanical study in the maxilla of miniature pigs. *J Biomed Mater Res* 45:75–83.

References

14. Buser D, Broggini N, Wieland M, Schenk RK, Denzer AJ, Cochran DL et al. (2004). Enhanced bone apposition to a chemically modified SLA titanium surface. *J Dent Res* 83:529–533.
15. Chiapasco M, Zaniboni M (2009). Clinical outcomes of GBR procedures to correct peri-implant dehiscences and fenestrations: a systematic review. *Clin Oral Implants Res* 20(Suppl 4):113–123.
16. Chikazu D, Tomizuka K, Ogasawara T, Saijo H, Koizumi T, Mori Y et al. (2007). Cyclooxygenase-2 activity is essential for the osseointegration of dental implants. *Int J Oral Maxillofac Surg* 36:441–446.
17. de Kok IJ, Peter SJ, Archambault M, van den Bos C, Kadiyala S, Aukhil I et al. (2003). Investigation of allogeneic mesenchymal stem cell-based alveolar bone formation: preliminary findings. *Clin Oral Implants Res* 14:481–489.
18. Dereka XE, Markopoulou CE, Mamalis A, Pepelassi E, Vrotsos IA (2006). Time- and dose-dependent mitogenic effect of basic fibroblast growth factor combined with different bone graft materials: an *in vitro* study. *Clin Oral Implants Res* 17:554–559.
19. Donos N, Kostopoulos L, Karring T (2002). Alveolar ridge augmentation using a resorbable copolymer membrane and autogenous bone grafts. An experimental study in the rat. *Clin Oral Implants Res* 13:203–213.
20. Egermann M, Goldhahn J, Schneider E (2005). Animal models for fracture treatment In osteoporosls. *Osteoporos Int* 16(Suppl 2):S129–S138.
21. Fonseca RJ, Nelson JF, Clark PJ, Frost DE, Olson RA (1983). Revascularization and healing of onlay particulate allogeneic bone grafts in primates. *J Oral Maxillofac Surg* 41:153–162.
22. Hanfelt JJ (1997). Statistical approaches to experimental design and data analysis of *in vivo* studies. *Breast Cancer Res Treat* 46:279–302.
23. Hanisch O, Sorensen RG, Kinoshita A, Spiekermann H, Wozney JM, Wikesjö UM (2003). Effect of recombinant human bone morphogenetic protein-2 in dehiscence defects with non-submerged immediate implants: an experimental study in Cynomolgus monkeys. *J Peridontol* 74:648–657.
24. Hazzard DG, Bronson RT, McClearn GE, Strong R (1992) Selection of an appropriate animal model to study aging processes with special emphasis on the use of rat strains. *J Gerontol* 47:B63–B64.
25. Hwang K, Schmitt JM, Hollinger JO (2000). Interface between titanium miniplate/screw and human calvaria. *J Craniofac Surg* 11:184–188.
26. Jensen SS, Terheyden H (2009). Bone augmentation procedures in localized defects in the alveolar ridge: clinical results with different bone grafts and bone-substitute materials. *Int J Oral Maxillofac Implants* 24(Suppl):218–236.
27. Jensen SS, Broggini N, Hjørting-Hansen E, Schenk R, Buser D (2006). Bone healing and graft resorption of autograft, anorganic bovine bone and beta-tricalcium phosphate. A histologic and histomorphometric study in the mandibles of minipigs. *Clin Oral Implants Res* 17:237–243.
28. Jensen SS, Bornstein MM, Dard M, Bosshardt DD, Buser D (2009). Comparative study of biphasic calcium phosphates with different HA/TCP ratios in mandibular bone defects. A long-term histomorphometric study in minipigs. *J Biomed Mater Res B Appl Biomater* 90B:171–181.
29. Karnowsky MJ (1965). A formaldehyde-glutaraldehyde fixation of high osmolarity for use in electron microscopy. *J Cell Biol* 27:137A–138A.
30. Katsaros C, Zissis A, Bresin A, Kiliaridis S (2006). Functional influence on sutural bone apposition in the growing rat. *Am J Orthod Dentofac Orthop* 129:352–357.
31. Kon K, Shiota M, Ozeki M, Yamashita Y, Kasugai S (2009). Bone augmentation ability of autogenous bone graft particles with different sizes: a histological and micro-computed tomography study. *Clin Oral Implants Res* 20:1240–1246.
32. Kostopoulos L, Karring T (1994). Augmentation of the rat mandible using guided tissue regeneration. *Clin Oral Implants Res* 5:75–82.
33. Liebschner MA (2004). Biomechanical considerations of animal models used in tissue engineering of bone. *Biomaterials* 25:1697–1714.
34. Mai R, Reinstorf A, Pilling E, Hlawitschka M, Jung R, Gelinsky M et al. (2008). Histologic study of incorporation and resorption of a bone cement-collagen composite: an *in vivo* study in the minipig. *Oral Surg Oral Med Oral Pathol Oral Radiol Endod* 105:e9–e14.
35. Maréchal M, Luyten F, Nijs J, Postnov A, Schepers E, van Steenberghe D (2005). Histomorphometry and micro-computed tomography of bone augmentation under a titanium membrane. *Clin Oral Implants Res* 16:708–714.
36. Miranda DA, Blumenthal NM, Sorensen RG, Wozney JM, Wikesjö UM (2005). Evaluation of recombinant human bone morphogenetic protein-2 on the repair of alveolar ridge defects in baboons. *J Peridontol* 76:210–220.
37. Muschler GF, Raut VP, Patterson TE, Wenke JC, Hollinger JO (2010). The design and use of animal models for translational research in bone tissue engineering and regenerative medicine. *Tissue Eng Part B Rev* 16:123–145.
38. Nanci A, Zalzal S, Smith CE (1990). Routine use of back-scattered electron imaging to visualize cytochemical and autoradiographic reactions in semi-thin plastic sections. *J Histochem Cytochem* 38:403–414.
39. O'Loughlin PF, Morr S, Bogunovic L, Kim AD, Park B, Lane JM (2008). Selection and development of preclinical models in fracture-healing research. *J Bone Joint Surg Am* 90(Suppl 1):79–84.
40. Olsen ML, Aaboe M, Hjørting-Hansen E, Hansen AK (2004). Problems related to an intraoral approach for experimental surgery on minipigs. *Clin Oral Implants Res* 15:333–338.
41. Orsini G, Scarano A, Piattelli M, Piccirilli M, Caputi S, Piattelli A (2006). Histologic and ultrastructural analysis of regenerated bone in maxillary sinus augmentation using a porcine bone-derived biomaterial. *J Periodontol* 7:1984–1990.

42. Pearce AI, Richards RG, Milz S, Schneider E, Pearce SG (2007). Animal models for implant biomaterial research in bone: a review. *Eur Cells Mater* 13:1–10.
43. Reinwald S, Burr D (2008). Review of nonprimate, large animal models for osteoporosis research. *J Bone Miner Res* 23:1353–1368.
44. Rocchietta I, Dellavia C, Nevins M, Simion M (2007). Bone regenerated via rhPDGF-bB and a deproteinized bovine bone matrix: backscattered electron microscopic element analysis. *Int J Periodontics Restorative Dent* 27:539–545.
45. Saffarzadeh A, Gauthier O, Bilban M, Bagot D'Arc M, Daculsi G (2009). Comparison of two bone substitute biomaterials consisting of a mixture of fibrin sealant (Tisseel) and MBCP (TricOs) with an autograft in sinus lift surgery in sheep. *Clin Oral Implants Res* 20:1133–1139.
46. Sawai T, Niimi A, Takahashi H, Ueda M (1996). Histologic study of the effect of hyperbaric oxygen therapy on autogenous free bone grafts. *J Oral Maxillofac Surg* 54:975–981.
47. Schenk RK, Olah AJ, Hermann W (1984). Preparation of calcified tissues for light microscopy. In: Methods of calcified tissue preparation, 1st ed. Dickson GR, editor. Amsterdam: Elsevier, pp. 1–56.
48. Schimandle JH, Boden SD (1994). Spine update. The use of animal models to study spinal fusion. *Spine* 19:1998–2006.
49. Schwarz F, Herten M, Ferrari D, Wieland M, Schmitz L, Engelhardt E *et al.* (2007). Guided bone regeneration at dehiscence-type defects using biphasic hydroxyapatite + beta tricalcium phosphate (Bone Ceramic) or a collagen-coated natural bone mineral (BioOss Collagen): an immunohistochemical study in dogs. *Int J Oral Maxillofac Surg* 36:1198–1206.
50. Schwarz F, Rothamel D, Herten M, Wüstefeld M, Sager M, Ferrari D *et al.* (2008a). Immunohistochemical characterization of guided bone regeneration at a dehiscence-type defect using different barrier membranes: an experimental study in dogs. *Clin Oral Implants Res* 19:402–415.
51. Schwarz F, Rothamel D, Herten M, Ferrari D, Sager M, Becker J (2008b). Lateral ridge augmentation using particulated or block bone substitutes biocoated with rhGDF-5 and rhBMP-2: an immunohistochemical study in dogs. *Clin Oral Implants Res* 19:642–652.
52. Schwarz F, Sager M, Ferrari D, Mihatovic I, Becker J (2009). Influence of recombinant human platelet-derived growth factor on lateral ridge augmentation using biphasic calcium phosphate and guided bone regeneration: a histomorphometric study in dogs. *J Periodontol* 80:1315–1323.
53. Stratton IM, Neil A (2005). How to ensure your paper is rejected by the statistical reviewer. *Diabet Med* 22:371–373.
54. Traini T, Degidi M, Sammons R, Stanley P, Piattelli A (2008). Histologic and elemental microanalytical study of anorganic bovine bone substitution following sinus floor augmentation in humans. *J Periodontol* 79:1232–1240.
55. Tung K, Fujita H, Yamashita Y, Takagi Y (2006). Effect of turpentine-induced fever during the enamel formation of rat incisor. *Arch Oral Biol* 51:464–470.
56. von Arx T, Cochran DL, Hermann JS, Schenk RK, Buser D (2001a). Lateral ridge augmentation using different bone fillers and barrier membrane application. A histologic and histomorphometric pilot study in the canine mandible. *Clin Oral Implants Res* 12:260–269.
57. von Arx T, Cochran DL, Hermann JS, Schenk RK, Higginbottom FL, Buser D (2001b). Lateral ridge augmentation and implant placement: an experimental study evaluating implant osseointegration in different augmentation materials in the canine mandible. *Int J Oral Maxillofac Implants* 16:343–354.
58. von Arx T, Cochran DL, Schenk RK, Buser D (2002). Evaluation of a prototype trilayer membrane (PTLM) for lateral ridge augmentation: an experimental study in the canine mandible. *J Oral Maxillofac Surg* 31:190–199.
59. Wang X, Mabrey JD, Agrawal CM (1998). An interspecies comparison of bone fracture properties. *Biomed Mater Eng* 8:1–9.
60. Whitley E, Ball J (2002a). Statistics review 3: hypothesis testing and P values. *Crit Care* 6:222–225.
61. Whitley E, Ball J (2002b). Statistics review 4: sample size calculations. *Crit Care* 6:335–341.
62. Ylinen P, Raekallio M, Toivonen T, Vihtonen K, Vainionpää S (1991). Preliminary study of porous hydroxylapatite particle containment with a curved biodegradable implant in the sheep mandible. *J Oral Maxillofac Surg* 49:1191–1197.

Vertical Ridge Augmentation

Isabella Rocchietta, David M. Kim, Khalid Al-Hezaimi, and Massimo Simion

11.1 General Overview

The evolution of osseointegrated implants required new regenerative concepts to increase the volume of bone to fulfill the basic tenet of the successful implant residing in bone. New concepts of guided bone regeneration (GBR) needed to be explored in preclinical models prior to human application as it is unethical to apply them without evidence of safety and efficacy. Proof of principle results are extended to small pilot and eventually to multicenter dosing and pivotal randomized controlled trials. Preclinical trials afford the opportunity to perform light microscopic and histomorphometric analyses by harvesting biopsy material (Yukna, 1976; Caton, 1980, 1994).

11.1.1 Advanced Osseous Defects

Horizontal and vertical ridge augmentation procedures are essential for restoring bone deformation following destructive periodontal disease, traumatic tooth extraction, endodontic infection, failing dental implant, or jaw trauma. Horizontal ridge augmentation procedures are routinely performed, but vertical ridge augmentation procedures are considered "elusive treatment" because of potential complications and limited success due to anatomic and technical difficulties. Conventional GBR, autogenous onlay bone grafting, and distraction osteogenesis have all been employed to correct severe bone loss (Nyman, 1991; Simion *et al.*, 1994; Jensen *et al.*, 2002; Levin *et al.*, 2007; Froum *et al.*, 2008). Each of these procedures has potential drawbacks relative to predictability (Simion *et al.*, 2009). Distraction osteogenesis for example may be associated with incomplete bone formation, which requires additional hard and soft tissue grafting and results in compromised esthetic outcome (Jensen *et al.*, 2002; Froum *et al.*, 2008). Autogenous bone grafts offer superior capacity to promote osteogenesis, but the graft harvesting is associated with undesirable morbidity as well as block graft shrinkage. Thus, extent and configurations of osseous deformity will dictate potential hard tissue augmentation procedures. Predictable treatment modalities that can treat advanced osseous defects require investigation in both preclinical and clinical models.

Recent advances in the areas of biomaterials, and the isolation and application of signaling devices along with technical advancements have enabled clinicians to attempt predictable vertical ridge augmentation in both preclinical and clinical settings (Simion *et al.*, 2006, 2007a–c, 2008, 2009; Wikesjö *et al.*, 2004, 2008). This chapter will introduce appropriate surgical protocols for application of biologics for vertical bone augmentation with and without simultaneous insertion of dental implant. We will suggest a proven defect model for preclinical animal studies that will allow various treatment modalities to succeed.

11.1.2 Construction of the Research Protocol

The eight steps described below should be taken into consideration before embarking on a new preclinical study to test the safety and efficacy of biologics or surgical techniques for vertical ridge augmentation.

Determine What Materials or Techniques are to be Tested
Proper study design and clinical application can minimize or prevent trial and error from occurring in the initial study submission phase. It is important to conduct preclinical trials that have clinical applicability and relevance.

Select Appropriate Model and Method and Become Familiar with Previous Publications
Review of previous publications will give insights regarding proper animal selection as well as limitations of certain animal models. In larger animal models such as nonhuman primates or canines, the oral anatomy and wound healing physiology are similar to humans, and these models might be better suited for reconstructive surgery.

Define Critical-size Defect
Creation of a bony defect that is reproducible and resembles the atrophic ridge in humans is essential. Large bony defects or critical-size defects need to be defined for each animal to prevent spontaneous bone regeneration and to minimize substantial native osteogenic potential. It is also important to realize the limitation of artificially created defects in animals because the results obtained from under-standardized defect conditions do not necessarily imply that the same treatment will produce equivalent results in humans (Selvig, 1994).

Option of Assembling With or Without Implant
Rigid fixation of device or bone grafting material is needed to obtain maximal bone regeneration response and for initial stabilization of the blood clot.

Determine Adequate Sample Size and Length of the Study
Consultation with a biostatistician is recommended to determine an appropriate sample size so that the study will have adequate power. The length of the study should be determined ahead of time to minimize study costs and for ethical considerations regarding use of animals.

Understand Appropriate Analysis of the Results
Potential endpoints of the study can include the rate and amount of new bone formation, resorption of graft particles, and any signs of foreign body reactions. Clinical data collection, radiographic data interpretation, histologic and histomorphometric analyses should all be considered.

Endpoint Assessments
Initial consultation with a histologist is recommended to assess the outcome of the study. Sample preparation is as important as surgical preparation, and different tissue processing,

embedding and sectioning techniques can be employed by the histologist to answer the study hypothesis.

Establishing Study Budget
Regulatory requirements as well as the high costs of animal maintenance can exponentially increase the cost of the study. A thoroughly planned out budget is a prerequisite to conduct large animal studies involving canines, pigs, or monkeys. Consultation with a veterinarian as well as animal facility coordinator is recommended before submitting a budget plan.

11.2 Selection of an Appropriate Animal Model

Preclinical research trials provide an estimate of potential osteogenic value of a biomaterial so it does not lead to unexpected complications and negative outcomes for patients. It is important for researchers and clinicians to select an appropriate animal model that has phylogenetically similar oral structures to humans, and develop an experimental defect that is suitable to establish validity of the scientific principle (Habal and Reddi, 1992). The rodent models are frequently used for early experimentation, but extrapolation of clinically relevant data is not optimal due to their high potential for innate bone regeneration (Habal and Reddi, 1992). Their small oral cavity also interferes with surgical access and the delivery of devices to be tested. The vestibular side of the rodents' mandibular ramus is often selected to test vertical bone augmentation in the so-called "capsule model" (Kostopoulous and Karring, 1994). The approach consists of space provision with a Teflon capsule with an internal diameter of 5 mm sutured to the mandibular ramus. According to Kostopoulous and Karring, 70% of the capsule was filled with newly formed bone within the first 4 months, and this would be completed within the first year. This type of bone regeneration is referred to as ectopic beyond the normal bony envelope, and not applicable to the human model.

Larger animal models such as sheep, alpine goats, pigs (normal and minipigs), canines, and nonhuman primates have oral anatomy and wound healing physiology that are similar to humans, and might be better suited for reconstructive surgery. The anatomy and physiology of the cutaneous blood supply and the wound healing characteristics have made the pig a standard model for plastic surgical and wound healing studies (Kerrigan et al., 1986; Mertz et al., 1986). Bone and implant studies in the swine oral cavity are frequently reported; however, long tooth roots and the difficult behavior management does not establish it as a preferred animal model (Ruehe et al., 2009). Sheep and goats are used for long bone defect repair (tibial mid-diaphysis is selected) (Giannoni et al., 2008) or maxillary sinuses to test biologics (Nevins et al., 1996; Gutwald et al., 2010). The majority of the studies in the international literature where vertical bone regeneration is evaluated, suggest the canine model (Foxhounds, mongrel, and Beagles). Some authors used Wistar rats' maxillae to test a tissue engineered block in vertical bone regeneration (Shimazu et al., 2006) while others (Tamimi et al., 2009) used New Zealand white rabbits.

11.2.1 Aim for the Use of the Canine Model

Canine or nonhuman primate models have strong applicability in the development of clinical guidelines and endpoints for the initiation of phase II and phase III human clinical trials. Economic considerations, demanding maintenance, as well as regulatory requirements may limit the use of nonhuman primates (Caton et al., 1994; Pellegrini et al., 2009). Hence, the canine emerges as the model of the choice for the vertical ridge augmentation. The investigative advantage of a preclinical model is an opportunity to create paired defects of equal size that may resemble bony defects in human (Selvig, 1994).

Table 11-1 Overview of animal models used in preclinical research on vertical ridge augmentation procedures

Animal model	Advantages	Disadvantages	Author/s
Nonhuman primates	Morphologic features similar to humans	Economics	Kleinschmidt and Hollinger, 1992; Pellegrini et al., 2009
	Phylogenetically similar oral structures to humans	Regulatory requirements	
	Minimal spontaneous repair	Demanding maintenance	
	Chronic and acute disease models	Small anatomic size of oral cavity hence technically challenging	
Dog	Morphologic features similar to humans	Economics	Rothamel et al., 2009; Simion et al., 2006, 2009; Wikesjö et al., 2004, 2008
	Microbiologic features similar to humans	Regulatory requirements in some countries	
	Oral cavity available to access		
	Favorable anatomic size of oral cavity		
	Easy maintenance		
	Minimal spontaneous repair		
	Reproducibly created		
	Chronic and acute disease models		
Pig	Oral cavity available to access	Demanding maintenance	Cestari et al., 2009
	Standard model for plastic surgical and wound healing studies	High self-regenerative bone healing potential	
		Long tooth roots	
Rabbit	Cost effective	Very high self-regenerative bone healing potential	Kon et al., 2009; Tamimi et al., 2009; Lundgren et al., 1995
	Easy maintenance		
	High number of animals per experiment	Oral cavity unable to access	
		Other anatomic structures available differ from human tissues	
		Raised mortality rate when general anesthesia is performed	
Mouse	Cost effective	Very high self-regenerative bone healing potential	Freilich et al., 2008; Shimazu et al., 2006
	Easy maintenance		
	High number of animals per experiment	Oral cavity difficult to access	
		Other anatomic structures available differ from human tissues	
		Small size of animal	

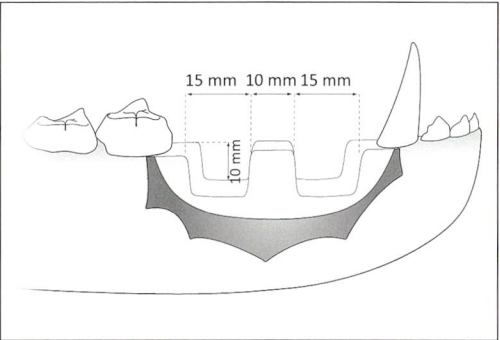 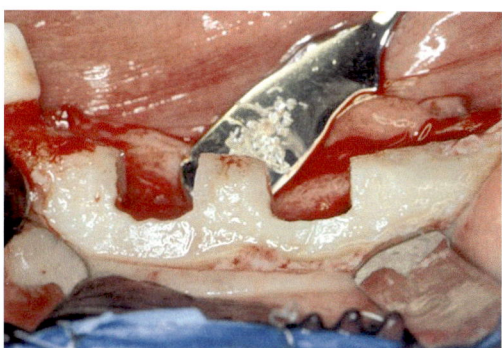

Fig 11-1 Schematic drawing of saddle-like defects in a canine mandible model.

Fig 11-2 Clinical image of saddle-like defects in a canine mandible model.

Canine as a Large Animal Defect Model
A critical-size defect is too large to anticipate spontaneous bone regeneration caused by the native osteogenic potential. The defect size for the bone-regeneration procedure should emulate the atrophic jaw and should explore biologic potential of a surgical procedure. The mandibular jaw is preferred over the maxillary jaw due to proximity of the maxillary sinus around premolars and molars. Vertical bone regeneration may be tested with various research protocols for reconstructive therapy (Table 11-1).

- **Saddle-like mandibular defects**: GBR following cell exclusionary biologic principles of periodontal guided tissue regeneration, i.e., using barrier membranes, has been thoroughly tested using saddle-like mandibular defects in a canine model (Schenk et al., 1994). With the advent of a multitude of barrier membranes to be tested, this model was used by many authors to evaluate their efficacy and potential (Dahlin et al., 1990; Simion et al., 1999). This defect was frequently used to test the barrier membrane. Two defects were created per mandible after extracting all four premolars and eliminating the buccal and lingual cortical plates. Spontaneous bone regeneration could be fostered from the mesial and distal walls as demonstrated by saddle-type defects (10 mm in depth and 15 mm in length, separated by 10 mm in length between two defects) in canine mandibles that achieved spontaneous bone fill of 60% in 3 months (Hunt et al., 2001; Jovanovic et al., 2007) (Fig 11-1 and Fig 11-2).

- **Supra-alveolar peri-implant defect model**: Investigators testing biologics for vertical bone regeneration may do so simultaneously with a dental implant or retention screw (Jensen et al., 1995; Jovanovic et al., 1995; Wikesjö et al., 2006). The Hound Labrador mongrel is selected, and the alveolar bone is removed around the circumference of the mandibular premolar teeth to a level approximately 6 mm from the cementoenamel junction. Then these teeth are extracted in addition to the first molar. On the same day, three dental implants are placed into the extraction site of the third (distal root) and fourth (mesial and distal roots) premolars. Then 10 mm long implants are placed to a depth of 5 mm (to the level of the reference notch), thus creating 5 mm supra-alveolar peri-implant defects. The maxillary first to fourth premolars are extracted to alleviate potential trauma from the maxillary teeth. The animals are euthanized at 8 weeks post surgery. This experimental model implies the use of a fresh wound with a high

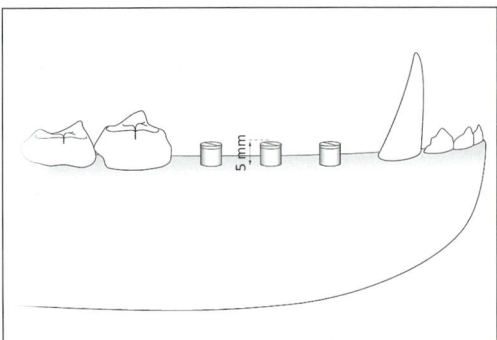

Fig 11-3 Schematic drawing of a supra-alveolar peri-implant defect model in a canine mandible. The implants are left protruding 5 mm from the bone crest.

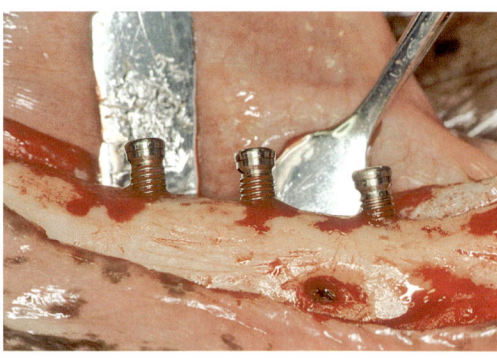

Fig 11-4 Clinical image of the supra-alveolar peri-implant defect model in a canine mandible.

self-regenerative potential of the alveolar bone. However, this condition never occurs in the clinical setting, in that patients present with chronic alveolar defects with no self-regenerative potential at all. The major advantage of this model is costs related to time duration of the experiment. The total duration is only 8 weeks (Fig 11-3 and Fig 11-4).

- **Chronic defect model**: A chronic defect model has been validated for the canine mandibular ridge defects to establish the appropriate biologics for vertical ridge augmentation (Simion et al., 2006, 2007a, 2009). It is proven to be reproducible and reliable for assessment of the potential of a three-dimensional scaffold in conjunction with dental implant placement (Simion et al., 2007b,c, 2008). A critical-size alveolar bone defect in foxhounds (weighing at least 25 kg) is created by bilateral removal of all four mandibular premolars (P1–P4) and surgical reduction of the ridge height and width with a carbide bur (size # 8) and a high-speed handpiece, or an acrylic bur and slow-speed handpiece. Adequate irrigation is required to avoid overheating the bone. The critical defect size dimensions of 20 to 25 mm mesiodistally, 7 to 8 mm apicocoronally and 10 mm buccolingually are created to mimic a flat atrophic ridge. A healing period of 3 months is allowed to create a chronic bony defect (Fig 11-5 and Fig 11-6).

11.2.2 Selection of the Species

In general, female foxhounds (aged between 8 to 24 months and weighing between 25 and 30 kg) that have been bred for research are recommended. Younger animals heal more completely and at a faster rate than their adult counterparts, thus false high expectations of the biologics or devices can occur (Kleinschmidt and Hollinger, 1992). Smaller animals usually present with small jaws and teeth, and larger animals are difficult to manage postoperatively (Wikesjö et al., 1994).

11.2.3 Timing

Selection of appropriate time points to determine the therapeutic efficacy window of a candidate therapeutic is important (Pellegrini et al., 2009). The limitation of the canine model described above is that this is not a naturally occurring bony defect, but an experimentally induced bony defect. Thus, it is very important to delay vertical ridge augmentation procedure up to 3 months post defect creation to diminish spontaneous bone regeneration potential and to confirm the chronicity of the created defects.

11.2 Selection of an Appropriate Animal Model

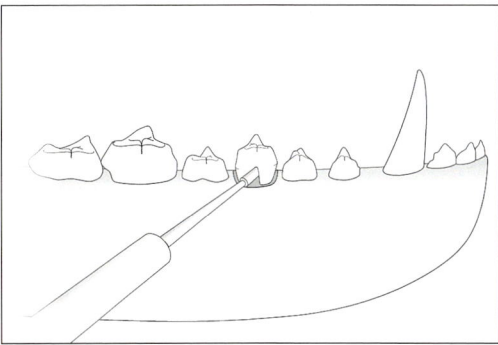

Fig 11-5 Schematic drawing of the canine mandible with the teeth present. The four premolars will be extracted to define the artificial defect.

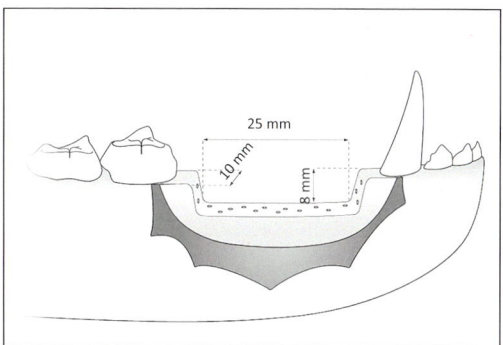

Fig 11-6 Schematic drawing of the created defect and its dimensions: 8 mm apicocoronally, 25 mm mesiodistally, and 10 mm buccolingually (the width of the canine mandible).

Longer healing times may cause the project to be very expensive due to prolonged animal care.

The appropriate healing time of the treated canine sites after the test procedure has been performed should be a minimum of 4 months. Schenk et al. (1994) have observed incomplete bone maturation and suggested a healing time of 5 months to be optimal.

11.2.4 Surgical Procedures – Selection of Appropriate Anesthesia

For premedication, ketamine hydrochloride (25 mg/kg) and atropine sulfate (0.04 to 0.05 mg/kg) can be used. Sodium pentothal (20 mg/kg) is given before intubation. The surgical procedure is similar to humans and a sterile technique should be used throughout the procedure. Consultation with a veterinarian is recommended to determine types and dosages of the medications.

11.2.5 Preparation – Determination and Creation of the Chronic Defect

The critical-size bone defect should be easy to produce and maintain and should be large enough to allow devices or biomaterials to be fitted. In order to simulate these defects, all four mandibular premolars should be removed (Fig 11-7) and the predetermined defect dimension should be outlined with a pencil to create identical defects in each animal. Then surgical reduction of the ridge height and width can be performed with a large round carbide bur (size # 8) in a high-speed handpiece or with an acrylic bur in a slow-speed handpiece. Water irrigation is crucial to reduce overheating of underlying bone.

The critical-size defect in mongrel dogs has been found to be 15 mm in length when the periosteum is removed and 50 mm when the periosteum is preserved (Huh et al., 2005). Thus, mandibular critical-size defect dimensions of 20 to 25 mm mesiodistally, 7 to 8 mm apicocoronally, and 10 mm buccolingually are adequate in the foxhound model (Fig 11-8). Removal or occlusal adjustment of maxillary teeth may be recommended to prevent trauma to the mandibular edentulous area testing underlying biologics. Primary wound closure must be achieved and sutures should be retained for 10 to 14 days.

11.2.6 Detailed Methodology and Surgical Procedure

A number of surgical procedures, devices, or biologics can be used to attempt vertical ridge augmentation. The rigid fixation of a grafting material is crucial to obtain maximal bone

Osteology Guidelines for Oral and Maxillofacial Regeneration

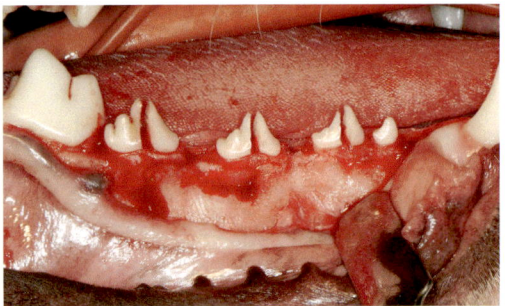

Fig 11-7 Clinical view of the canine mandible with teeth in place. A full thickness flap is elevated to create the osseous defect and allow tooth extraction. The four premolars are separated along their longitudinal axis and extracted.

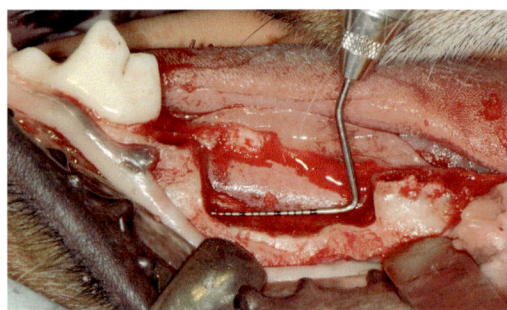

Fig 11-8 The surgical reduction of the ridge height and width is performed according to the defined measurements.

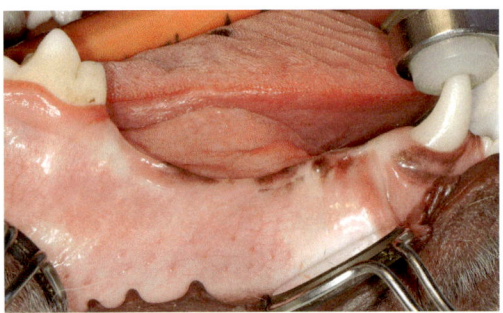

Fig 11-9 Clinical view of the canine mandible after tooth extraction and defect creation. Three months have passed and the main surgery may be performed at this time point.

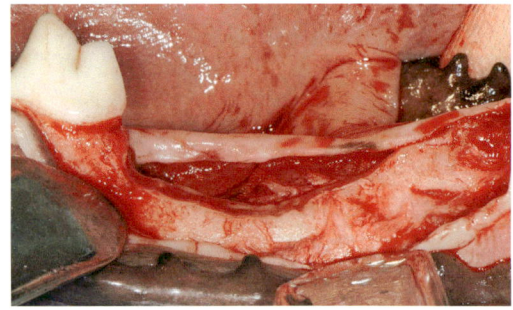

Fig 11-10 A full thickness mid-crestal incision is performed from the distal aspect of the cuspid to the mesial aspect of the molar. The flaps are elevated and the mandibular crest is exposed. The mandible appears atrophic with a flat bone defect.

regeneration. The first days of healing are critical for chemotaxis, differentiation, and proliferation of osteoclasts (Kleinschmidt and Hollinger, 1992). The following protocol has been successfully used to assess the vertical bone gain when applying a tissue engineered block graft to a mandibular chronic defect in a canine model.

A mid-crestal incision within the keratinized tissue is made from the mesial aspect of the canine to the distal aspect of the first molar. Full-thickness mucoperiosteal flaps are elevated on both buccal and lingual sides, and all soft tissue remnants are removed from the bone crest with a back-action chisel to prepare for the block placement (Fig 11-9 and Fig 11-10). Cortical perforations are made with a round carbide bur (size # 2) to provide an avenue for the progenitor cells to move in and for angiogenesis.

A pre-formed tissue-engineered block measuring 20 × 10 × 10 mm should be closely adapted to the alveolar crest and assembled with dental implants or screws. It is necessary to exercise extreme caution to avoid breaking the block. If the protocol includes the infusion of the growth factor, the block is placed in a sterile syringe

11.2 Selection of an Appropriate Animal Model

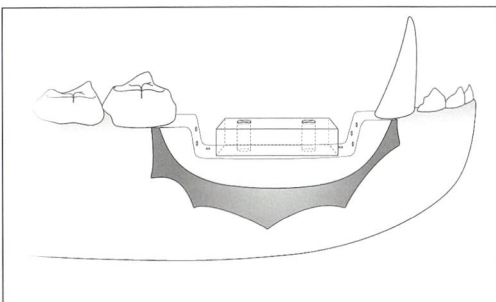

Fig 11-11 Schematic drawing of the canine mandible on reopening after defect creation (3 months). A three-dimensional block graft is positioned over the crest and stabilized by means of two titanium dental implants.

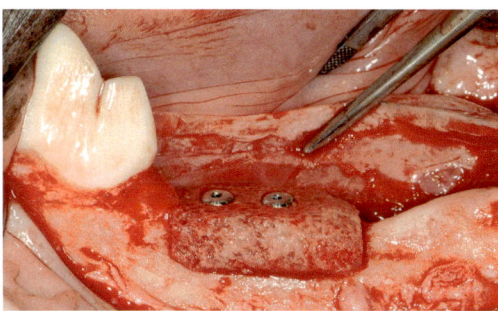

Fig 11-12 Clinical view of the block graft adapted to the atrophic bone crest and stabilized by means of two titanium dental implants. If the protocol involves the use of a growth factor, the latter is infused prior to positioning the block to the canine bone crest.

loaded with growth factor and infused under pressure for 5 minutes. The block is then adapted and stabilized to the alveolar crest by titanium implants or screws that penetrate both the block and the native mandibular cortical bone. The choice of the implant diameter and length will be dependent on the size of the block. Cover screws are placed for the implants (Fig 11-11 and Fig 11-12).

Depending on the protocol applied, a barrier membrane may be adapted (Fig 11-13). Flap management is a crucial factor for successful bone regeneration. A single periosteal incision is performed along the entire length of the buccal flap. The lingual flap may need to be coronally positioned. Both buccal and lingual flaps should be coronally positioned via partial thickness dissection to release tension and muscular pull. It should be done with care so not to perforate tissue. Primary tension-free wound closure can be achieved with a double line of sutures. Initially horizontal mattress sutures are placed to adapt the buccal and lingual connective tissue. The second line of interrupted sutures is performed to seal the buccal and lingual flaps on its most coronal portion (Fig 11-14 and Fig 11-15). The suturing is performed with nonresorbable sutures, which should be removed in 10 to 14 days.

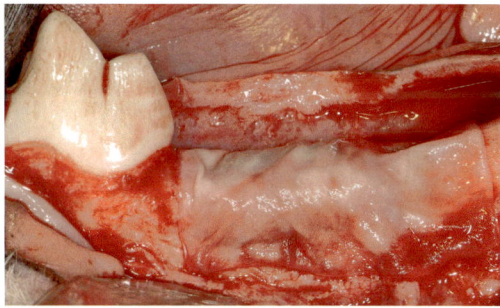

Fig 11-13 Clinical view of the block graft covered by a resorbable collagen membrane. The barrier completely covers the block and the surrounding tissues.

11.2.7 Postoperative Care and Sacrifice

Periapical radiographs are taken prior to and immediately following surgery. We have administered antimicrobial prophylaxis consisting of spiramycin 750 000 IU and metronidazole 125 mg one tablet/10 kg per day orally beginning at least 5 days before and continuing for at least 14 days after surgery. Consultation with a veterinarian is required for an appropriate choice of antibiotics and analgesics.

Oral hygiene is maintained with chlorhexidine digluconate wipes three times a week for 2 weeks. Animals should be kept on a soft diet

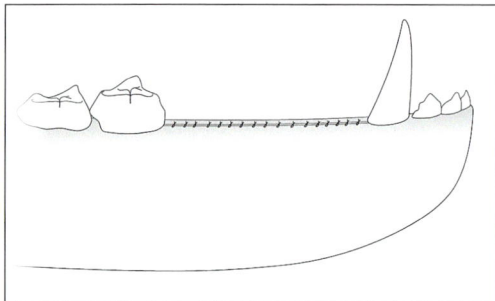 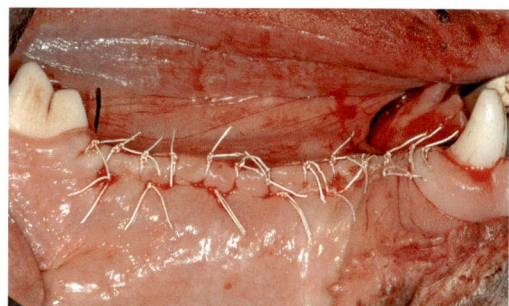

Fig 11-14 Schematic drawing of the tension-free suture. Two lines of sutures are performed, i.e., a horizontal mattress suture and interrupted sutures in the most coronal portion.

Fig 11-15 Clinical view of the flaps sutured after the augmentation procedure. A completely tension-free passive suture is mandatory to achieve successful healing. The two lines of sutures (horizontal mattress and interrupted coronal sutures) are clearly visible.

and water (*ad libitum*) to prevent food causing injury to the wound area. Surgical sites should be prevented from any mechanical trauma, thus careful inspection of the animal cage is important to reduce the risk of trauma to the jaw during the early healing phase.

Periapical radiographs and other necessary data collection should be obtained prior to euthanizing the animals. Animals can be euthanized by a lethal overdose of sodium phenobarbital or the association of 0.3 ml/kg embutane 200 mg, mebenzonium iodide 50 mg, and tetracaine HCl 5 mg intravenously.

11.2.8 Endpoint Measures – Assessment of Outcomes

Evaluation of the results often includes interpretation of clinical and radiographic findings. It is important to validate the outcome via definitive qualitative and quantitative analyses such as histologic and histomorphometric assessments that identify new bone formation, residual matrix, and connective tissue/marrow space. When implants are involved, it will also provide bone-to-implant contact of the area of the regenerated bone. The limitation of two-dimensional radiographic imaging is that it does not allow detailed descriptions of the healing process (Murphey et al., 1992). Bone graft failure can be assessed by the progressive resorption of the block or graft material by decrease in the size, and radiodensity of the graft material or increasing radiolucency around fixation screws. The applied graft may eventually disappear, with replacement by fibrous tissue (Murphey et al., 1992). Soft tissue swelling, host bone destruction, marginal irregularity, and increasing irregular and aggressive-appearing periosteal reaction are additional radiographic and clinical signs, suggesting infection (Murphey et al., 1992). The following analyses can be employed to assess the outcomes.

- **Micro-computed tomography** allows good information about the contour and position of the graft and its placement. Qualitative and quantitative analyses of the regenerated bone are possible in three dimensions (Fig 11-16).
- **Back-scattered electron microscopy** (BSE) is a powerful technique for investigating cancellous bone structure. Its main function is to offer information regarding the degree of mineralization of the tissue within individual trabeculae (Fig 11-17 and Fig 11-18). In addition, element analysis can be done to identify whether the regenerated bone is similar or

11.2 Selection of an Appropriate Animal Model

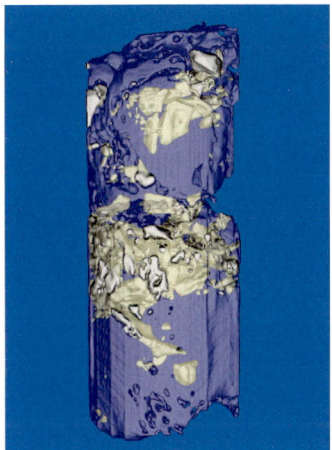

Fig 11-16 Micro-computed tomographic image of a bone core. The hard tissue volumes are clearly visible in this three-dimensional image. The blue portion represents all the newly regenerated bone and the gray portion represents the scaffold.

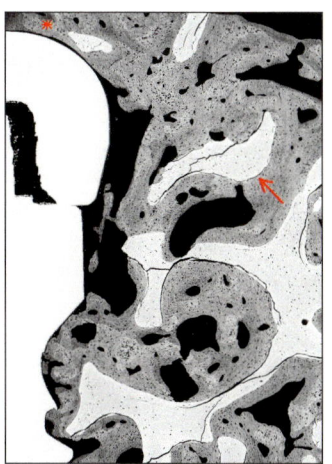

Fig 11-17 Back-scattered electron microscopic image of regenerated bone in proximity to an oxidized implant. The scaffold particles are clearly visible (arrow). Magnification ×106.

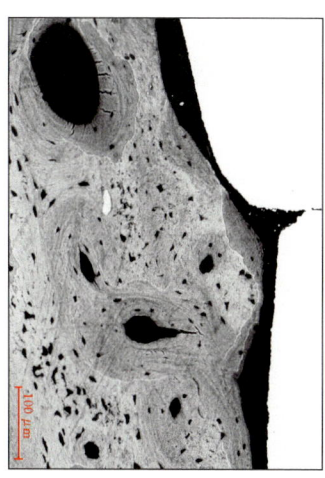

Fig 11-18 High magnification of a back-scattered electron microscopic image of reg enerated bone adjacent to a dental implant. Lacunae of osteocytes are visible and different degrees of mineralization are present in its internal portion. Magnification ×106.

identical to the native bone. The BSE imaging technique can be utilized to identify waves of new bone formations to illustrate the qualitative information (Rocchietta et al., 2007).

- **Histologic/histomorphometric evaluations.** The final biopsies can be embedded and prepared for conventional histologic investigations. Sections can be examined to identify the new bone, the residual graft particles, and the soft tissue (Fig 11-19 to Fig 11-24). Vital bone can be distinguished from nonvital grafted bone by the presence of nuclei in the lacunae of the bone samples. Histomorphometric parameters can include the amount of newly formed bone, remnant graft materials, connective tissue and height of the newly formed bone, and the amount of osseointegration. Histomorphometric analysis can be done by dividing the specific tissue area by the total sample area to calculate percentage of soft tissue, residual particle area, and new bone.

The number of animals in the investigation will determine the amount and variability of the differences in performing a power analysis. Data from the sample can be recorded for statistical analysis, but will be limited by sample size.

Histologic Preparation and Processing
Block sections are dissected free, fixed in 10% neutral buffered formalin, dehydrated and processed for light microscopy without demineralization. The blocks are embedded in Kulzer Technovit 7200 VLC-resin and sliced on an Exakt cutting unit (Exakt, Norderstedt, Germany). The slices are reduced using an Exakt grinding unit to an even thickness of 30 to 40 µm and stained with toluidine blue/pyronine G and examined with a Leica DM6000B light microscope (Leica, Glattbrugg, Switzerland). Ground sections are prepared in a mesiodistal direction.

Osteology Guidelines for Oral and Maxillofacial Regeneration

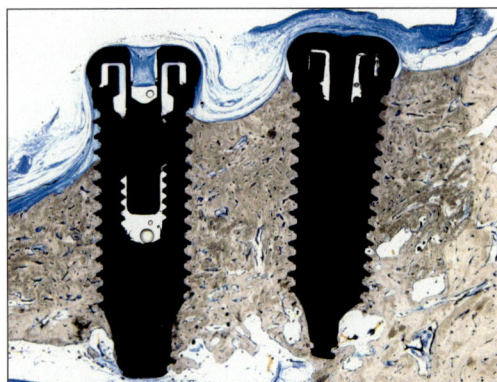

Fig 11-19 Histologic specimen of the vertical bone regeneration achieved using a tissue-engineered scaffold in the canine model (magnification ×8). The new bone, the residual graft particles, and the soft tissue can be identified.

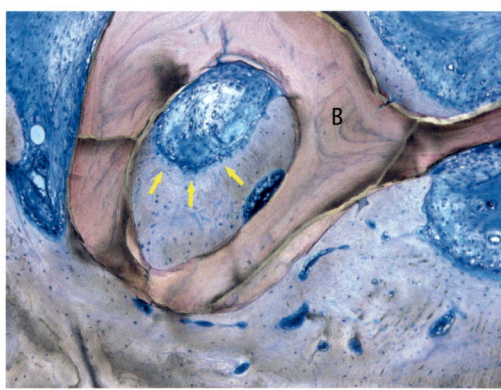

Fig 11-20 High magnification of a histologic specimen of regenerated bone and a scaffold. Ongoing bone formation is visible in the central portion of the scaffold (B). Note the lacunae in the central portion of the scaffold (arrows) filled with new bone and an osteoblast lining. Magnification ×160.

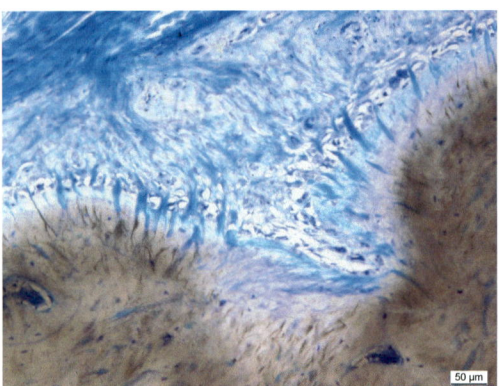

Fig 11-21 Higher magnification of the osteoblast lining in contact with the newly formed bone (magnification ×160).

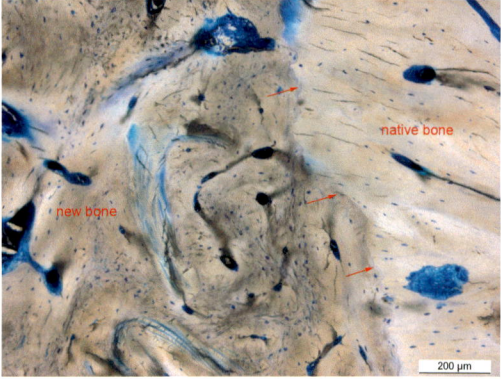

Fig 11-22 Light microscopic view of the border (arrows) between native bone and newly formed bone in an specimen with the scaffold infused with rhPDGF-BB without membrane (magnification ×160). Note the high remodeling activity in newly formed bone (ground section, toluidine blue).

11.2.9 Statistical Analysis Plan

The Mann-Whitney U test ($P < 0.05$) is used for statistical comparison of the histomorphometry results. The Wilcoxon signed rank test for paired samples is used to calculate statistical differences between the groups. Vertical bone height is compared between groups or structures and periods by two-way analysis of variance (ANOVA).

11.2.10 Materials and Consumables

The surgical instruments used to perform the above-mentioned canine study should be the same as utilized in the daily practice. Instruments must be sterile and in the operating room the animal should be prepared with sterile drapes in the same manner as for patients. All consumables to be tested (scaffold/barrier

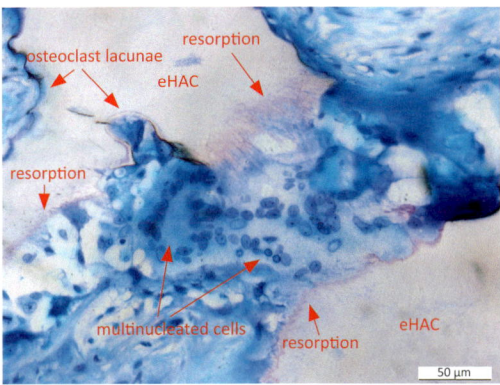

Fig 11-23 Light microscopic view of ongoing resorption phenomena in the scaffold (eHAC) particle areas (magnification ×160). Note the presence of multinucleated giant cells forming resorption seams, as well as osteoclastic activity resulting in osteoclastic lacunae (ground section, toluidine blue).

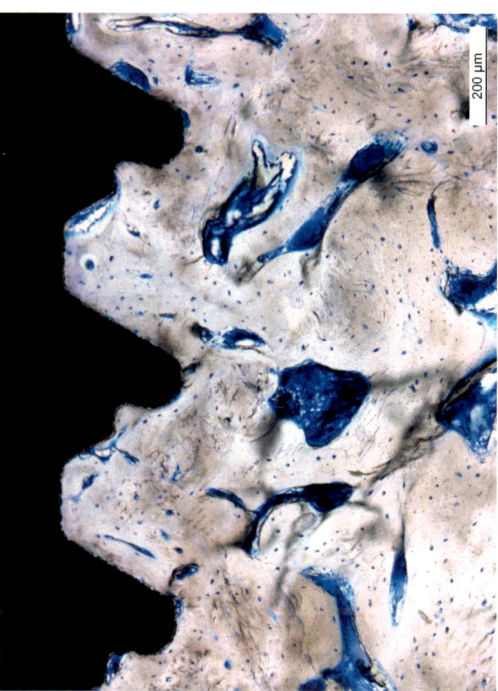

Fig 11-24 Light microscopic view of the osseointegration of an implant by newly formed woven bone (NB) formation in a scaffold (eHAC) specimen with rhPDGF-BB without membrane (magnification ×160). Note the high remodeling activity in woven bone (ground section, toluidine blue).

membrane or other) must be kept closed in their appropriate sterile packs until needed on the operating table, avoiding contamination. Sutures should be nonresorbable and preferably with low plaque retention.

11.3 Conclusion

The translations of vertical ridge augmentation techniques from preclinical models to clinical application have been possible due to innovative scientific advances and technological improvements (Simion et al., 2006, 2007a–c, 2008, 2009). The vertical ridge block augmentation technique described by Simion et al. is a novel method that allows in a single operation, the placement of both block and implant, and surgical morbidity can be reduced. The alternative is to place supra-alveolar implants and select graft material with or without growth factor and with or without a barrier membrane (Wikesjö et al., 1994).

Proper study design and clinical judgment can minimize or prevent trial and error from occurring in the initial application phase. Sometimes the data driven from the preclinical trials cannot be replicated in clinical trials due to high costs and ethical considerations. Thus, it is important to select a well-studied preclinical investigation that can be later replicated in human studies.

References

1. Caton J, Nyman S (1980). Histometric evaluation of periodontal surgery. I. The modified Widman flap procedure. *J Clin Periodontol* 7:212–223.
2. Caton J, Mota L, Gandini L, Laskaris B (1994a). Non-human primate models for testing the efficacy and safety of periodontal regeneration procedures. *J Periodontol* 65:1143–1150.
3. Cestari TM, Granjeiro JM, de Assis GF, Garlet GP, Taga R (2009). Bone repair and augmentation using block of sintered bovine-derived anorganic bone graft in cranial bone defect model. *Clin Oral Implants Res* 20:340–350.
4. Dahlin C, Gottlow J, Linde A, Nyman S (1990). Healing of maxillary and mandibular bone defects using a membrane technique. An experimental study in monkeys. *Scand J Plast Reconstr Surg Hand Surg* 24:13–19.
5. Freilich M, M Patel C, Wei M, Shafer D, Schleier P, Hortschansky P, Kompali R, Kuhn L (2008). Growth of new bone guided by implants in a murine calvarial model. *Bone* 43:781–788.
6. Froum SJ, Rosenberg ES, Elian N, Tarnow D, Cho SC (2008). Distraction osteogenesis for ridge augmentation: prevention and treatment of complications. Thirty case reports. *Int J Periodontics Restorative Dent* 28:337–345.
7. Giannoni P, Mastrogiacomo M, Alini M, Pearce SG, Corsi A, Santolini F et al. (2008). Regeneration of large bone defects in sheep using bone marrow stromal cells. *J Tissue Eng Regen Med* 2:253–262.
8. Gutwald R, Haberstroh J, Stricker A, Rüther E, Otto F, Xavier SP et al. (2010). Influence of rhBMP-2 on bone formation and osseointegration in different implant systems after sinus-floor elevation. An in vivo study on sheep. *J Craniomaxillofac Surg* 38:501–504.
9. Habal MB, Reddi AH (1992). Preface. In: Bone grafts and bone substitutes. Habal MB, Reddi AH, editors. Philadelphia: WB Sauders, pp. xv–xvi.
10. Huh JY, Choi BH, Kim BY, Lee SH, Zhu SJ, Jung JH (2005). Critical size defect in the canine mandible. *Oral Surg Oral Med Oral Pathol Oral Radiol Endod* 100:296–301.
11. Hunt DR, Jovanovic SA, Wikesjö UM, Wozney JM, Bernard GW (2001). Hyaluronan supports recombinant human bone morphogenetic protein-2 induced bone reconstruction of advanced alveolar ridge defects in dogs. A pilot study. *J Periodontol* 72:651–658.
12. Jensen OT, Greer RO Jr, Johnson L, Kassebaum D (1995). Vertical guided bone-graft augmentation in a new canine mandibular model. *Int J Oral Maxillofac Implants* 10:335–344.
13. Jensen OT, Cockrell R, Kuhike L, Reed C (2002). Anterior maxillary alveolar distraction osteogenesis: a prospective 5-year clinical study. *Int J Oral Maxillofac Implants* 17:52–68.
14. Jovanovic SA, Schenk RK, Orsini M, Kenney EB (1995). Supracrestal bone formation around dental implants: an experimental dog study. *Int J Oral Maxillofac Implants* 10:23–31.
15. Jovanovic SA, Hunt DR, Bernard GW, Spiekermann H, Wozney JM, Wikesjö UM (2007). Bone reconstruction following implantation of rhBMP-2 and guided bone regeneration in canine alveolar ridge defects. *Clin Oral Implants Res* 18:224–230.
16. Kerrigan CL, Zelt RG, Thomson JG, Diano E (1986). The pig as an experimental animal in plastic surgery research for the study of skin flaps, myocutaneous flaps and fasciocutaneous flaps. *Lab Anim Sci* 36(4):408–412.
17. Kleinschmidt JC, Hollinger JO (1992). Animal models in bone research. In: Bone grafts and bone substitutes. Habal MB, Reddi AH, editors. Philadelphia: WB Sauders, pp. 133–146.
18. Kon K, Shiota M, Ozeki M, Yamashita Y, Kasugai S (2009). Bone augmentation ability of autogenous bone graft particles with different sizes: a histological and microcomputed tomography study. *Clin Oral Implants Res* 20:1240–1246.
19. Kostopoulous L, Karring T (1994). Augmentation of the rat mandible using guided tissue regeneration. *Clin Oral Implants Res* 5:75–82.
20. Levin L, Nitzan D, Schwartz-Arad D (2007). Success of dental implants placed in intraoral block bone grafts. *J Periodontol* 78:18–21.
21. Lundgren D, Lundgren AK, Sennerby L, Nyman S (1995). Augmentation of intramembraneous bone beyond the skeletal envelope using an occlusive titanium barrier. An experimental study in the rabbit. *Clin Oral Implants Res* 6:67–72.
22. Mertz PM, Hebda PA, Eaglstein WH (1986). A porcine model for evaluation of epidermal wound healing. In: Swine in biomedical research, Vol 1. Tumbleson ME, editor. New York: Plenum Press, pp. 291–302.
23. Murphey MD, Sartoris DJ, Bramble JM (1992). Radiographic assessment of bone grafts. In: Bone grafts and bone substitutes. Habal MB, Reddi AH, editors. Philadelphia: WB Sauders, pp. 9–36.
24. Nevins M, Kirker-Head C, Nevins M, Wozney JA, Palmer R, Graham D (1996). Bone formation in the goat maxillary sinus induced by absorbable collagen sponge implants impregnated with recombinant human bone morphogenetic protein-2. *Int J Periodontics Restorative Dent* 16:8–19.
25. Nyman S (1991). Bone regeneration using the principle of guided tissue regeneration. *J Clin Periodontol* 18:494–498.
26. Pellegrini G, Seol YJ, Gruber R, Giannobile WV (2009). Pre-clinical models for oral and periodontal reconstructive therapies. *J Dent Res* 88:1065–1076.
27. Rocchietta I, Dellavia C, Nevins M, Simion M (2007). Bone regenerated via rhPDGF-bB and a deproteinized bovine bone matrix: backscattered electron microscopic element analysis. *Int J Periodontics Restorative Dent* 27:539–545.
28. Rothamel D, Schwarz F, Herten M, Ferrari D, Mischkowski RA, Sager M, Becker J (2009). Vertical ridge augmentation using xenogenous bone blocks: a histomorphometric study in dogs. *Int J Oral Maxillofac Implants* 24:243-50.

References

29. Ruehe B, Niehues S, Heberer S, Nelson K (2009). Miniature pigs as an animal model for implant research: bone regeneration in critical-size defects. *Oral Surg Oral Med Oral Pathol Oral Radiol Endod* 108:699–706.
30. Schenk RK, Buser D, Hardwick WR, Dahlin C (1994). Healing pattern of bone regeneration in membrane-protected defects: a histologic study in the canine mandible. *Int J Oral Maxillofac Implants* 9:13–29.
31. Selvig KA (1994). Discussion: animal models in reconstructive therapy. *J Periodontol* 65:1169–1172.
32. Shimazu C, Hara T, Kinuta Y, Moriya K, Maruo Y, Hanada S et al. (2006). Enhanced vertical alveolar bone augmentation by recombinant human bone morphogenetic protein-2 with a carrier in rats. *J Oral Rehabil* 33:609–618.
33. Simion M, Trisi P, Piattelli A (1994). Vertical ridge augmentation using a membrane technique associated with osseointegrated implants. *Int J Periodontics Restorative Dent* 14:496–511.
34. Simion M, Dahlin C, Blair K, Shenk R (1999). Effect of 3 different types of titanium reinforced e-PTFE membranes on bone regeneration in surgically created defects: A histological study in canine mandible. *Clin Oral Implants Res* 10:73–84.
35. Simion M, Rocchietta I, Kim D, Nevins M, Fiorellini J (2006). Vertical ridge augmentation by means of deproteinized bovine bone block and recombinant human platelet-derived growth factor-BB: a histologic study in a dog model. *Int J Periodontics Restorative Dent* 26:415–23.
36. Simion M, Dahlin C, Rocchietta I, Stavropoulos A, Sanchez R, Karring T (2007a). Vertical ridge augmentation with guided bone regeneration in association with dental implants: an experimental study in dogs. *Clin Oral Implants Res* 18:86–94.
37. Simion M, Fontana F, Rasperini G, Maiorana C (2007b). Vertical ridge augmentation by expanded-polytetrafluoroethylene membrane and a combination of intraoral autogenous bone graft and deproteinized anorganic bovine bone (Bio Oss). *Clin Oral Implants Res* 18:620–629.
38. Simion M, Rocchietta I, Dellavia C (2007c). Three-dimensional ridge augmentation with xenograft and recombinant human platelet-derived growth factor-BB in humans: report of two cases. *Int J Periodontics Restorative Dent* 27:109–115.
39. Simion M, Rocchietta I, Monforte M, Maschera E (2008). Three-dimensional alveolar bone reconstruction with a combination of recombinant human platelet-derived growth factor BB and guided bone regeneration: a case report. *Int J Periodontics Restorative Dent* 28:239–243.
40. Simion M, Nevins M, Rocchietta I, Fontana F, Maschera E, Schupbach P et al. (2009). Vertical ridge augmentation using an equine block infused with recombinant human platelet-derived growth factor-BB: a histologic study in a canine model. *Int J Periodontics Restorative Dent* 29:245–255.
41. Tamimi F, Torres J, Gbureck U, Lopez-Cabarcos E, Bassett DC, Alkhraisat MH et al. (2009). Craniofacial vertical bone augmentation: a comparison between 3D printed monolithic monetite blocks and autologous onlay grafts in the rabbit. *Biomaterials* 30:6318–6326.
42. Wikesjö UM, Kean CJ, Zimmerman GJ (1994). Periodontal repair in dogs: supraalveolar defect models for evaluation of safety and efficacy of periodontal reconstructive therapy. *J Periodontol* 65:1151–1157.
43. Wikesjö UM, Qahash M, Thomson RC, Cook AD, Rohrer MD, Wozney JM et al. (2004). rhBMP-2 significantly enhances guided bone regeneration. *Clin Oral Implants Res* 15:194–204.
44. Wikesjö UM, Susin C, Qahash M, Polimeni G, Leknes KN, Shanaman RH et al. (2006). The critical-size supraalveolar peri-implant defect model: characteristics and use. *Clin Periodontol* 33:846–854.
45. Wikesjö UM, Qahash M, Polimeni G, Susin C, Shanaman RH, Rohrer MD et al. (2008). Alveolar ridge augmentation using implants coated with recombinant human bone morphogenetic protein-2: histologic observations. *Clin Periodontol* 35:1001–1010.
46. Yukna RA (1976). A clinical and histologic study of healing following the excisional new attachment procedure in rhesus monkeys. *J Periodontol* 47:701–709.

CHAPTER 12

Sinus Floor Augmentation

K. Andreas Schlegel, Rainer Lutz, and Falk Wehrhan

12.1 General Overview

12.1.1 Maxillary Sinus

Maxillary sinus floor augmentations allow improvement of vertical bone height to achieve primary stability of endosseous implants in the severely resorbed posterior maxilla. This technique has been shown to be a safe technique with high predictability of success (Adell *et al.*, 1990; Hirsch and Ericsson, 1991; Smiler *et al.*, 1992; Raghoebar *et al.*, 1993; Blomqvist, 1998; Schlegel *et al.*, 2008). In humans, as well as in all other mammals, the maxillary sinus is a structure that grows with age. In humans the biggest dimension is found in the edentulous adult, with an approximate size of 15 cm^3. The maxilla normally extends from the second premolar area to the area of the wisdom teeth. On one hand, this explains the high rate of interest in this region as an augmentation area in order to place implants for the replacement of teeth lost in the main masticatory zone. On the other hand this already indicates one major problem in the choice of the animal model. In general, mammals are appropriate specimens since they all show similar anatomic features as humans. When using mammals it is mandatory to ensure the animals have achieved full growth prior to the experiment due to the above-mentioned fact, as the maxillary sinus is a structure which only exists as an anatomic landmark at the time of birth.

12.1.2 Choice of Animal

Anatomic Considerations
The animal model should have:
- Appropriate cortical thickness of the lateral wall (important for creating a bone window because of the resistance). A thin cortical bone is necessary because of two main reasons: the animal model is to be used in teaching, and so it has to be easy to reach the antrum; on the other hand, the cortical bone

is very thin in edentulous patients, even transparent under a transmitted light
- Similar morphology and resistance of the Schneiderian membrane to that in humans
- Ability for an oral approach.

Considering the third criterion, the number of animal models that can be used for research is quite easy to overview. It is only in the goat (see below for details), using some surgical dexterity, that the maxillary sinus can be accessed from the oral cavity and more importantly, that implants can be placed in the alveolar crest with the possibility of extending into the sinus and also the possibility of being loaded. Although one can find numerous articles on sinus lift in the literature, which claim to have used animal models and which describe the loading of implants placed in sinus, it will become clear on closer reading that instead of using the described maxillary sinus model the authors used nasal augmentation.

Biologic Considerations
Basically the choice of animal is frequently influenced by exogenous factors, such as the cost of acquiring and of care for animals, availability, tolerance to captivity and ease of housing, i.e., the kind of animal facility available, and the expertise and preference of the working group. Also the lifespan of the species chosen should be suitable for the duration of the study. Hazzard et al. (1992) commented that within a field of study, neither will a single animal model be appropriate for all purposes, nor can a model be dismissed as inappropriate for all purposes.

Furthermore, the selection of an appropriate animal test model with a high degree of biologic similarity to human bone repair is a prerequisite for the transferability of the experimental results to the clinical situation (Chapter 1). Briefly, one could say that the smaller a mammalian model, the harder it is to give predictable answers for the clinical applicability of the model in humans. Nevertheless, when starting testing of new biomaterials and/or indications one tends to go chronologically from *in vitro* testing models to small *in vivo* models, on to more specific models with a high degree of similarity to human biologic behavior. The established international standards regarding the species suitable for testing implantation of materials in bone, state that dogs, sheep, goats, pigs, and rabbits are suitable (International Standards Organization, 2007: ISO 10993-6:2007). As Pearce et al. (2007) quoted in their article "the rat is one of the most commonly used species in medical research, it will not be discussed here due to significant dissimilarities between rat and human bone and the limitations of size making rats unsuitable for testing multiple implants simultaneously". Table 12-1 summarizes the advantages and disadvantages of the different animal models.

Dog
The dog is one of the more frequently used large animal species for musculoskeletal and implant research. One of the most favored dog species in *in vivo* investigation of implants and bone substitution materials is Beagles.
- **Macrostructure**
  The bone exhibits a secondary osteon structure, which is also found in humans (Eitel et al., 1981).
- **Microstructure**
  Furthermore, both human and dog cortical and cancellous bone are similar in terms of water fraction, organic fraction, volatile inorganic fraction, and ash fraction (Gong et al., 1964). In terms of bone density the dog and pig most closely resemble the human situation (Aerssens et al., 1998). While there are structural similarities in trabecular bone turnover between dogs and humans, it is difficult to make an exact comparison of bone turnover between these species from the published data (Kimmel and Jee, 1982).
- **Sinus**
  Wetzel et al. (1995) and HJ Lee et al. (2007) performed sinus-floor augmentation on sev-

Table 12-1 Pros and cons of the different animal models

Quality of similarity Model	Bone macro-structure	Bone micro-structure	Bone remodeling	Time of remodeling	Anatomic location	De novo bone formation comparable to human findings
Dog						
Sinus augmentation	++	++	+++	++	++++	+++
Nasal augmentation	++	++	+++	++	+++++++	+++
Sheep	++++++	++++++	++++	+++	++	++++
Goat	+++++	+++++	+++++	++++	+++++++	++++
Pig						
Sinus augmentation	++++	++++	+++++++	+++++++	++	+++++++
Nasal augmentation	++++	++++	+++++++	+++++++	+++++++	+++++++
Forehead	++++	++++	+++++++	+++++++	+	+++++++
Minipig						
Sinus augmentation	++++	++++	+++++++	+++++++	++	+++++++
Nasal augmentation	++++	++++	+++++++	+++++++	+++++++	+++++++

+ least similar, +++++++ most similar.

eral dogs and reported that the sinus membranes were found to be intact (SH Lee et al., 2007). However, Haas et al. (1998a, b) have suggested that the Wetzel experiment is not comparable with sinus lift surgery in human subjects because the nasal sinus of dogs differs significantly from the human maxillary sinus in that it lacks the Schneiderian membrane and does not undergo pneumatization. These reasons and other ethical and economic reasons confer a secondary role to the dog as a model in this technique.

Sheep
The sheep is a commonly used animal model and has proven its suitability for experimental research on fracture healing.

- **Macrostructure**
The primary bone healing and the remodeling of the Haversian system of the sheep have already been described extensively (Nunamaker, 1998). For orthopedic research on long bones of the lower extremity the sheep is a useful animal model since the tibia is practically in the same carrying axle compared with humans.
- **Microstructure**
Sheep bone shows a significantly higher density and subsequently greater strength than humans. In a study on trabecular bone density it was found that the density of sheep bone was 1.5 to 2 times greater than that of humans (Turner et al., 2001; Liebschner, 2004). On the other hand, the sheep seems

to be a valuable animal model for osteoporosis research since the bone volume, osteoid volume, and mineral apposition rates of 9- to 10-year-old ewes are comparable with those of men and post-menopausal women in their sixth to seventh decade of life.

- **Sinus**

  The sheep is a useful animal model because the general nasal anatomy – the paranasal sinus anatomy – is similar to humans in appearance and orientation (Brumund et al., 2004). The approach to the maxillary sinus in sheep from the buccal vestibule requires prior surgical preparation because of the small size of the mouth, which just allows reaching the first molar. Releasing and elevating the Schneiderian membrane from the sinus floor is relatively easy (Estaca et al., 2008).

Goat

Goats are a popular large animal model because they can be easily obtained and bred, and exhibit minimal genetic variation. In comparison with sheep, goats tend to have a more inquisitive and interactive nature which may make confinement for long durations more challenging. However, in certain regions such as Southeast Asia, where the temperatures and humidity are often high, goats are reported to be more tolerant to ambient conditions than other species such as sheep (Leung et al., 2001).

- **Macrostructure**

  Goats have a body size suitable for the implantation of multiple implants per goat or of larger, human implants and prostheses (Anderson et al., 1999; van der Donk et al., 2001).

- **Microstructure**

  Goat bones do not have uniformly dispersed Haversian systems. Similar to the sheep, where the Haversian systems are nonuniformly distributed throughout the individual bones, in the goat bone, the Haversian systems are located primarily in the cranial, cranio-lateral, and medial sectors of the tibial diaphysis, while the caudal sector mainly consists of lamellar bone (where the collagen fibers are arranged in sheets and do not contain a central blood vessel) (Qin et al., 1999).

- **Sinus**

  The maxillary sinus of a goat is similar to that of humans:

  – It pneumatizes the entire maxilla

  – It is situated superior to the alveolar process and inferior to the orbital floor, extending laterally to the lateral wall of the maxilla and protruding into the palatine bone bilaterally.

  – The diameter of the goat infraorbital canal, however, is about 3 to 6 mm, and the sinus lateral floor still has enough width for maxillary sinus augmentation with implant placement through the maxillary alveolar process in this model. There is enough space in the lateral floor of the maxillary sinus for dental implantation, and the third premolar area might be a suitable position suggested for maxillary sinus augmentation with simultaneous implant placement in a goat model (Derong et al., 2010).

  – The goat maxillary sinus is similar to that in humans, with a slender pyramidal shape that pneumatizes the entire maxilla, and a sinus wall covered with a mucosal lining. The maxillary sinus floor increases towards the posterior area, where the maxillary sinus floor is close to the related teeth roots. A goat model is considered one of the suitable larger animal models for sinus elevation studies, as the size and the morphologic anatomy of the goat sinus as well as bone physiology and structure are similar to that in humans (Kirker-Head et al., 1997; Grageda et al., 2005).

Pig

Remodeling processes in porcine bone are similar to those in humans, comprising both trabecular and intracortical bone metabolic unit (BMU)-based remodeling (Laiblin and Jaeschke, 1979; Mosekilde and Danielsen, 1987; Mosekilde, 1993). Studies on the effects of fluoride on cortical bone remodeling in growing pigs showed that control animals have a similar cortical bone mineralization rate to that in humans (Kragstrup et al., 1989).

- **Macrostructure**
  The pig seems to be a desirable animal for the investigation of vascular disease and bone formation as well as the biologic behavior of bone substitution materials (BSMs) and dental implants due to its advantages in comparative experimental medicine. In addition, it has already been recognized as a valuable model in biomedical research because of its anatomic, physiologic, and metabolic similarities with humans (Beddoe, 1978; Laiblin and Jaeschke, 1979; Eitel et al., 1981; Swindle et al., 1988).

- **Microstructure**
  The pig has also become a popular animal model in investigations of the mechanisms underlying bone formation (Schlegel et al., 2006a). The rate of bone regeneration (1.2 to 1.5 mm per day) is comparable with that of humans (1.0 to 1.5 mm per day); that is, closest to the clinical situation in comparison to all other animal models (Laiblin and Jaeschke, 1979; Aerssens et al., 1998). The domestic pig has already proven its suitability for the testing of medical implants, BSM as well as conventional, and biologically active coatings for implants (Schlegel et al., 2006b; Park et al., 2007).

Schlegel et al. (2009) compared bone regeneration in a porcine experimental forehead model with the clinical outcome in humans after application of autogenous bone and two different bone substitutes in the maxillary sinus. Their results clearly demonstrated that the porcine morphologic and anatomic bone characteristics yield results which are comparable with humans

- **Sinus**
  The porcine cortical bone is very dense and difficult to trephine. In pigs, the maxillary sinus is located caudally, even within the zygomatic bone in adult animals. It is also a smaller cavity compared with that in sheep and goats. For the pig model, the implants cannot be inserted from the alveolar process because the infraorbital nerve canal, which is approximately 9 mm in diameter, is interposed between the process and the sinus (Fig 12-1) (Terheyden et al., 1999).

Minipigs
Minipigs were first used as experimental models (Honig and Merten, 1993). These authors found the minipigs to be quite similar to humans in terms of platelet count, clotting parameters, and long bone structure. The structure of maxillary bone is also reported to be quite similar to that in humans (Buser et al., 1998). The minipig sinus is pneumatized with comparable shape and size to humans, and the Schneiderian membrane is also thin. Minipigs also are not eligible for implant placement other than through the facial sinus wall, because the course of the infraorbital nerve does not permit implant insertion via an intraoral access (Terheyden et al., 1999).

12.1.3 Summary
From the present knowledge it can be stated that no animal model fulfills the ideal experimental setting. The choice of the model will depend on the experimental design of the *in vivo* study and the defined research question.

12.2 Animal Model – Sheep

12.2.1 Aim of the Sheep Model
The anatomic features of the sheep make an intraoral approach difficult, unless the mouth is enlarged surgically by an incision at the angle of the mouth. Therefore the *in vivo* trials available are restricted to an extraoral approach to the maxillary sinus, via an infraorbital incision

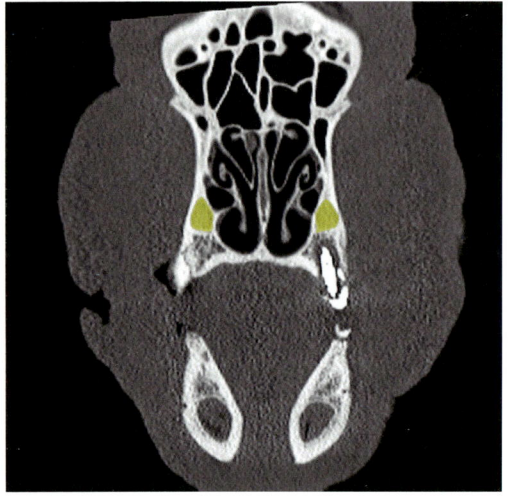
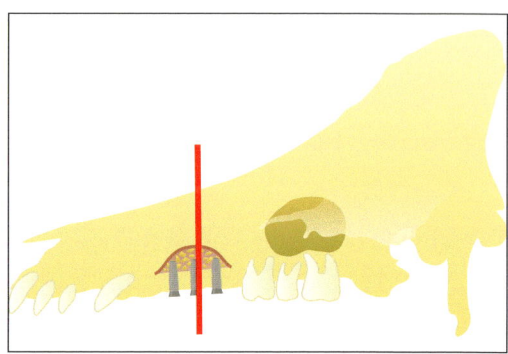
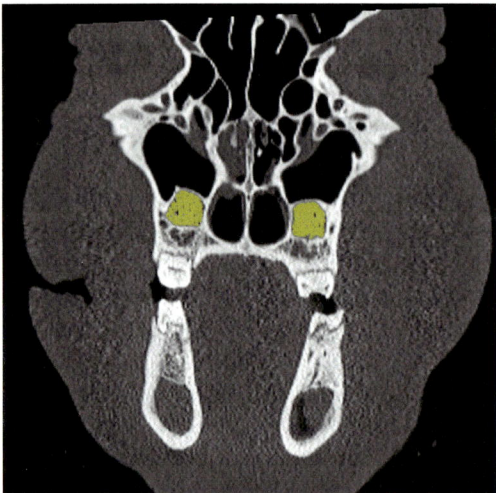
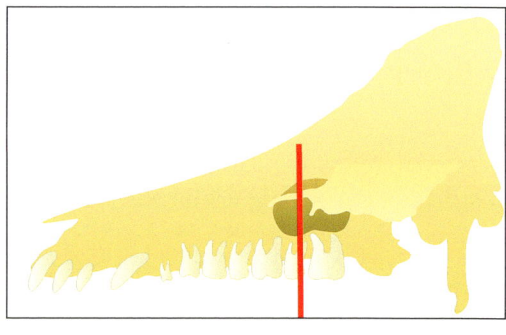

Fig 12-1 CT image of minipig showing the position of the infraorbital nerve bundle (yellow). Right panel shows the position of the sagittal slice.

without communication with the oral cavity. The indication which can be simulated in this animal model is augmentation of the maxillary sinus with autogenous bone or bone substitutes. Implants can be inserted simultaneously with augmentation or at second-stage surgery and heal without loading. Table 12-2 displays a summary of the sheep model for sinus elevation.

12.2.2 Advantages/Disadvantages of the Sheep Model

The sheep model is a large animal model, which shows similar bone regeneration to humans. The maxillary sinus has an adequate size to be augmented.

The location and anatomy of the maxillary sinus favors an extraoral approach, which limits the model as it cannot then be used for testing

Table 12-2 Overview of the sheep animal model for sinus elevation

Breed	Approach	Extraction of teeth (healing period)	Implants inserted	Unloaded vs. loaded implants	Characteristics	Reference
Mountain sheep	Extraoral	–	Simultaneously with sinus elevation	–	Location of the maxillary sinus in sheep, with a small mediodorsal and a large ventrolateral part, favors an extraoral surgical approach (Estaca et al., 2008)	Haas et al., 1998a,b, 2002a,b,c, 2003
Western sheep	Extraoral	–	–	–		Grageda et al., 2005
Traditional Sheep	Extraoral		6 months after augmentation	–		Saffarzadeh et al., 2009
	Extraoral	–	Simultaneously with sinus elevation	–	Maxillary sinus has an adequate size to be augmented	Gutwald et al., 2010a,b
	Extraoral	–	–	–	Inserted implants have no correlation to the oral cavity and cannot be loaded functionally	Jakse et al., 2003

functionally loaded implants in the augmented area (Grageda et al., 2005).

12.2.3 Timing

Figure 12-2 gives an overview of timing of the procedures for the sheep model.

12.2.4 Surgical Procedures

To visualize the surgical landmarks (angular vein of the eye and transverse artery of the face) the infraorbital skin of the sheep is shaved (Grageda et al., 2005).

The surgical site is prepared with iodine and the incision line is located and marked with a sterile pencil (Fig 12-3). Local anesthetic (e.g., Polocaine 2%, 1:20,000 or Ultracain (R) D-S forte 1:100,000) is administered in the surgical site. Then an oblique caudodorsal, rostroventral, or a paramedian sagittal extraoral incision, approximately 5 to 6 cm in length, is made over the most ventral aspect of the maxillary sinus. The subcutaneous tissue is divided and one-third of the masseter muscle is detached to expose the maxillary periosteum, which is incised and elevated dorsally. A bone window (sized 1 × 1 cm to 5 × 1.5 cm) is created at the lateral wall of the sinus under copious irrigation with saline solution. The antrum window is removed by fracturing along the osteotomy with a chisel. The antral membrane is elevated from the buccal bony wall and displaced dorsocranially with variably bent blunt dissectors. Care is taken during this procedure to avoid damage to the sinus membrane. The sinus is augmented with autogenous bone or bone substitutes. Implants can be inserted simultaneously or after the healing of the augmented area, in a second surgical approach with the same type of incision. The masseter muscle and skin flap are reapproximated in a simple continu-

Osteology Guidelines for Oral and Maxillofacial Regeneration

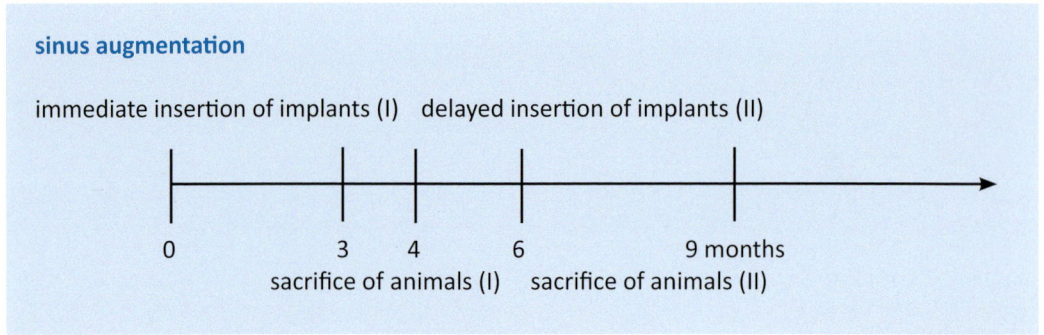

Fig 12-2 Overview of timing of the procedures in the sheep model.

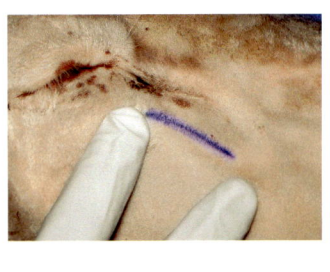
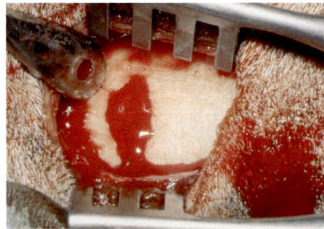
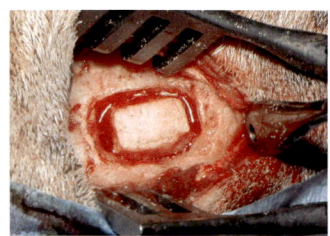
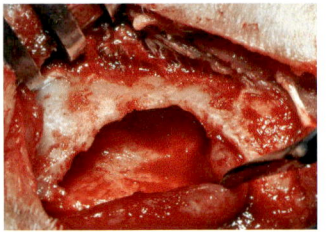
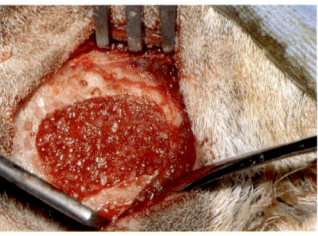

Fig 12-3 (a–e) Elevation of the maxillary sinus in the sheep model. Reproduced from Grageda et al. (2005) with permission from Allen Press.

ous pattern. Subcutaneous tissue and the skin are also sutured separately with 3-0 Vicryl (Haas et al., 1998a; Grageda et al., 2005; Saffarzadeh et al., 2009).

12.2.5 Preparation

The surgical procedures were performed under general anesthesia induced by diazepam, 1 mg/kg, and ketamine, 8 mg/kg, followed by intubation and supply of halothane or isoflurane.

During surgery, the sheep can receive 1 g amoxicillin intravenously to prevent perioperative infections (Haas et al., 1998a; Grageda et al., 2005; Saffarzadeh et al., 2009).

12.2.6 Detailed Methodology

To guarantee a clear allocation of the animals and specimens to the experimental groups, the animals additionally can be marked with a transponder (e.g., Alvic® complete, Alvetra, Neumünster, Germany), which is fixed in the bone or soft tissue structure beside the augmented area.

12.2.7 Postoperative Care

To avoid postoperative inflammation, the animals are administered amoxicillin (2 g/day) for 5 days postoperatively (Saffarzadeh et al., 2009). Due to the extraoral approach no special diet is required (Haas et al., 1998a).

12.3 Animal Model – Dog

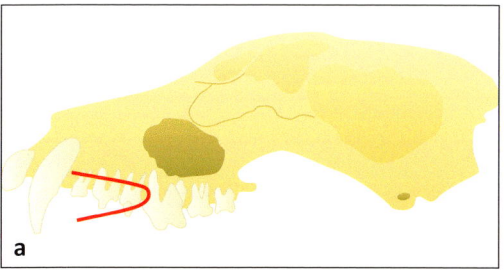
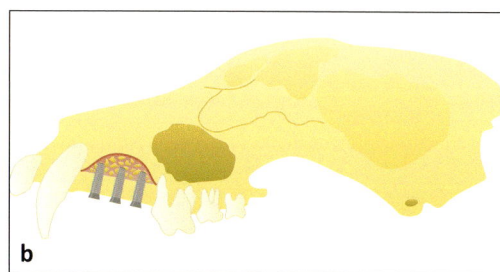
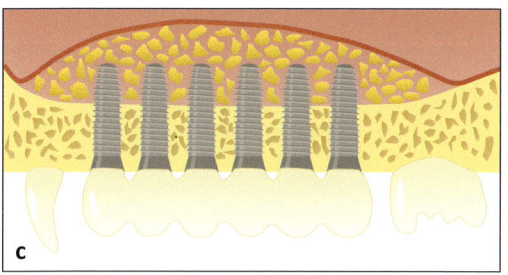
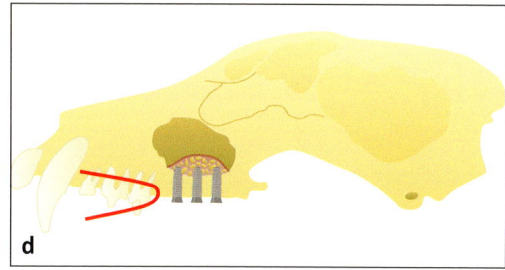

Fig 12-4 Schematic drawing of an adult dog skull indicating the position of **(a)** the lip angle, **(b)** a nasal augmentation **(c)** close-up of a nasal augmentation, and **(d)** the possible sinus augmentation (requires a temporary cheek incision).

12.3 Animal Model – Dog

12.3.1 Aim of the Dog Model
The dog model allows an intraoral approach for sinus elevation (Fig 12-4) and thus good simulation of sinus augmentation. Additionally, there is the possibility of functional loading of the inserted implants. Table 12-3 displays a summary of the dog model for sinus elevation.

12.3.2 Advantages/Disadvantages of the Dog Model
The posterior location of the maxillary sinus makes the intraoral surgical approach more difficult compared with humans, and due to the anatomic configuration not more than two implants can be inserted.

12.3.3 Timing
Figure 12-5 gives an overview of timing of the procedures for the dog model.

12.3.4 Surgical Procedures
After extraction of the maxillary premolars and molars (see Table 12-3), the alveolar ridges are allowed to heal between 42 and 180 days. The access to maxillary sinus is performed by a crestal incision in the edentulous region, accompanied by a mesial releasing incision. A full thickness mucoperiosteal flap is prepared extending from the first maxillary premolar to the second maxillary molar (Fig 12-4). With a round bur or a Lindemann bur a bony window (1 × 1 cm to 1 × 2 cm) is created, taking care to avoid perforation of the antral membrane. The sinus is augmented with autogenous bone or bone substitutes. The implants can be inserted simultaneously with augmentation. The remaining cortical bone allows insertion with primary stability (Wetzel *et al.*, 1995; Schlegel *et al.*, 2003; HJ Lee *et al.*, 2007; SH Lee *et al.*, 2007; Sul *et al.*, 2008a,b).

12.3.5 Preparation
The surgical procedures are performed under systemic anesthesia with ketamine (5 mg/kg)

Table 12-3 Overview of the canine animal model for sinus elevation

Breed	Approach	Extraction of teeth (healing period)	Implants inserted	Unloaded vs. loaded implants	Characteristics	Reference
Beagle dogs	Intraoral	P3, M1 (180 days)	Simultaneously with sinus elevation	Unloaded	Elevation of maxillary sinus	Wetzel et al., 1995
	Intraoral	P1, P2, P3 (42 days)	Simultaneously with sinus elevation	Unloaded	Elevation of the nasal floor	Schlegel et al., 2003
	Intraoral	Maxillary posterior teeth (56 days)	–	–	Elevation of maxillary sinus	Wang et al., 2010
Mongrel dogs	Intraoral	Maxillary premolars and molars (90 days)	Simultaneously with sinus elevation	Unloaded	Elevation of maxillary sinus	HJ Lee et al., 2007; SH Lee et al., 2007; Sul et al., 2008a,b; Kim et al., 2010

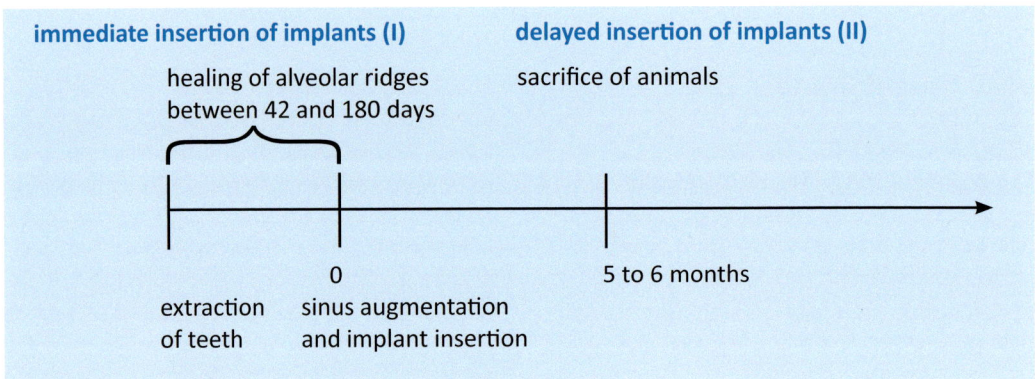

Fig 12-5 Overview of timing of the procedures in the dog model.

and xylazine (2 mg/kg) intramuscularly (HJ Lee et al., 2007; SH Lee et al., 2007; Sul et al., 2008a,b).

12.3.6 Detailed Methodology

Before insertion of the dental implants the bone of the maxillary sinus floor can be reduced to a thickness of 5 mm for standardization (HJ Lee et al., 2007; SH Lee et al., 2007; Sul et al., 2008a,b).

12.3.7 Postoperative Care

To avoid postoperative inflammation, the animals are administered penicillin for 5 days postoperatively; the animals receive professional oral hygiene treatment of tooth brushing, and local application of chlorhexidine gel (Wetzel et al., 1995). Postoperative analgesic treatment can consist of buprenorphine (Schlegel et al., 2003).

Table 12-4 Overview of the goat animal model for sinus elevation

Breed	Approach	Extraction of teeth (healing period)	Implants inserted	Unloaded vs. loaded implants	Characteristics	Reference
Chaanene goats	Extraoral	–	–	–	Location of the maxillary sinus in goat, with a small mediodorsal and a large venterolateral region, favors an extraoral surgical approach	Bravetti et al., 1998
Alpine-saanen goats	Extraoral	–	–	–		Nevins et al., 1996

12.4 Animal Model – Goat

12.4.1 Aim of the Goat Model

The anatomic situation of the goat is similar to sheep. Therefore, the *in vivo* studies available are restricted to an extraoral approach to the maxillary sinus by an infraorbital incision without correlation to the oral cavity. The indication which can be simulated in this animal model is the augmentation of the maxillary sinus with autogenous bone or bone substitutes. Implants can be inserted simultaneously with augmentation or at second-stage surgery and heal without loading. Table 12-4 displays a summary of the goat model for sinus elevation.

12.4.2 Advantages/Disadvantages of the Goat Model

The size and the morphologic anatomy of the goat sinus, as well as the bone physiology and structure are similar to humans. The location and anatomy of the maxillary sinus favor an extraoral approach, which limits the model, as it cannot be used for testing functionally loaded implants in the augmented area (Grageda *et al.*, 2005).

12.4.3 Timing

Figure 12-6 gives an overview of timing of the procedures for the goat model.

12.4.4 Surgical Procedures

After shaving the skin, the extraoral access to the maxillary sinus is performed orientating on the following landmarks: the angular vein of the eye, the transverse artery of the face, and a hypothetical line passing through the external angle of the eye (Fig 12-7) (Bravetti *et al.*, 1998). A horizontal incision at its posterior is supplemented by a vertical incision following the maxilla to the zygoma arch. Then a full thickness mucoperiosteal flap is raised, and the lateral wall of the maxillary sinus fully exposed. With a Lindemann bur a rectangular bony window is created (Fig 12-7). The sinus is augmented with autogenous bone or bone substitutes. Implants can be inserted simultaneously, or after the healing of the augmented area in a second surgical approach with the same type of incision. Subcutaneous tissue and the skin are also sutured separately with 3-0 Vicryl (Bravetti *et al.*, 1998).

12.4.5 Preparation

Surgery is performed under general anesthesia. The goats are therefore anesthetized by an injection of ketamine (2.5 mg/kg) in the jugular (Bravetti *et al.*, 1998).

12.4.6 Postoperative Care

Postoperatively, to prevent infections the animals are given subcutaneous injections of a mixture of benzylpenicillin-procaine (5 Um/d)

Osteology Guidelines for Oral and Maxillofacial Regeneration

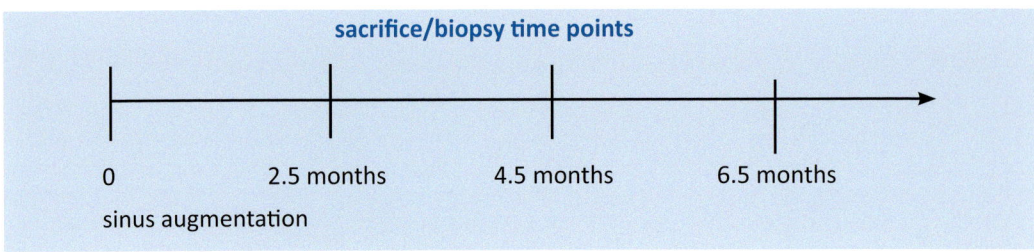

Fig 12-6 Overview of timing of the procedures in the goat model.

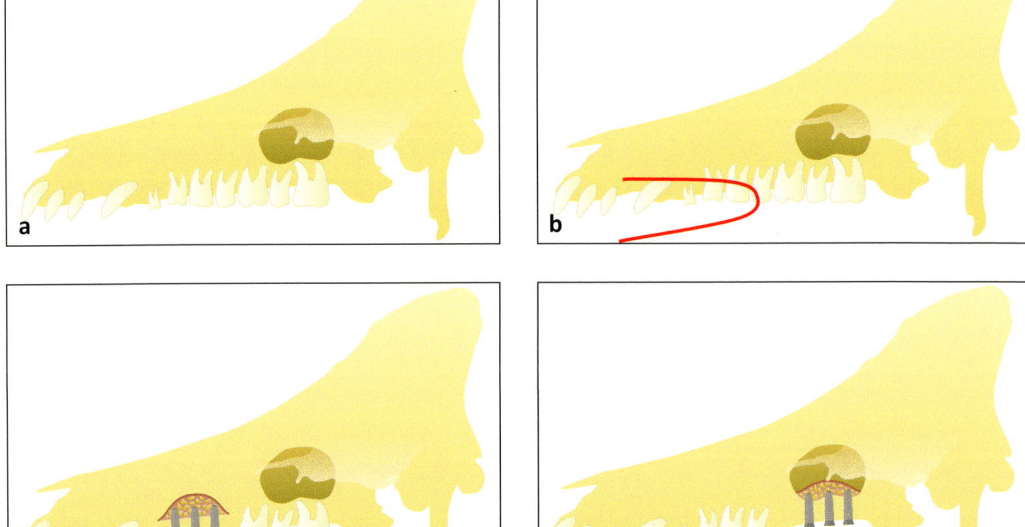

Fig 12-7 Schematic drawing of an adult pig skull indicating the position of **(a)** the maxillary sinus, **(b)** the lip angle, **(c)** a nasal augmentation, and **(d)** the possible sinus augmentation (requires a temporary cheek incision).

and dihydrostreptomycin (5 g/d) and ketoprofen (4 mg/kg) for postoperative pain management for 10 days (Bravetti *et al.*, 1998).

12.5 Animal Model – Pig/Minipig

12.5.1 Aim

The minipig has similar bone regeneration rates to humans. Sinus augmentation can be performed with an extraoral approach, in combination with the insertion of dental implants. Thus the minipig model allows testing new materials for augmentation and the parameters of osseointegration for unloaded implants. Another approach is to test the materials in defects of the pig's calvaria, which has been shown to have bone regeneration and material degradation rates comparable with human sinus augmentation (Schlegel *et al.*, 2009). Table 12-5 displays a summary of the pig/minipig model for sinus elevation.

12.5 Animal Model – Pig/Minipig

Table 12-5 Overview of the minipig/pig animal model for sinus elevation

Breed	Approach	Extraction of teeth (healing period)	Implants inserted	Unloaded vs. loaded implants	Characteristics	Reference
Goettingen minipigs	Intraoral	P2, P3, P4 (60 days)	Simultaneously with sinus elevation	Unloaded and loaded	Maxillary sinus is located within the maxilla and zygomatic bones	Klongnoi et al., 2006a,b; Schlegel et al., 2007a
	Intraoral	P2, P3, P4, M1, M2 on one side (90 days)	Simultaneously with sinus elevation	Unloaded and loaded		Nkenke et al., 2005; Fenner et al., 2009a,b
	Extraoral	–	–	–	Due to the infraorbital nerve an intraoral approach is not possible	Pieri et al., 2008
	Extraoral	–	Simultaneously with sinus elevation	Unloaded	The intraoral approaches presented here are elevations of the nasal floor	Terheyden et al., 1999; Roldan et al., 2004, 2008; Gruber et al., 2008, 2009; Liu et al., 2008
Domestic pigs	Frontal bone	–	–	–	Alternative model, study compares results with sinus augmentation in humans	Schlegel et al., 2009

12.5.2 Advantages/Disadvantages of the Pig/Minipig Model

The anatomic situation of the minipig (Fig 12-1) with the interposition of the infraorbital nerve between the alveolar ridge and the maxillary sinus makes an intraoral approach for sinus elevation impossible. However, there are the alternatives involving an extraoral approach (Table 12-5) or the elevation of the nasal floor. An extraoral approach has the advantage of better access, as the implants are not at risk of becoming infected with the bacteria of the oral cavity and there is no risk of losing implants due to inadequate loading (Terheyden et al., 1999; Roldan et al., 2004; Gruber et al., 2008, 2009; Liu et al., 2008; Pieri et al., 2008; Roldan et al., 2008).

In the intraoral approach, which allows loading of the implants, the nasal floor is elevated instead of the maxillary sinus (Nkenke et al., 2005; Klongnoi et al., 2006a,b; Schlegel et al., 2007a; Fenner et al., 2009a,b). In both cases implants can be inserted simultaneously with augmentation or at a second-stage surgery.

12.5.3 Timing

Figure 12-9 gives an overview of timing of the procedures for the pig/minipig model.

12.5.4 Surgical Procedures

Intraoral Approach

Before performing nasal floor elevation the maxillary premolars are extracted and the

Osteology Guidelines for Oral and Maxillofacial Regeneration

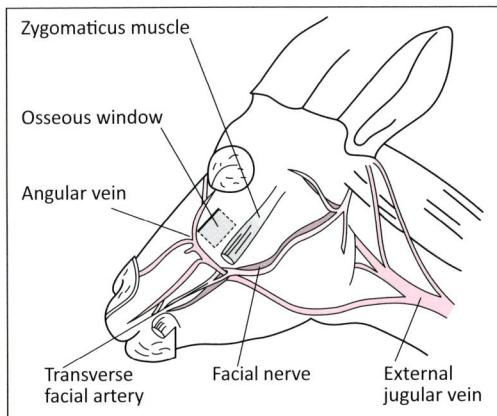

Fig 12-8 Location of osteotomies in the goat model. Reproduced from Bravetti et al. (1998) with permission.

alveolar ridges are allowed to heal for 60 days. In the area of the extracted teeth the facial antral wall is exposed by a crestal incision with a mesial relaxing incision. A bony window (3.5 cm × 1 cm) is created with a Lindemann bur. The nasal membrane is carefully elevated with bent dissectors. The sinus is augmented with autogenous bone or bone substitutes. Implants can be inserted simultaneously or after the healing of the augmented area in a second surgical approach (Nkenke et al., 2005; Klongnoi et al., 2006a,b; Schlegel et al., 2007a; Fenner et al., 2009a,b).

Extraoral Approach

The facial maxillary sinus wall is exposed through a 5 cm long sagittal skin incision below the lower lid, followed by a subperiosteal preparation of the facial maxillary bone, the crista zygomaticoalveolaris and the malar prominence. Access to the sinus is achieved by thinning the facial wall with a diamond bur. The membrane within the sinus is elevated carefully below the malar prominence using blunt elevators to avoid perforations. The sinus is augmented with autogenous bone or a bone substitute material. Afterwards a dental implant can then be inserted in latero-cranial direction. To approximate the clinical situation the malar bone is reduced to a height of 5 mm (Terheyden et al., 1999; Roldan et al., 2004, 2008; Gruber et al., 2008, 2009; Liu et al., 2008; Pieri et al., 2008)

12.5.5 Preparation

All surgical interventions are performed under general anesthesia. Anesthesia is induced with azaperone (5 mg/kg intramuscularly) and thiopental (7 mg/kg intravenously) and maintained with gaseous anesthesia (4% by volume halothane) after intubation with an endotracheal tube with a cuff.

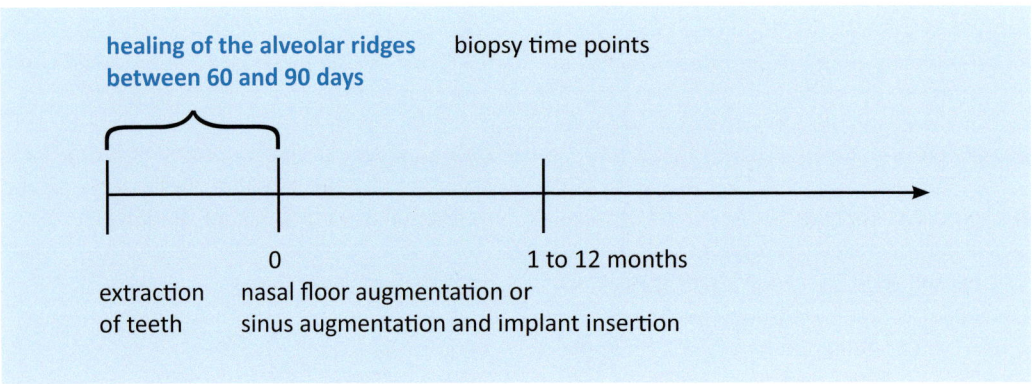

Fig 12-9 Overview of timing of the procedures in the pig/minipig model.

12.5.6 Detailed Methodology

Perforation of the Sinus Membrane
When a perforation of the nasal membrane or maxillary sinus membrane occurs, a bovine collagen sponge is applied to cover the perforation (Nkenke *et al.*, 2005; Klongnoi *et al.*, 2006a,b; Schlegel *et al.*, 2007a; Fenner *et al.*, 2009a,b).

12.5.7 Postoperative Care

To prevent postoperative infections, streptomycin 0.5 g/kg/day (I) is administered. Analgesic treatment involves administration of buprenorphine (0.3 mg/day subcutaneously) for the first three postoperative days. In the intraoral approach the animals receive a liquid diet during the first week after the surgical procedures.

12.5.8 Endpoint Measurements

Assessment of bone regeneration in critical-size defects comprises traditional two-dimensional radiographic evaluations and three-dimensional methods of computed tomography (CT) to address bone density, shape, and continuity during the maturation process. Sophisticated imaging methods of micro-CT and *in vivo* CT provide quantitative data of bone structure and mineralized volume changes. They can be used to estimate skeletal effects of pharmacologic or regenerative interventions. Histomorphologic analysis and histologic data provide the most sensitive description of bone formation and remodeling. Immunohistochemistry and molecular biology measures represent tools to differentiate temporary and spatial changes of bone formation regulating proteins and bone remodeling itself.

Radiographic Analysis

Radiographs and Microradiographic Analysis
Radiographs and microradiographs are produced by the summation of attenuation of radiation along a single scanning direction. Advantages of the methods are rapid, relatively inexpensive, visualization, and data gathering of morphology (Christiansen, 1995; Hassager and Christiansen, 1995). It should be noted that radiographs are limited to two-dimensional evaluations. Comparison of microradiographic analysis and histochemistry of guided bone regeneration in the calvarial critical-size defect model revealed no significant quantitative differences between these methods (Thorwarth *et al.*, 2007). These findings suggest that microradiography is appropriate to evaluate the quantitative extent of newly formed bone in *critical-size* defects. Microradiography represents a simple, inexpensive, alternative method to evaluate the progress of *de novo* bone formation. The microradiographs, as used in our previous work, are X-rayed in a Faxitron® cabinet (Faxitron, Rohde and Schwarz, Köln, Germany) for 6 min at 13 kV and 2.5 mA. The radiographs (Kodak, Stuttgart, Germany) are digitized with an Epson scanner (Epson Perfection 4900 Photo) at 2400 dpi and 8-bit grayscale, stored in TIFF format, and evaluated with imaging software.

CT
CT is used for assessment of bone geometry and volumetric analysis. The commercially available CT devices achieve resolutions of ~70 µm per voxel. This resolution does not allow effective imaging of trabecular structures but it enables excellent quantitative assessment of compartment-specific changes in bone composition. Since the voxel size (~70 µm) is relatively large compared with the bone compartment thickness in small animals such as mice and rats (thickness of the femur ~300 µm), quantitative CT measurement of such small structures has an innate error of at least 15 % in density analysis (Brodt *et al.*, 2003).

Micro-CT
Micro-CT is the gold standard for evaluation of bone morphology and bone architecture of animal models *ex vivo*. Current micro-CT scanners achieve a resolution of voxel size of 6 to

10 µm (Martin-Badosa et al., 2003a,b). This enables the nondestructive measurement of bone morphology much faster than typical histologic analyses of undecalcified bone specimens. Furthermore, when in vivo, combined with a perfused contrast agent, micro-CT can image three-dimensional vascular architecture within the bone compartment (Bolland et al., 2008a,b).

Micro-CT does not provide biologic data describing cellular composition, or protein or mRNA expression patterns, therefore substitution of sophisticated and time-consuming histologic and molecular biology tissue analysis by micro-CT is not likely.

MRI
Although magnetic resonance imaging (MRI) is widely used for assessment of nonmineralized, free-proton-containing tissue, a few studies have performed analysis and morphometry of bone trabecular structure using MRI (Gardner et al., 2001). If used in large animal models or humans, results of MRI analysis are highly correlated with those from two-dimensional histology assessment (Weber et al., 2005).

Histomorphologic Analysis

Labeling of Bone by Tetracycline
Labeling of the bone during the regeneration process allows precisely to quantify the extent of bone formation within a given time schedule (Ott, 1993; Sasaki et al., 1994; Vitorovic et al., 1995; Pautke et al., 2010). For labeling in therapeutic and experimental approaches, tetracyclines, preferentially known as bacteriostatic antibiotics, are used. Tetracycline binds irreversibly to recently formed hydroxyapatite crystals at sites undergoing new bone matrix deposition. Commonly used fluorochromes in experimental bone labeling of the pig model are oxytetracyline, alizarine-complex, calcein blue and xylenol orange (Nkenke et al., 2002) Subjected to ultraviolet light, microscopy of tetracycline labeled sections present fluorescence at the topographic position corresponding to the time point of tetracycline application during bone formation.

Bone Sample Preparation for Histomorphologic Assessment
Following the harvesting of the samples, immersion fixation should be performed using 4% paraformaldehyde. Paraformaldehyde fixation has been shown to enable a variety of further analytic procedures including immunohistochemistry. If tetracycline labeling of the bone samples is of special importance, 70% ethanol fixation should be performed. More aqueous fixatives might leach the tetracycline from the bone (Baron et al., 1983). For preparation for histologic analysis, samples are embedded in specified methacrylate resin (e.g., Technovit 9100, Heraeus Kulzer, Werheim, Germany). For the microradiographic examination the embedded bone samples are cut down to thin sections of 180 µm thickness using a precision saw and grinding machine (Exakt Gerätebau, Norderstedt, Germany). For histologic and immunohistochemical analysis, 5 µm thick histologic sections are prepared using a hard tissue microtome (Leica, Nussloch, Germany).

Histomorphometric Analysis
For the evaluation of tissue samples in guided bone regeneration approaches, the trabecular/bone volume (TV/BV) is commonly evaluated. For assessment of BV and the differentiation of newly formed bone, toluidine blue staining has been developed (Baron et al., 1983; Schlegel et al., 2006b, 2007b, 2009). It enables differentiation of newly formed bone matrix from mature, calcified bone. Histologic sections of 5 µm thickness are stirred in 10% H_2O_2 for 20 minutes and rinsed under cold running water. After drying, the section is stained with toluidine blue solution for 15 minutes. Excess staining solution is removed

by rinsing with water, and the stained sections are examined under a bright field microscope at ×50 magnification.

Masson's trichrome staining represents an alternative method to distinguish different stages of mineralization within one bone sample in one histologic examination (Schwarz et al., 2007a,b). Mineralized bone matrix and collagen are stained bright green, calcified cartilage matrix light green, osteoid red, and cell cores blue.

Immunohistochemical Analysis
Immunohistochemistry, using autostaining devices, has been developed to provide reproducible information about protein expression within tissue sections. Specific proteins can be visualized, exploring their localization within tissues and cell compartments, and relative quantitative comparisons are possible. Prior to suggested research applications, the availability of specific antibodies for the animal species intended to be used should be considered. For osteoimmunologic studies the domestic pig serves as an excellent model considering the homology of bone homeostasis regulating cytokines and transcription factors. In particular, mechanisms of bone remodeling, mediated by the Rank-Rank(L)/OPG-axis are highly conserved. Therefore a broad variety of antibodies, designed for targeting human tissue, can be used in pig experimental approaches. Different immunohistochemistry staining kits are available at present; for automated staining devices, alkaline phosphatase antialkaline phosphatase (APAAP)-based kits have been recommended due to their relatively constant staining intensity, independent from influences such as room temperature. Usually monoclonal or affinity purified polyclonal antibodies of different species than the tissue section are used as primary, epitope-mapping antibodies. Secondary antibodies are raised against the species of the primary antibody and linked to enzyme complexes mediating color reactions.

For immunohistochemical analysis of protein expression, sections are qualitatively evaluated under a bright-field microscope at ×100 to ×400 magnification. For semiquantitative assessment the method of systematic randomized subsampling has been demonstrated to be appropriate for estimating cytokine and matrix protein expressions (Weibel, 1982, 1989; Wehrhan et al., 2004). Five visual fields per section for each sample are digitized at ×200 magnification. The relative expression of a specifically marked protein is determined by counting the number of positively stained cells and the total number of cells within each visual field. For each visual field the labeling index is given as the ratio (number of positively stained cells/total number of cells ×100).

Since immunohistochemistry is a highly sensitive method, it can be used to trace the distribution of protein within tissue sections even when occurring in very small concentrations.

12.5.9 Statistical Analysis Plan (see also Chapter 4)

Testing statistical significance in histomorphometric and immunohistochemistry analysis can be performed by using several test algorithms appropriate for multiple independent test data. Multiple measurements per study group are aggregated prior to analysis. The mineralization rate and labeling indices can be sufficiently described as the median (ME) and the interquartile range (IQR). Graphical diagrams should represent the median, the interquartile range, minimum (Min), and maximum (Max) values. Confirmatory comparisons between treatment and control groups are performed. Multiple P values are adjusted according to Bonferroni by multiplying each P value obtained by the number of confirmatory tests performed (n = 10). Alternatively, an analysis of variance (ANOVA) test is possible. Two-sided adjusted P values ≤ 0.05 are considered significant.

Table 12-6 Overview of the nonhuman primate animal model for sinus elevation

Breed	Approach	Extraction of teeth (healing period)	Implants inserted	Unloaded vs. loaded implants	Reference
Macaca fascicularis	Intraoral	Second premolar and all molars (42 days)	12 weeks after sinus elevation	Unloaded	Hanisch et al., 1997
Cebus paella	Intraoral	P1, P2, P3, M1 (120 days)	Simultaneously with sinus elevation	Unloaded	Palma et al., 2006; Cricchio et al., 2009a,b
Macaca mulatta	Intraoral	M1, M2, M3 (90 days)	Simultaneously with sinus elevation and 4 months after sinus elevation	Unloaded and loaded	Hürzeler et al., 1997a,b; Quinones et al., 1997a,b

12.6 Animal Model – Nonhuman Primates

12.6.1 Aim

The anatomic situation in nonhuman primates is the nearest to the circumstances found in humans. The model provides an intraoral approach and the possibility to compare loaded with unloaded implants. Table 12-6 displays a summary of the nonhuman primate model for sinus elevation.

12.6.2 Advantages/Disadvantages of the Nonhuman Primate Model

This animal model is nearest to the clinical situation found in patients. Disadvantages include restricted availability due to ethical reasons.

12.6.3 Timing

Figure 12-10 gives an overview of timing of the procedures for the nonhuman primate model.

12.6.4 Surgical Procedures

After extraction of the teeth in the maxilla (see Table 12-6) the alveolar ridges are allowed to heal for between 42 and 120 days. Then a palatal or mid-crestal incision from the canine area to the maxillary tuberosity with a mesial vertical releasing incision is chosen, and a full thickness mucoperiosteal flap is raised. The access to the maxillary (1 cm × 0.8 cm) sinus is created with a round bur. Then the membrane is elevated with specially designed elevators (Friatec™, Friedrichsfeld, Germany) (Hanisch et al., 1997; Hurzeler et al., 1997a,b; Palma et al., 2006).

12.6.5 Preparation

Anesthesia is induced by administration of ketamine (10 mg/kg intramuscularly) and maintained with pentobarbital sodium (30 mg/kg) or isoflurane after intubation. The anesthesia is supplemented with 2% mepivacaine HCl or with epinephrine by local administration at the surgical site (Hanisch et al., 1997; Hurzeler et al., 1997a,b; Palma et al., 2006).

12.6.6 Detailed Methodology

During the postoperative healing period, systematic periodontal care is carried out, accomplished by the local application of 0.12% chlorhexidine solution (Hanisch et al., 1997).

12.6.7 Postoperative Care

The animals are fed a soft diet during the first 15 postoperative days. For postoperative pain control the animals receive buprenorphine (0.01 mg/kg intramuscularly) every 12 hours for 2 days. To prevent infections the animals are given cefazolin sodium (50 mg/kg intramuscularly every 8 hours for 1 week) (Hanisch et al., 1997; Palma et al., 2006).

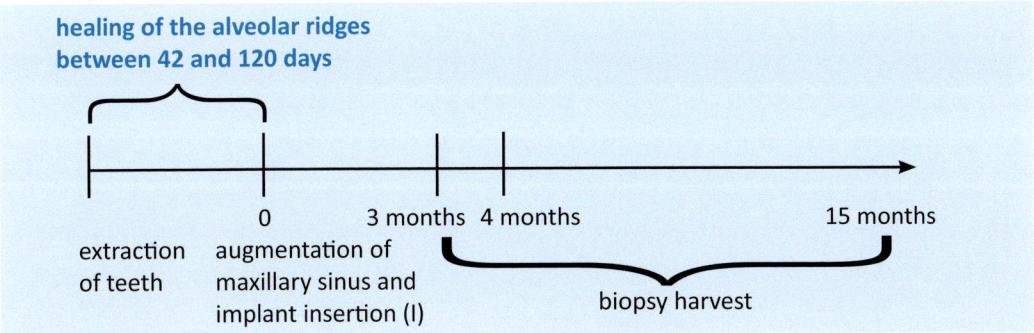

Fig 12-10 Overview of timing of the procedures in the nonhuman primate model.

References

1. Adell R, Lekholm U, Grondahl K, Branemark PI, Lindstrom J, Jacobsson M (1990). Reconstruction of severely resorbed edentulous maxillae using osseointegrated fixtures in immediate autogenous bone grafts. *Int J Oral Maxillofac Implants* 5:233–246.
2. Aerssens J, Boonen S, Lowet G, Dequeker J (1998). Interspecies differences in bone composition, density, and quality: potential implications for *in vivo* bone research. *Endocrinology* 139:663–70.
3. Anderson ML, Dhert WJ, de Bruijn JD, Dalmeijer RA, Leenders H, van Blitterswijk CA et al. (1999). Critical size defect in the goat's os ilium. A model to evaluate bone grafts and substitutes. *Clin Orthop Relat Res* 364:231–239.
4. Baron R, Gertner JM, Lang R, Vignery A (1983). Increased bone turnover with decreased bone formation by osteoblasts in children with osteogenesis imperfecta tarda. *Pediatr Res* 17:204–207.
5. Beddoe AH (1978). A quantitative study of the structure of trabecular bone in man, rhesus monkey, beagle and miniature pig. *Calcif Tissue Res* 25:273–281.
6. Blomqvist JE (1998). Aspects of maxillary sinus reconstruction with endosseous implants. *Swed Dent J Suppl* 130:7–48.
7. Bolland BJ, Kanczler JM, Dunlop DG, Oreffo RO (2008a). Development of *in vivo* muCT evaluation of neovascularisation in tissue engineered bone constructs. *Bone* 43:195–202.
8. Bolland BJ, Kanczler JM, Ginty PJ, Howdle SM, Shakesheff KM, Dunlop DG, et al. (2008b). The application of human bone marrow stromal cells and poly(dl-lactic acid) as a biological bone graft extender in impaction bone grafting. *Biomaterials* 29:3221–3227.
9. Bravetti P, Membre H, Marchal L, Jankowski R (1998). Histologic changes in the sinus membrane after maxillary sinus augmentation in goats. *J Oral Maxillofac Surg* 56:1170–1176; discussion 1177.
10. Brodt MD, Pelz GB, Taniguchi J, Silva MJ (2003). Accuracy of peripheral quantitative computed tomography (pQCT) for assessing area and density of mouse cortical bone. *Calcif Tissue Int* 73:411–418.
11. Brumund KT, Graham SM, Beck KC, Hoffman EA, McLennan G (2004). The effect of maxillary sinus antrostomy size on xenon ventilation in the sheep model. *Otolaryngol Head Neck Surg* 131:528–533.
12. Buser D, Nydegger T, Hirt HP, Cochran DL, Nolte LP (1998). Removal torque values of titanium implants in the maxilla of miniature pigs. *Int J Oral Maxillofac Implants* 13:611–619.
13. Christiansen C (1995). Osteoporosis: diagnosis and management today and tomorrow. *Bone* 17: 513S–516S.
14. Cricchio G, Palma VC, Faria PE, de Oliveira JA, Lundgren S, Sennerby L et al. (2009a). Histological findings following the use of a space-making device for bone reformation and implant integration in the maxillary sinus of primates. *Clin Implant Dent Relat Res* 11(Suppl 1):e14–22.
15. Cricchio G, Palma VC, Faria PE, de Olivera JA, Lundgren S, Sennerby L et al. (2009b). Histological outcomes on the development of new space-making devices for maxillary sinus floor augmentation. *Clin Implant Dent Relat Res* 3 August [Epub ahead of print].
16. Derong Z, Lian G, Jiayu L, Xiuli Z, Zhiyuan Z, Xinquan J (2010). Anatomic and histological analysis in a goat model used for maxillary sinus floor augmentation with simultaneous implant placement. *Clin Oral Implants Res* 21:65–70.
17. Eitel F, Klapp F, Jacobson W, Schweiberer L (1981). Bone regeneration in animals and in man. A contribution to understanding the relative value of animal experiments to human pathophysiology. *Arch Orthop Trauma Surg* 99:59–64.
18. Estaca E, Cabezas J, Uson J, Sanchez-Margallo F, Morell E, Latorre R (2008). Maxillary sinus-floor elevation: an animal model. *Clin Oral Implants Res* 19:1044–1048.
19. Fenner M, Vairaktaris E, Fischer K, Schlegel KA, Neukam FW, Nkenke E (2009a). Influence of residual alveolar bone height on osseointegration of implants in the maxilla: a pilot study. *Clin Oral Implants Res* 20:555–559.
20. Fenner M, Vairaktaris E, Stockmann P, Schlegel KA, Neukam FW, Nkenke E (2009b). Influence of residual alveolar bone height on implant stability in the maxilla: an experimental animal study. *Clin Oral Implants Res* 20:751–755.

21. Gardner JR, Hess CP, Webb AG, Tsika RW, Dawson MJ, Gulani V (2001). Magnetic resonance microscopy of morphological alterations in mouse trabecular bone structure under conditions of simulated microgravity. *Magn Reson Med* 45:1122–1125.
22. Gong JK, Arnold JS, Cohn SH (1964). Composition of trabecular and cortical bone. *Anat Rec* 149:325–331.
23. Grageda E, Lozada JL, Boyne PJ, Caplanis N, McMillan PJ (2005). Bone formation in the maxillary sinus by using platelet-rich plasma: an experimental study in sheep. *J Oral Implantol* 31:2–17.
24. Gruber RM, Ludwig A, Merten HA, Achilles M, Poehling S, Schliephake H (2008). Sinus floor augmentation with recombinant human growth and differentiation factor-5 (rhGDF-5): a histological and histomorphometric study in the Goettingen miniature pig. *Clin Oral Implants Res* 19:522–529.
25. Gruber RM, Ludwig A, Merten HA, Pippig S, Kramer FJ, Schliephake H (2009). Sinus floor augmentation with recombinant human growth and differentiation factor-5 (rhGDF-5): a pilot study in the Goettingen miniature pig comparing autogenous bone and rhGDF-5. *Clin Oral Implants Res* 20:175–182.
26. Gutwald R, Haberstroh J, Kuschnierz J, Kister C, Lysek DA, Maglione M et al. (2010a). Mesenchymal stem cells and inorganic bovine bone mineral in sinus augmentation: comparison with augmentation by autologous bone in adult sheep. *Br J Oral Maxillofac Surg* 48:285–290.
27. Gutwald R, Haberstroh J, Stricker A, Ruther E, Otto F, Xavier SP et al. (2010b). Influence of rhBMP-2 on bone formation and osseointegration in different implant systems after sinus-floor elevation. An *in vivo* study on sheep. *J Craniomaxillofac Surg* 38:501–504.
28. Haas R, Donath K, Fodinger M, Watzek G (1998a). Bovine hydroxyapatite for maxillary sinus grafting: comparative histomorphometric findings in sheep. *Clin Oral Implants Res* 9:107–116.
29. Haas R, Mailath G, Dortbudak O, Watzek G (1998b). Bovine hydroxyapatite for maxillary sinus augmentation: analysis of interfacial bond strength of dental implants using pull-out tests. *Clin Oral Implants Res* 9:117–122.
30. Haas R, Baron M, Donath K, Zechner W, Watzek G (2002a). Porous hydroxyapatite for grafting the maxillary sinus: a comparative histomorphometric study in sheep. *Int J Oral Maxillofac Implants* 17:337–346.
31. Haas R, Haidvogl D, Donath K, Watzek G (2002b). Freeze-dried homogeneous and heterogeneous bone for sinus augmentation in sheep. Part I: histological findings. *Clin Oral Implants Res* 13:396–404.
32. Haas R, Haidvogl D, Dortbudak O, Mailath G (2002c). Freeze-dried bone for maxillary sinus augmentation in sheep. Part II: biomechanical findings. *Clin Oral Implants Res* 13:581–586.
33. Haas R, Baron M, Zechner W, Mailath-Pokorny G (2003). Porous hydroxyapatite for grafting the maxillary sinus in sheep: comparative pullout study of dental implants. *Int J Oral Maxillofac Implants* 18:691–696.
34. Hanisch O, Tatakis DN, Rohrer MD, Wohrle PS, Wozney JM, Wikesjo UM (1997). Bone formation and osseointegration stimulated by rhBMP-2 following subantral augmentation procedures in nonhuman primates. *Int J Oral Maxillofac Implants* 12:785–792.
35. Hassager C, Christiansen C (1995). Measurement of bone mineral density. *Calcif Tissue Int* 57:1–5.
36. Hazzard DG, Bronson RT, McClearn GE, Strong R (1992). Selection of an appropriate animal model to study aging processes with special emphasis on the use of rat strains. *J Gerontol* 47:B63–64.
37. Hirsch JM, Ericsson I (1991). Maxillary sinus augmentation using mandibular bone grafts and simultaneous installation of implants. A surgical technique. *Clin Oral Implants Res* 2:91–96.
38. Honig JF, Merten HA (1993). Subperiosteal versus epiperiosteal forehead augmentation with hydroxylapatite for aesthetic facial contouring: experimental animal investigation and clinical application. *Aesthetic Plast Surg* 17:93–98.
39. Hürzeler MB, Quinones CR, Kirsch A, Gloker C, Schupbach P, Strub JR et al. (1997a). Maxillary sinus augmentation using different grafting materials and dental implants in monkeys. Part I. Evaluation of anorganic bovine-derived bone matrix. *Clin Oral Implants Res* 8:476–486.
40. Hürzeler MB, Quinones CR, Kirsch A, Schupbach P, Krausse A, Strub JR et al. (1997b). Maxillary sinus augmentation using different grafting materials and dental implants in monkeys. Part III. Evaluation of autogenous bone combined with porous hydroxyapatite. *Clin Oral Implants Res* 8:401–411.
41. International Standards Organization (2007). Biological evaluation of medical devices – Part 6: Tests for local effects after implantation. ISO 10993-6.
42. Jakse N, Tangl S, Gilli R, Berghold A, Lorenzoni M, Eskici A et al. (2003). Influence of PRP on autogenous sinus grafts. An experimental study on sheep. *Clin Oral Implants Res* 14:578–583.
43. Kim HR, Choi BH, Xuan F, Jeong SM (2010). The use of autologous venous blood for maxillary sinus floor augmentation in conjunction with sinus membrane elevation: an experimental study. *Clin Oral Implants Res* 21:346–9.
44. Kimmel DB, Jee WS (1982). A quantitative histologic study of bone turnover in young adult beagles. *Anat Rec* 203:31–45.
45. Kirker-Head CA, Nevins M, Palmer R, Nevins ML, Schelling SH (1997). A new animal model for maxillary sinus floor augmentation: evaluation parameters. *Int J Oral Maxillofac Implants* 12:403–411.
46. Klongnoi B, Rupprecht S, Kessler P, Thorwarth M, Wiltfang J, Schlegel KA (2006a). Influence of platelet-rich plasma on a bioglass and autogenous bone in sinus augmentation. An explorative study. *Clin Oral Implants Res* 17:312–320.
47. Klongnoi B, Rupprecht S, Kessler P, Zimmermann R, Thorwarth M, Pongsiri S et al. (2006b). Lack of beneficial effects of platelet-rich plasma on sinus augmentation using a fluorohydroxyapatite or autogenous bone: an explorative study. *J Clin Periodontol* 33:500–509.

48. Kragstrup J, Shijie Z, Mosekilde L, Melsen F (1989). Effects of sodium fluoride, vitamin D, and calcium on cortical bone remodeling in osteoporotic patients. *Calcif Tissue Int* 45:337–341.
49. Laiblin C, Jaeschke G (1979). Clinical chemistry examinations of bone and muscle metabolism under stress in the Gottingen miniature pig: an experimental study. *Berl Munch Tierarztl Wochenschr* 92:124–128.
50. Lee HJ, Choi BH, Jung JH, Zhu SJ, Lee SH, Huh JY et al. (2007). Maxillary sinus floor augmentation using autogenous bone grafts and platelet-enriched fibrin glue with simultaneous implant placement. *Oral Surg Oral Med Oral Pathol Oral Radiol Endod* 103:329–333.
51. Lee SH, Choi BH, Li J, Jeong SM, Kim HS, Ko CY (2007). Comparison of corticocancellous block and particulate bone grafts in maxillary sinus floor augmentation for bone healing around dental implants. *Oral Surg Oral Med Oral Pathol Oral Radiol Endod* 104:324–328.
52. Leung KS, Siu WS, Cheung NM, Lui PY, Chow DH, James A et al. (2001). Goats as an osteopenic animal model. *J Bone Miner Res* 16:2348–2355.
53. Liebschner MA (2004). Biomechanical considerations of animal models used in tissue engineering of bone. *Biomaterials* 25:1697–1714.
54. Liu Y, Springer IN, Zimmermann CE, Acil Y, Scholz-Arens K, Wiltfang J et al. (2008). Missing osteogenic effect of expanded autogenous osteoblast-like cells in a minipig model of sinus augmentation with simultaneous dental implant installation. *Clin Oral Implants Res* 19:497–504.
55. Martin-Badosa E, Amblard D, Nuzzo S, Elmoutaouakkil A, Vico L, Peyrin F (2003a). Excised bone structures in mice: imaging at three-dimensional synchrotron radiation micro CT. *Radiology* 229:921–928.
56. Martin-Badosa E, Elmoutaouakkil A, Nuzzo S, Amblard D, Vico L, Peyrin F (2003b). A method for the automatic characterization of bone architecture in 3D mice microtomographic images. *Comput Med Imaging Graph* 27:447–458.
57. Mosekilde L (1993). Vertebral structure and strength *in vivo* and *in vitro*. *Calcif Tissue Int* 53(Suppl 1):S121–125; discussion S125–126.
58. Mosekilde L, Danielsen CC (1987). Biomechanical competence of vertebral trabecular bone in relation to ash density and age in normal individuals. *Bone* 8:79–85.
59. Nevins M, Kirker-Head C, Wozney JA, Palmer R, Graham D (1996). Bone formation in the goat maxillary sinus induced by absorbable collagen sponge implants impregnated with recombinant human bone morphogenetic protein-2. *Int J Periodontics Restorative Dent* 16:8–19.
60. Nkenke E, Kloss F, Wiltfang J, Schultze-Mosgau S, Radespiel-Troger M, Loos K et al. (2002). Histomorphometric and fluorescence microscopic analysis of bone remodelling after installation of implants using an osteotome technique 30. *Clin Oral Implants Res* 13:595–602.
61. Nkenke E, Lehner B, Fenner M, Roman FS, Thams U, Neukam FW et al. (2005). Immediate versus delayed loading of dental implants in the maxillae of minipigs: follow-up of implant stability and implant failures. *Int J Oral Maxillofac Implants* 20:39–47.
62. Nunamaker DM (1998). Experimental models of fracture repair. *Clin Orthop Relat Res* 355(Suppl):S56–65.
63. Ott SM (1993). Bone formation periods studied with triple tetracycline labels in women with postmenopausal osteoporosis. *J Bone Miner Res* 8:443–450.
64. Palma VC, Magro-Filho O, de Oliveria JA, Lundgren S, Salata LA, Sennerby L (2006). Bone reformation and implant integration following maxillary sinus membrane elevation: an experimental study in primates. *Clin Implant Dent Relat Res* 8:11–24.
65. Park J, Lutz R, Felszeghy E, Wiltfang J, Nkenke E, Neukam FW et al. (2007). The effect on bone regeneration of a liposomal vector to deliver BMP-2 gene to bone grafts in peri-implant bone defects. *Biomaterials* 28:2772–2782.
66. Pautke C, Bauer F, Bissinger O, Tischer T, Kreutzer K, Steiner T et al. (2010). Tetracycline bone fluorescence: a valuable marker for osteonecrosis characterization and therapy. *J Oral Maxillofac Surg* 68:125–129.
67. Pearce AI, Richards RG, Milz S, Schneider E, Pearce SG (2007). Animal models for implant biomaterial research in bone: a review. *Eur Cell Mater* 13:1–10.
68. Pieri F, Lucarelli E, Corinaldesi G, Iezzi G, Piattelli A, Giardino R et al. (2008). Mesenchymal stem cells and platelet-rich plasma enhance bone formation in sinus grafting: a histomorphometric study in minipigs. *J Clin Periodontol* 35:539–546.
69. Qin L, Mak AT, Cheng CW, Hung LK, Chan KM (1999). Histomorphological study on pattern of fluid movement in cortical bone in goats. *Anat Rec* 255:380–387.
70. Quinones CR, Hurzeler MB, Schupbach P, Arnold DR, Strub JR, Caffesse RG (1997a). Maxillary sinus augmentation using different grafting materials and dental implants in monkeys. Part IV. Evaluation of hydroxyapatite-coated implants. *Clin Oral Implants Res* 8:497–505.
71. Quinones CR, Hurzeler MB, Schupbach P, Kirsch A, Blum P, Caffesse RG et al. (1997b). Maxillary sinus augmentation using different grafting materials and osseointegrated dental implants in monkeys. Part II. Evaluation of porous hydroxyapatite as a grafting material. *Clin Oral Implants Res* 8:487–496.
72. Raghoebar GM, Brouwer TJ, Reintsema H, Van Oort RP (1993). Augmentation of the maxillary sinus floor with autogenous bone for the placement of endosseous implants: a preliminary report. *J Oral Maxillofac Surg* 51:1198–1203; discussion 1203–1205.
73. Roldan JC, Jepsen S, Schmidt C, Knuppel H, Rueger DC, Acil Y et al. (2004). Sinus floor augmentation with simultaneous placement of dental implants in the presence of platelet-rich plasma or recombinant human bone morphogenetic protein-7. *Clin Oral Implants Res* 15:716–723.
74. Roldan JC, Knueppel H, Schmidt C, Jepsen S, Zimmermann C, Terheyden H (2008). Single-stage sinus augmentation with cancellous iliac bone and anorganic bovine bone in the presence of platelet-rich plasma in the miniature pig. *Clin Oral Implants Res* 19:373–378.

75. Saffarzadeh A, Gauthier O, Bilban M, Bagot D'Arc M, Daculsi G (2009). Comparison of two bone substitute biomaterials consisting of a mixture of fibrin sealant (Tisseel) and MBCP (TricOs) with an autograft in sinus lift surgery in sheep. *Clin Oral Implants Res* 20:1133–1139.
76. Sasaki T, Ramamurthy NS, Golub LM (1994). Bone cells and matrix bind chemically modified non-antimicrobial tetracycline. *Bone* 15:373–375.
77. Schlegel A, Hamel J, Wichmann M, Eitner S (2008). Comparative clinical results after implant placement in the posterior maxilla with and without sinus augmentation. *Int J Oral Maxillofac Implants* 23:289–298.
78. Schlegel KA, Fichtner G, Schultze-Mosgau S, Wiltfang J (2003). Histologic findings in sinus augmentation with autogenous bone chips versus a bovine bone substitute. *Int J Oral Maxillofac Implants* 18:53–58.
79. Schlegel KA, Lang FJ, Donath K, Kulow JT, Wiltfang J (2006a). The monocortical critical size bone defect as an alternative experimental model in testing bone substitute materials. *Oral Surg Oral Med Oral Pathol Oral Radiol Endod* 102:7–13.
80. Schlegel KA, Thorwarth M, Plesinac A, Wiltfang J, Rupprecht S (2006b). Expression of bone matrix proteins during the osseus healing of topical conditioned implants: an experimental study. *Clin Oral Implants Res* 17:666–672.
81. Schlegel KA, Zimmermann R, Thorwarth M, Neukam FW, Klongnoi B, Nkenke E et al. (2007a). Sinus floor elevation using autogenous bone or bone substitute combined with platelet-rich plasma. *Oral Surg Oral Med Oral Pathol Oral Radiol Endod* 104:e15–25.
82. Schlegel KA, Zimmermann R, Thorwarth M, Neukam FW, Klongnoi B, Nkenke E et al. (2007b). Sinus floor elevation using autogenous bone or bone substitute combined with platelet-rich plasma. *Oral Surg Oral Med Oral Pathol Oral Radiol Endod* 103:e8–12.
83. Schlegel KA, Rupprecht S, Petrovic L, Honert C, Srour S, von Wilmowsky C et al. (2009). Preclinical animal model for de novo bone formation in human maxillary sinus. *Oral Surg Oral Med Oral Pathol Oral Radiol Endod* 108:e37–44.
84. Schwarz F, Herten M, Ferrari D, Wieland M, Schmitz L, Engelhardt E et al. (2007a). Guided bone regeneration at dehiscence-type defects using biphasic hydroxyapatite + beta tricalcium phosphate (Bone Ceramic) or a collagen-coated natural bone mineral (BioOss Collagen): an immunohistochemical study in dogs. *Int J Oral Maxillofac Surg* 36:1198–1206.
85. Schwarz F, Herten M, Sager M, Wieland M, Dard M, Becker J (2007b). Histological and immunohistochemical analysis of initial and early osseous integration at chemically modified and conventional SLA titanium implants: preliminary results of a pilot study in dogs. *Clin Oral Implants Res* 18:481–488.
86. Smiler DG, Johnson PW, Lozada JL, Misch C, Rosenlicht JL, Tatum OH Jr et al. (1992). Sinus lift grafts and endosseous implants. Treatment of the atrophic posterior maxilla. *Dent Clin North Am* 36:151–186; discussion 187–188.
87. Sul SH, Choi BH, Li J, Jeong SM, Xuan F (2008a). Histologic changes in the maxillary sinus membrane after sinus membrane elevation and the simultaneous insertion of dental implants without the use of grafting materials. *Oral Surg Oral Med Oral Pathol Oral Radiol Endod* 105:e1–5.
88. Sul SH, Choi BH, Li J, Jeong SM, Xuan F (2008b). Effects of sinus membrane elevation on bone formation around implants placed in the maxillary sinus cavity: an experimental study. *Oral Surg Oral Med Oral Pathol Oral Radiol Endod* 105:684–687.
89. Swindle MM, Smith AC, Hepburn BJ (1988). Swine as models in experimental surgery. *J Invest Surg* 1:65–79.
90. Terheyden H, Jepsen S, Moller B, Tucker MM, Rueger DC (1999). Sinus floor augmentation with simultaneous placement of dental implants using a combination of deproteinized bone xenografts and recombinant human osteogenic protein-1. A histometric study in miniature pigs. *Clin Oral Implants Res* 10:510–521.
91. Thorwarth M, Wehrhan F, Srour S, Schultze-Mosgau S, Felszeghy E, Bader RD et al. (2007). Evaluation of substitutes for bone: comparison of microradiographic and histological assessments. *Br J Oral Maxillofac Surg* 45:41–47.
92. Turner CH, Roeder RK, Wieczorek A, Foroud T, Liu G, Peacock M (2001). Variability in skeletal mass, structure, and biomechanical properties among inbred strains of rats. *J Bone Miner Res* 16:1532–1539.
93. van der Donk S, Buma P, Aspenberg P, Schreurs BW (2001). Similarity of bone ingrowth in rats and goats: a bone chamber study. *Comp Med* 51:336–340.
94. Vitorovic D, Nikolic Z, Cvetkovic D (1995). In vivo tetracycline labelling as a measure of rearing-system influence on chicken-bone dynamics. *Anat Histol Embryol* 24:85–86.
95. Wang S, Zhang Z, Xia L, Zhao J, Sun X, Zhang X et al. (2010). Systematic evaluation of a tissue-engineered bone for maxillary sinus augmentation in large animal canine model. *Bone* 46:91–100.
96. Weber MH, Sharp JC, Latta P, Sramek M, Hassard HT, Orr FW (2005). Magnetic resonance imaging of trabecular and cortical bone in mice: comparison of high resolution in vivo and ex vivo MR images with corresponding histology. *Eur J Radiol* 53:96–102.
97. Wehrhan F, Rodel F, Grabenbauer GG, Amann K, Bruckl W, Schultze-Mosgau S (2004). Transforming growth factor beta 1 dependent regulation of Tenascin-C in radiation impaired wound healing. *Radiother Oncol* 72:297–303.
98. Weibel ER (1982). Biomorphometry in physiological and pathological research. *Acta Med Pol* 23:115–125.
99. Weibel ER (1989). Measuring through the microscope: development and evolution of stereological methods. *J Microsc* 155:393–403.
100. Wetzel AC, Stich H, Caffesse RG (1995). Bone apposition onto oral implants in the sinus area filled with different grafting materials. A histological study in beagle dogs. *Clin Oral Implants Res* 6:155–163.

CHAPTER 13

Peri-implantitis Defect Model

Frank Schwarz, Martin Sager, and Jürgen Becker

13.1 General Overview

The cause and effect relationship between microbial plaque colonization and the pathogenesis of peri-implant diseases was originally investigated in preclinical animal studies by means of an experimental breakdown of the implant-supporting soft and hard tissues (Lindhe *et al.*, 1992; Lang *et al.*, 1993). In this model, peri-implantitis lesions were induced by stopping the plaque control regimen, along with submarginal placement of cotton ligatures, thus establishing a pocket around titanium implants. This resulted in a plaque-associated progressive inflammation and the subsequent rapid breakdown of the peri-implant soft and hard tissues (Lindhe *et al.*, 1992; Lang *et al.*, 1993) (Fig 13-1). In the same observation period, the inflammatory infiltrate at natural teeth was separated from the alveolar bone by an intact subepithelial connective tissue (Lindhe *et al.*, 1992), implying that the progression of peri-implant diseases is pronounced in comparison with chronic periodontal disease.

Basically, this specific defect model was originally described by Rovin *et al.* (Rovin *et al.*, 1966) and proven to cause microorganism-associated, progressive periodontal lesions in rats. In subsequent years, this principle was successfully adopted to investigate the pathogenesis of periodontal diseases in larger animals such as monkeys (Kennedy and Polson, 1973) and dogs (Ericsson *et al.*, 1975).

Until today, the ligature-induced defect model remains the gold standard experimental setting to investigate both pathogenesis and therapy (Renvert *et al.*, 2009) of peri-implantitis lesions (Fig 13-1; Table 13-1).

Osteology Guidelines for Oral and Maxillofacial Regeneration

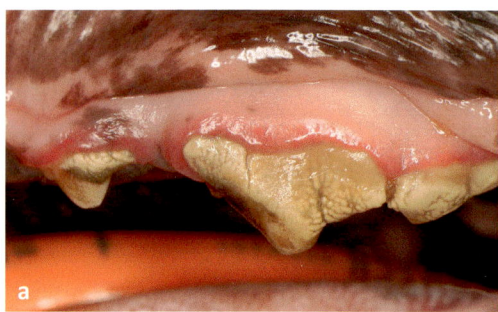
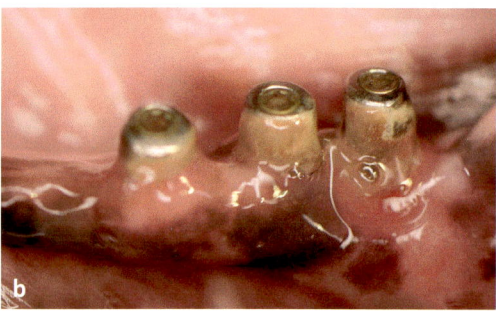
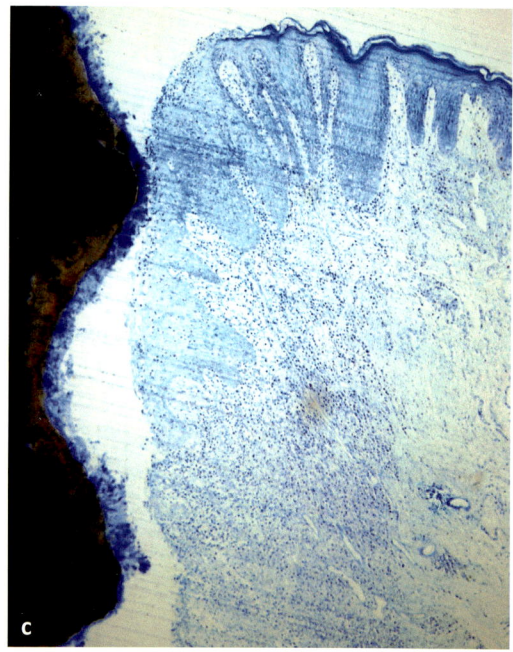

Fig 13-1 Periodontitis and peri-implantitis in canine. (**a**) Naturally occurring periodontal disease. (**b**) Ligature-induced peri-implantitis. (**c**) Histologic view of supra- and subgingival formation of mineralized plaque biofilms with secondary infiltration of the bordering peri-implant tissue. Toluidine blue stain, original magnification ×200.

Table 13-1 Pre-clinical large-animal peri-implantitis defect models

Characteristics	Defect type	Animal species	Advantages	Disadvantages
Chronic disease model	Intrabony (mainly circumferential) + supracrestal	Canine	Configuration and sizes of peri-implantitis bone defects (dogs) seemed to resemble naturally occurring lesions in humans	Time consuming
		Nonhuman primate		Technically demanding
Ligature-induced bone resorption around titanium implants				Non-standardized defect configuration and sizes
	Defect components (Schwarz et al., 2007)	Minipig		
			No tendency towards spontaneous regeneration	
Acute/chronic disease model	Dehiscence (Takasaki et al., 2007)	Canine	Less time consuming than ligature-induction	Do not closely resemble naturally occurring lesions in humans
Surgically created acute defects at titanium implants	Circumferential (Jovanovic, 1993; Jovanovic et al., 1993)		Standardization of defect configuration and sizes	
Secondary plaque infection				Tendency towards spontaneous regeneration

13.2 Animal Models

13.2.1 Aim of Using Canine, Nonhuman Primate, and Minipig Animal Models

Canine
It is well documented that most canines (i.e., Beagle, fox, Labrador) exhibit a natural susceptibility to periodontal disease (Weinberg and Bral, 1999). While periodontal health could be maintained in case of a meticulous plaque control, the induction of progressive inflammatory reactions in the periodontal tissues was simply correlated with an undisturbed plaque accumulation (see Fig 7-1a), which could be accelerated by a soft-food diet and submarginal placement of ligatures (Ericsson *et al.*, 1975; Lindhe *et al.*, 1975). These findings have been successfully transferred to the peri-implant tissues (Berglundh *et al.*, 1992; Ericsson *et al.*, 1992; Lindhe *et al.*, 1992). Accordingly, the dog is the most frequently used large-animal model to investigate both the pathogenesis of peri-implant diseases and the efficacy of nonsurgical and surgical/regenerative treatment approaches to control disease progression with the aim of reestablishing the lost tissue structures (Faggion *et al.*, 2009; Renvert *et al.*, 2009). Probably due to their docile character, convenient size, and maintenance, Beagle dogs are most commonly used in the dental literature (Table 13-2). While the macro- and microstructure of canine bone is moderately similar to human bone, bone composition (i.e., water fraction, organic fraction, volatile inorganic fraction, ash fraction) most closely represents the human situation (similar for pigs – see below). It is important to emphasize that bone remodeling in the mandible has been reported to be twofold greater than in the maxilla (51%/year vs. 25.5%/year), and remained high with animal age (Huja and Beck, 2008), but still being moderately similar to human bone (dog: 1.5 to 2.0 μm/day vs. human: 1.0 to 1.5 μm/day) (Pearce *et al.*, 2007). The specific anatomical characteristics of the canine jaw bone usually facilitates the insertion of common dental implants (e.g., length: 10 mm; diameter: 3 to 4 mm). A potential advantage of most canines is related to their easy manageability during postoperative oral hygiene procedures, thus facilitating infection control. This issue is particularly relevant to the ligature-induced peri-implantitis defect model.

Nonhuman Primate
Nonhuman primates possess similar oral structures to humans and also exhibit naturally occurring bacterial plaque biofilms and a certain susceptibility to develop periodontitis (Samuel and Woodall, 1988). However, in case of undisturbed plaque accumulation, spontaneous progression of the inflammatory cell infiltrate and subsequently an ongoing attachment loss is limited to implants and ankylosed teeth and does not occur in relation to control teeth exhibiting an intact periodontal ligament (Schou *et al.*, 1993a,b, 1996). Accordingly, nonhuman primates (i.e., macaque, baboon, and cynomolgus macaque) have been frequently used species in the ligature-induced peri-implant mucositis and peri-implantitis defect model (Table 13-3). The specific anatomic characteristics of the nonhuman primate jaw bone does require the insertion of diameter-reduced dental implants. Due to strict regulatory requirements, difficulty in acquisition and maintenance costs, as well as difficulties in controlling postsurgical infections and trauma (Weinberg and Bral, 1999), nonhuman primates are nowadays rarely used in dental research.

Minipig
The breeding of miniature and micro-pigs has overcome some potential disadvantages commonly encountered with domestic pigs (i.e., large growth rate, excessive body weight, demanding manageability). Both, the macro- and the microstructure of pig bone are moderately similar to human bone. Most similarities between pig and human bone have been

Table 13-2 Pre-clinical ligature-induced peri-implantitis defect model: canine

Aim	Animals	Healing period I	Healing period II	Active breakdown period	Progression period	Bone loss
Patho-genesis	Beagle dogs (Leonhardt et al., 1992; Lindhe et al., 1992; Tillmanns et al., 1997, 1998; Gotfredsen et al., 2002; Sennerby et al., 2005; Schwarz et al., 2006; Berglundh et al., 2007b)	13.2 ± 7.7 weeks	TPI: submerged: 13.2 ± 2.7 weeks Abutment: 8.8 ± 6.3 weeks OPI: 13.2 ± 4.0 weeks	12.2 ± 5.2 weeks Ligature replacement: 3.8 ± 1.8 weeks	21.1 ± 19.9 weeks	41.2 ± 16.8%*
	Labrador dogs (Zitzmann et al., 2004; Albouy et al., 2008, 2009)					
	Mongrel dogs (Nociti et al., 2001a; Shibli et al., 2003a; Martins et al., 2004, 2005; Zechner et al., 2004)					
Therapy	Beagle dogs (Grunder et al., 1993; Jovanovic, 1993; Jovanovic et al., 1993; Hurzeler et al., 1995, 1997; Machado et al., 1999, 2000; Persson et al., 1999, 2001a,b, 2004; Wetzel et al., 1999; Deppe et al., 2001, 2002; Stubinger et al., 2005; Schwarz et al., 2007)	13.2 ± 7.7 weeks	TPI: submerged: 13.2 ± 2.7 weeks Abutment: 8.8 ± 6.3 weeks OPI: 13.2 ± 4.0 weeks	14.3 ± 6.4 weeks Ligature replacement: 2.3 ± 2.2 weeks	5.5 ± 10.4 weeks	40.0 ± 14.0%*
	Labrador dogs (Marinello et al., 1995; Ericsson et al., 1996b; Persson et al., 1996; Hayek et al., 2005)					
	Mongrel dogs (Nociti et al., 2000, 2001b; Shibli et al., 2003b, 2003c, 2006; You et al., 2007; Parlar et al., 2009)					

Pathogenesis = available studies assessing pathogenesis of peri-implantitis.
Therapy = available studies assessing treatment of peri-implantitis.
*Calculated from the data provided in the original papers.
OPI, one-part implant; TPI, two-part implant.

13.2 Animal Models

Table 13-3 Pre-clinical ligature-induced peri-implantitis defect model: nonhuman primate (for key see Table 13-2)

Aim	Animals	Healing period I	Healing period II	Active breakdown period	Progression period	Bone loss
Pathogenesis	*Macaca fuscata* (Akagawa et al., 1993)	3.0 ± 0.0 weeks	TPI: (Warrer et al., 1995)	30.0 ± 13.2 weeks	0.7 ± 1.5 weeks	27.0 ± 16.3%
	Macaca fascicularis (Lang et al., 1993; Schou et al., 1993a,b; Warrer et al., 1995)		Submerged: 12 weeks Abutment: 20 weeks	Ligature replacement: 2.8 ± 3.3		
	Macaca mulatta (Hanisch et al., 1997a; Eke et al., 1998)		OPI: 11.4 ± 5.4 weeks			
Therapy	*Macaca fascicularis* (Schou et al., 2003a,b,c)			59.0 ± 19.0 weeks	3.5 ± 0.5 weeks	37.5 ± 12.5%
	Macaca mulatta (Hanisch et al., 1997b)			Ligature replacement: 16.0 ± 6.0		

observed for bone composition and bone remodeling (pig: 1.2 to 1.5 µm/day vs. human: 1.0 to 1.5 µm/day) (Pearce et al., 2007). Accordingly, miniature and micro-pigs are frequently used animal models to evaluate the safety and efficacy of biomaterials related to implant dentistry. For the time being, the ligature-induced peri-implantitis defect model has been employed in only two animal studies (Table 13-4). However, these limited data also pointed to a successful experimental breakdown of the peri-implant tissues, which was associated with a microbiological shift from Gram-positive facultative to Gram-negative obligate anaerobes (Hickey et al., 1991). The specific anatomic characteristics of the pig jaw bone also facilitates the insertion of common dental implants (e.g., length: 10 mm; diameter: 3 to 4 mm).

Box 13-1
The ligature-induced defect model must be considered as the gold standard experimental setting to investigate both pathogenesis and therapy of peri-implantitis lesions. This defect model was predominantly employed in canine, which will in turn serve as the basic animal species in the following sections. With reference to the existing literature, alternative animal species (i.e., nonhuman primates and minipigs) will also be mentioned.

13.2.2 Advantages/Disadvantages of the Presented Model

To the best of our knowledge, only one publication has employed surgically created buccal dehiscence-type defects around titanium implants, which were subsequently plaque infected by the application of a stainless steel mesh (Takasaki et al., 2007). Since configurations and sizes of ligature-induced peri-implantitis bone defects (Schwarz et al., 2007) as well as the associated microflora in dogs (Nociti et al., 2001a) seemed to closely resemble naturally occurring lesions in humans, this preclini-

Table 13-4 Pre-clinical ligature-induced peri-implantitis defect model: **swine**

Aim	Animals	Healing period I	Healing period II	Active breakdown period	Progression period	Bone loss
Pathogenesis	Micropig (Hickey et al., 1991)	3.5 ± 0.5 weeks	TPI: submerged: 8 weeks	45 days singular ligature application	No	Not indicated
			Abutment: 2 weeks			
Therapy	Micropig (Singh et al., 1993)			6 weeks singular ligature application	No	Not indicated

Pathogenesis = available studies assessing pathogenesis of peri-implantitis.
Therapy = available studies assessing treatment of peri-implantitis.
TPI, two-part implant

cal model may be favored prior to more definitive studies in humans. In this context, one must keep in mind the potential clinical relevance of an experimentally induced chronic-type defect model, since it features no tendency towards spontaneous regeneration (Zitzmann et al., 2004) and therefore possesses similarities to the biologic environment of a true peri-implantitis lesion. However, a potential disadvantage is related to difficulties in the standardization of the defect configuration and sizes (i.e., Class I and II defect components) subsequent to the chronification period (Schwarz et al., 2007) (Table 13-1). This might be particularly true for the horizontal dimension of the adjacent alveolar bone, which has been reported to be an important determinant of bone regeneration (Polimeni et al., 2004). An extensive evaluation of the available literature on the ligature-induced peri-implantitis defect model, as conducted for the present chapter, clearly revealed that the methodological approaches varied considerably among these publications, thus implying that a standardized protocol is still missing. Interestingly, only a minority of the publications presented below (see Tables 13-2, 13-3, and 13-4) referred to the original literature, but commonly ignored the specific methodological procedures reported herein. Accordingly, the following sections will critically evaluate the methodological procedures previously employed for an experimental breakdown of peri-implant soft and hard tissues. Particular emphasis will be given to specific methodological procedures employed in different animal species.

13.2.3 Timing of the Surgical Procedure

The basic methodological procedure and all corresponding experimental phases are presented in Figures 13-2 and 13-3. Briefly, these include:
1. Tooth extraction
2. Healing period I
3. Placement of endosseous implants
4. Healing period II (plaque control)

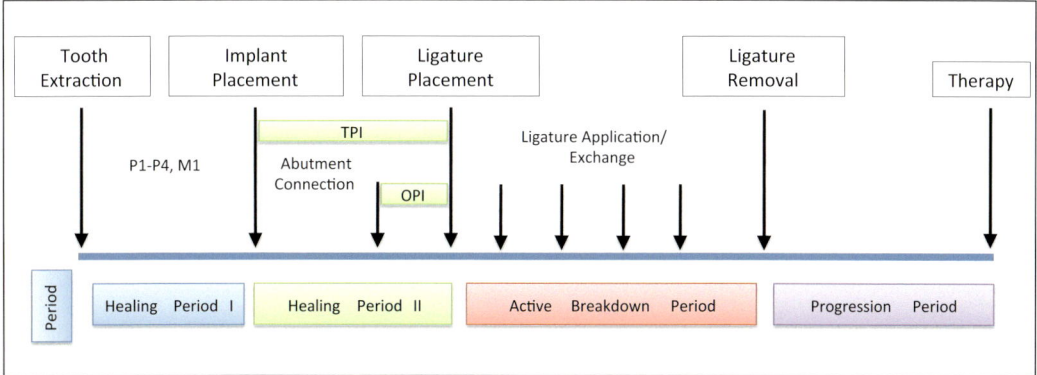

Fig 13-2 Protocol for ligature-induced peri-implantitis. M, molar; P, premolar; OPI, one-part implant; TPI, two-part implant. Healing Period II includes submerged healing + implant uncovering + abutment connection.

5. Implant uncovering + healing period III (plaque control) in the case of two-part implants and a submerged healing procedure
6. Active breakdown period: ligature placement – progression period: after ligature removal (plaque control).

13.2.4 Surgical Procedures

For the detailed surgical procedures, see Section 13.2.6.

13.2.5 Preparation – Animal Care and General Anesthesia

Animal Care

Usually, the experimental segment of a study starts after an animal adaption period of 4 weeks. During the experiment, the animals are fed once per day with a soft-food diet and water ad libitum.

General Anesthesia (Canine)

General anesthesia is mandatory for all surgical interventions (i.e., phases 1, 3, and 5) and should include initial intramuscular sedation, which is usually accomplished with acepromazine (e.g., 0.17 mg/kg). Subsequently, anesthesia is initiated using thiopental-sodium (e.g., 21.5 mg/kg). During all surgical procedures, inhalation anesthesia is performed by use of oxygen and nitrous oxide and isoflurane. To maintain hydration, each animal receives a constant rate infusion of lactated Ringer's solution while anesthetized. Intraoperative analgesia is performed by intravenous injection of piritramide (e.g., 0.4 mg/kg) and carprofen (e.g., 4.5 mg/kg). For postoperative treatment, piritramide and carprofen are usually applied subcutaneously for 3 days in the same dose.

13.2.6 Detailed Methodology

Tooth Extraction
Canine

The permanent dentition in dogs comprises three incisors, one canine, four premolars, and three molars in the mandible (two molars in the maxilla). Most authors defined the mandibular premolar (P1 to P4) and molar (M1) region as the primary experimental unit (Fig 13-4). Since the maxilla merely has sufficient alveolar bone height and width in the molar region (M1 to M2), these areas are usually not considered for this experimental model. However, some authors have decided to remove the maxillary premolars and molars in order to avoid any traumatic injury to the primary experimental sites (Table 13-2).

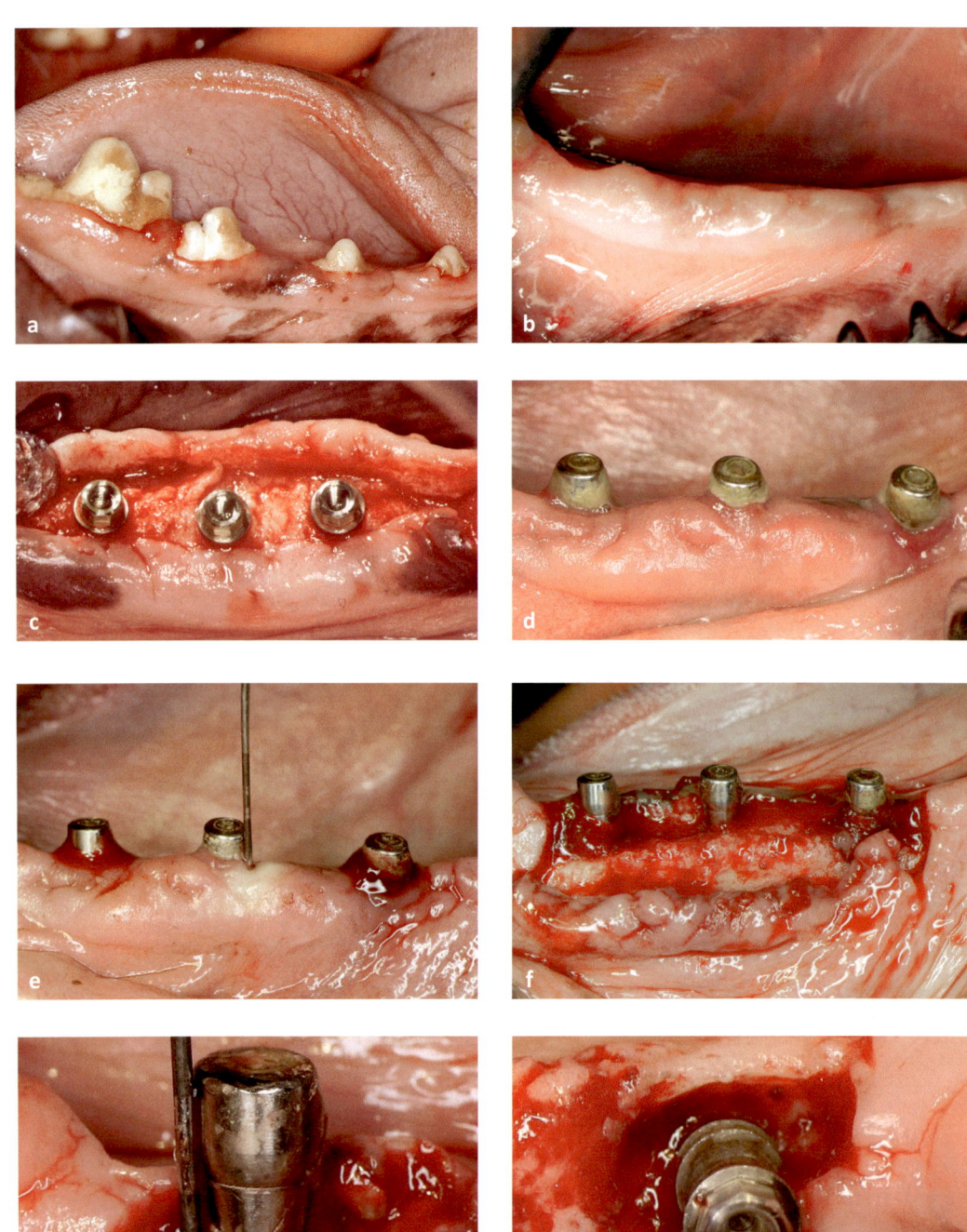

Fig 13-3 *(left page)* Ligature induced peri-implantitis in canine – basic methodologic procedure. (**a**) Phase 1: tooth extraction. At the beginning of the experiment, the first, second, and third mandibular premolars as well as the first molar are extracted. Prior to tooth extraction, meticulous plaque removal should be performed. (**b**) Phase 2: healing period I. Clinical situation at 12 weeks, indicating an undisturbed healing of the alveolar ridge. (**c**) Phase 3: placement of endosseous implants. After 12 weeks of healing, installation of diameter-reduced (3.3 mm) screw-type titanium implants was performed in a one-stage procedure. Phase 4 (healing period II) is supported by meticulous plaque control. (**d**) Phase 5: induction of peri-implantitis. Peri-implantitis lesions were induced by ligature placement and subsequent plaque accumulation. (**e**) Clinical situation 3 months after application of cotton ligatures in a submarginal position. The progression period is initiated by ligature removal and the renewal of meticulous plaque control. (**f**) Situation at 4 weeks after ligature removal and plaque control. The elevation of a mucoperiosteal flap clearly indicates that the peri-implantitis bone defects are filled with granulation tissue. (**g1**) Removal of the granulation tissue revealed the circumferential-type intrabony defect component (i.e., Class Ie [see Box 13-1]), which was combined with a supracrestal exposure (i.e., Class II) of structured aspects of the titanium implant. (**g2**) Occlusal view showing the ligature-induced circumferential-type bone resorption.

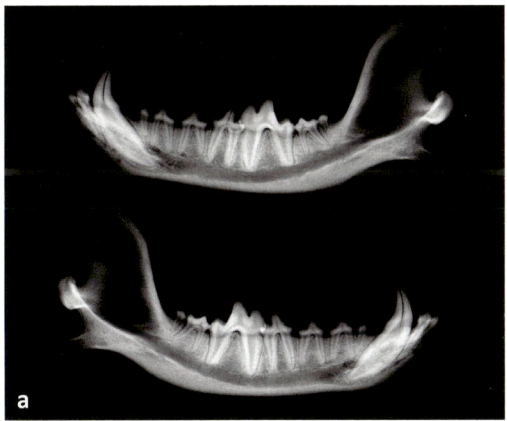
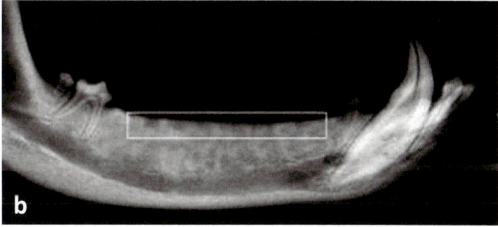
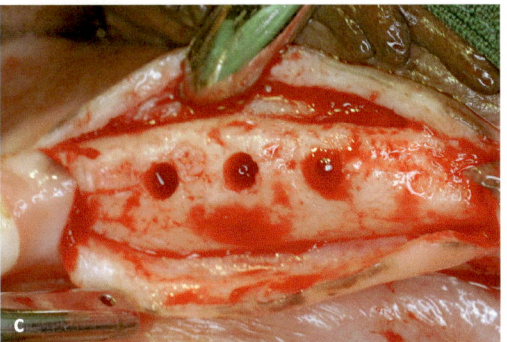
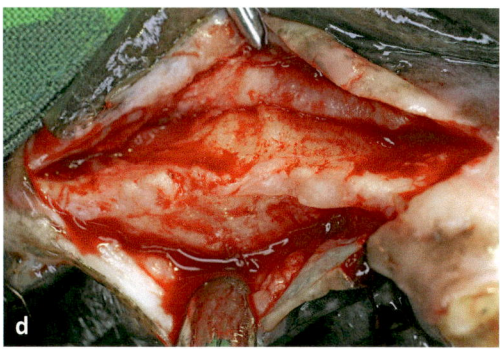

Fig 13-4 Permanent dentition in canine – tooth extraction. (**a**) The permanent dentition in dogs comprises three incisors, one canine, four premolars, and three molars in the mandible. (**b**) The mandibular premolar (P1 to P4) and molar (M1) region (boxed area) is the most frequent experimental unit for the ligature-induced peri-implantitis defect model. (**c**) After healing period I, the resulting width of the mandibular alveolar ridge in the premolar and molar areas usually varies between 5 to 6 mm and 6 to 8 mm, respectively. The final diameter of the implant bed is 3.3 mm. (**d**) The maxillary alveolar ridge usually features an uneven and sharp-edged contour, which in turn complicates implant placement and subsequently the induction of peri-implantitis defects.

Nonhuman primate
All strains exhibit a similar primary and permanent dentition as humans. However, the size of the teeth is considerably smaller. While most authors defined the mandibular premolar and molar region as primary experimental units, others have extended these areas to the corresponding maxillary regions (Table 13-3).

Minipig
The pig dentition has three incisors, one canine (without root), four premolars, and three molars in both the mandible and the maxilla. Both published studies have defined the mandibular premolar region as primary experimental unit (Table 13-4).

Surgical Procedure
In the second surgery, mucoperiosteal flaps are reflected bilaterally in each jaw and the respective teeth (e.g., P1 to M2) are carefully removed after gentle tooth separation. This should be accomplished by means of a straight fissure carbide bur under copious irrigation with sterile 0.9% physiological saline. Wound closure is usually accomplished by means of resorbable mattress sutures. Prophylactic administration of clindamycin (e.g., 11.0 mg/kg) is recommended intra- and postoperatively for 10 days.

Note: in this phase, it is of utmost importance to avoid any injury to the buccal or lingual bone plate (i.e., iatrogenic caused dehiscence). This will be associated with a pronounced remodeling at the respective site, thus compromising the width of the alveolar bone after healing period I.

Healing Period I
Canine
The mean healing period following tooth extraction is 13.2 ± 7.7 weeks (Table 13-2).

Nonhuman Primate
The mean healing period following tooth extraction is 3.0 ± 0.0 months (Table 13-3).

Minipig
The mean healing period following tooth extraction is 3.5 ± 0.5 months (Table 13-4).

Postoperative Care
A plaque control program including tooth and implant cleaning just with the use of a toothbrush is usually performed twice per week. While this procedure can easily be performed without sedation/anesthesia in dogs, postsurgical infection control is obviously more demanding in nonhuman primates and minipigs.

Implant Placement
Canine
The mean implant diameter and length is 4.0 ± 1.4 mm and 8.8 ± 1.8 mm, respectively.

Note: It must be considered that after healing period I, the resulting width of the alveolar ridge in the premolar and molar areas may vary between 5 to 6 mm and 6 to 8 mm, respectively (Fig 13-4). Since the circumferential width s(c) of the peri-implantitis defect usually is 1 to 2 mm (Schwarz et al., 2007), the diameter-reduced (3.3 to 3.75 mm) endosseous implants should be favored in order to account for these biologic conditions.

Nonhuman Primate
The mean implant diameter and length was 2.8 ± 0.2 mm and 8.0 ± 1.4 mm, respectively.

Minipig
The implant diameter and length has not been reported in the available literature.

Surgical Procedure
In the second surgery, midcrestal incisions are made and mucoperiosteal flaps reflected to expose the experimental sites for implant insertion in the respective jaws. Surgical implant sites are usually prepared bilaterally, at a distance of 10 mm apart, using a low-trauma surgical technique under copious irrigation with sterile 0.9% physiological saline (Fig 13-3c).

Only one study (two publications: Jovanovic, 1993; Jovanovic et al., 1993) employed a surgical widening of the marginal portion of the implant channel by means of a specially designed step drill. Accordingly, following implant placement, a circumferential gap about 0.6 mm wide and 4 mm deep was present at the experimental implants. Basically, all implants must be inserted with good primary stability (i.e., lack of clinical mobility) in a way that the borderline between the machined and structured aspects coincides with the alveolar crest, as suggested in the surgical protocol of the manufacturer. Implants can be left to heal in either a submerged or a non-submerged position.

In the case of a nonsubmerged healing procedure (two-part implants with connected abutment component), mucoperiosteal flaps are usually repositioned with resorbable mattress sutures. Periosteal-releasing incisions are mandatory to obtain a tension-free primary wound closure at submerged sites. Subsequently, the mucoperiosteal flaps are advanced, repositioned coronally and fixed with vertical or horizontal resorbable mattress sutures.

Healing Period II
Canine
Most authors favor a submerged healing procedure. The mean healing period following implant placement is 13.2 ± 2.7 weeks for submerged, and 13.2 ± 4.0 weeks for nonsubmerged implants (Table 13-2).

Nonhuman Primate
Employing this animal model, most authors favor a nonsubmerged healing procedure with a mean healing period of 11.4 ± 5.4 weeks. Only one study reported on a submerged approach with a healing time of 12 weeks (Table 13-3).

Minipig
Both available studies employed a submerged healing procedure following implant placement with a healing period of 8 weeks, as elucidated in only one publication (Table 13-3).

Postoperative Care
In order to prevent trauma to the peri-implant mucosa, oral hygiene procedures should be omitted during the initial healing period of 7 days. Thereafter, a plaque control program including tooth and implant cleaning just with a toothbrush should be initiated and performed at least twice per week. This is a mandatory requirement in case of a nonsubmerged healing procedure.

Basically, healing period II should result in a proper and equal osseointegration of all experimental implants. When considering the available evidence derived from experimental animal studies reporting on the osseointegration of recent titanium implant surface modifications (Junker et al., 2009), a healing period of 10 to 12 weeks seems to be appropriate to predictably achieve this objective.

Implant Uncovering + Healing Period III (Optional)
Canine
The mean healing period following implant uncovering is 8.8 ± 6.3 weeks (Table 13-2).

Nonhuman Primate
The only study (two publications: Hanisch et al., 1997a,b), employing a submerged healing procedure reported that a 3-month plaque control measure was initiated at 2 months after abutment connection (Table 13-3).

Minipig
Only one study (Hickey et al., 1991) reported on a 2-week healing period following implant uncovering (Table 13-3).

Postoperative Care
See procedure reported in Section 13.2.6. Previous experimental animal studies have indi-

cated that the transmucosal attachment revealed a junctional epithelium and connective tissue, resulting in a 3 to 4 mm wide zone of biological soft tissue coverage of the implant-supporting bone (Berglundh et al., 1991; Abrahamsson et al., 1996; Berglundh and Lindhe, 1996; Abrahamsson et al., 1998). The formation of peri-implant tissues was not dependent on the surgical approach (i.e., submerged healing + abutment connection vs. nonsubmerged healing) (Abrahamsson et al., 1996; Ericsson et al., 1996a; Weber et al., 1996). However, it was demonstrated that maturation of the barrier epithelium and organization of the collagen fibers in the subepithelial connective tissue around nonsubmerged moderately rough implants with a transmucosal machined surface may require a healing period of at least 6 to 8 weeks in Beagle dogs (Berglundh et al., 2007a). Based on these findings, healing period III should not be less than 6 to 8 weeks at submerged implants.

At the end of the plaque control period (i.e., healing period II or III), the conditions of the peri-implant tissues must be documented, either by means of clinical and/or radiographic examinations.

Clinical Parameters
The following clinical parameters may be considered.

Index System for Plaque Biofilms
The original plaque index (PI) according to Silness and Löe (1964), or the modified PI of Mombelli et al. (1987), which has been adapted to the marginal situation of titanium dental implants.

Index system for the Assessment of the Condition of the Peri-implant Mucosa
The original gingiva index (GI) according to Löe and Silness (1963), or the modified GI of Mombelli et al. (1987) (mGI), adapted to the marginal situation of titanium dental implants.

Bleeding On Probing (BOP)
If possible, the probe is inserted in the peri-implant pocket at six aspects per implant: mesio-vestibular, mid-vestibular, disto-vestibular, mesio-oral, mid-oral and disto-oral. As a dichotomous index, it determines whether bleeding occurs after a period of 15 seconds (Y/N). A high index value is accordingly associated with a strong likelihood of a peri-implant inflammatory condition. Although a negative BOP index could be correlated with healthy periodontal conditions (Lang et al., 1990; Joss et al., 1994), the sensitivity and specificity at implant sites are controversially discussed. Lekholm et al. (1986) were not able to determine a correlation between a positive BOP and histologic, microbiologic, or radiological alterations at implants. The authors suspected that the bleeding could be induced by traumatization of the peri-implant tissue. These observations were confirmed in an experimental animal study (Ericsson and Lindhe, 1993). On the contrary, Lang et al. (1994) showed in an animal model that healthy peri-implant conditions could be correlated with negative BOP values since peri-implant mucositis was related to a significantly increased index value of 67% and a peri-implantitis of 91%. These results were confirmed in a prospective clinical study (Jepsen et al., 1996). The differences between these results are best explained with probe pressure, which should not exceed 0.25 N.

Probing Depth, Gingival Recession, Clinical Attachment Level
From a histologic point of view, the transmucosal attachment at submerged and nonsubmerged implants consists of a junctional epithelium (JE) with a length of approximately 2 mm and a connective tissue zone with a height of approximately 1 to 2 mm, thus resulting in a 3 to 4 mm wide zone of biological soft tissue coverage of the implant-supporting bone (Berglundh et al., 1991).

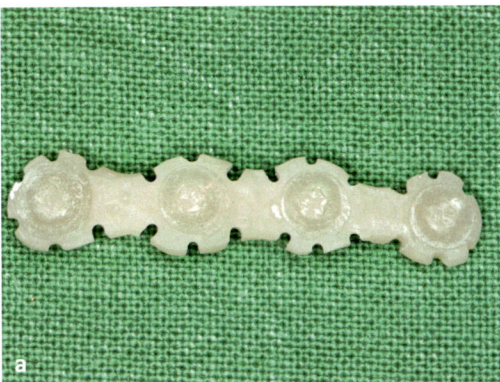 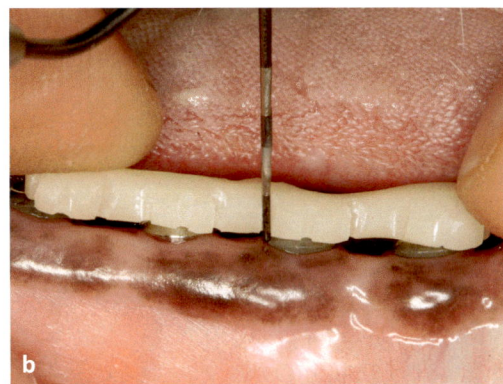

Fig 13-5 Clinical soft tissue in the canine – reproducibility. Custom-made acrylic stents exhibiting six vertical grooves per implant (i.e., mesiobuccal, midbuccal, distobuccal, mesiolingual, midlingual and distolingual) should be employed to ensure reproducible clinical probing (i.e., in a direction and angulation parallel to the long axis of the implant).

Previous clinical and experimental studies have indicated that peri-implant tissues are sensitive to force variation (Ericsson and Lindhe, 1993; Mombelli et al., 1997). A single conventional probing using a light force of 0.2 to 0.25 N was associated with a complete re-establishment of the mucosal seal after 5 days of healing (Etter et al., 2002). However, frequent clinical probing of healthy implants (i.e., 2, 4, 8, and 12 weeks) was associated with dimensional and structural changes of the mucosal seal (Schwarz et al., 2010).

One must realize that the probing pressure may be of crucial importance in the presence of inflammation in the peri-implant mucosa (Schou et al., 2002). While at healthy and mucositis sites, the probe penetration tended to stop at the histological level of connective tissue adhesion, it reached the base of the inflammatory lesion at peri-implantitis sites (Lang et al., 1994). With reduced probing pressure (0.25 N) however, the histologic attachment could almost be exactly defined in healthy conditions as well as in the presence of a peri-implant mucositis (Lang et al., 1994).

The following reference points are used for the clinical assessment of probing depth, gingival recession and attachment level:

- Probing depth (PD): distance (mucosal margin – bottom of pocket)
- Mucosal recession/hyperplasia (GR/GH): distance (implant shoulder – marginal mucosa)
- Clinical attachment level (CAL): distance (implant shoulder – bottom of pocket).

Clinical probing is usually performed using a pressure-sensitive probe. It is recommended to use individual acrylic stents with six vertical grooves per implant (i.e., mesiobuccal, midbuccal, distobuccal, mesiolingual, midlingual and distolingual) (Fig 13-5). The grooves allow the exact reproducibility of both direction and parallel angulation of the probe along with the long axis of the implant at each specific site. For all probing procedures, intramuscular sedation should be initiated and followed by short-acting anesthesia. All probing procedures must be performed by an experienced investigator masked to the specific experimental conditions.

Intraexaminer Reproducibility
Prior to the start of the experimental part of the study, a clinical calibration procedure should be initiated. This can be accomplished on five patients, each having two implants with probing depths ≥ 4 mm on at least one aspect. The exam-

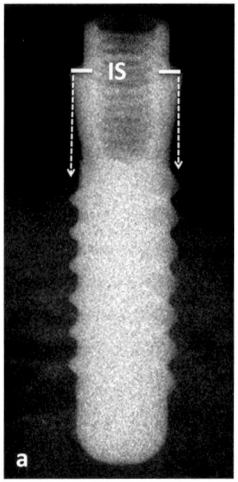
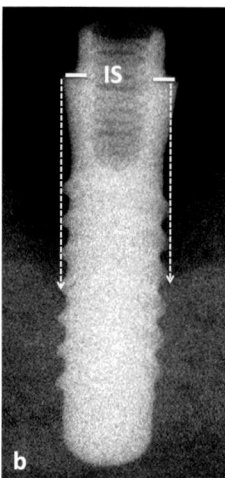

Fig 13-6 Radiographic assessment of peri-implant bone loss in canine. Standardized radiographs (end of phase 6) should be used to assess the distance between the implant shoulder (IS) and the bottom of the bone defect (arrow) next to the implant at the mesial and distal surfaces.

iner should evaluate the patients on two separate occasions, 48 hours apart. Calibration can be accepted if measurements at baseline and at 48 hours are within 1 mm at >90% of the time.

Radiological Parameters
The following radiographic parameters may be considered:
- Standardized radiographs should be obtained from each implant site using individually adjustable film holder devices (e.g., Eggen).
- Digital images of the radiographs should be evaluated using:
  – A software program to assess the distance between the implant shoulder and the bottom of the bone defect at the mesial and distal surfaces (Schwarz *et al.*, 2006) (Fig 13-6)
  – Subtraction radiography (Schou *et al.*, 2003a).

Recommended time intervals are:
- End of healing period II/III
- At each ligature exchange
- End of active breakdown period
- End of progression period (baseline)
- End of scheduled healing interval after therapy.

Active Breakdown and Progression Periods
The original protocol, as reported by (Lindhe *et al.*, 1992), described termination of the plaque control regimen and forcing cotton ligatures into a position immediately apical of the peri-mucosal margin in Beagle dogs. The ligatures were replaced after 3 weeks in the pocket of a receded mucosal margin. The second set of ligatures was removed after 3 weeks.

This active breakdown period was followed by a progression period of 4 weeks and supported by renewal of the plaque control regimen (i.e., teeth and abutments were cleaned with a toothbrush and dentifrice) (Lindhe *et al.*, 1992).

In an experimental study employing a progression period of 12 months without plaque control, it was observed that 16 out of 21 implants revealed varying amounts of additional radiographic bone loss, thus pointing to a spontaneous progression of ligature-induced peri-implantitis in dogs (Zitzmann *et al.*, 2004). Interestingly, subsequent to a 2-month plaque control regimen, histologic analysis revealed a separation of the inflammatory cell infiltrate from the adjacent alveolar bone by healthy connective tissue (Zitzmann *et al.*, 2004). Similar findings have also been reported by other authors employing the same animal model (Marinello *et al.*, 1995; Albouy *et al.*, 2008, 2009).

The following practical implications may be derived from these basic findings:
- Renewal of a plaque control regimen seems to be mandatory during the progression period
- The end of the progression period must be defined as the baseline point for studies aimed at investigating any therapeutic intervention of ligature-induced peri-implantitis lesions.

13.2 Animal Models

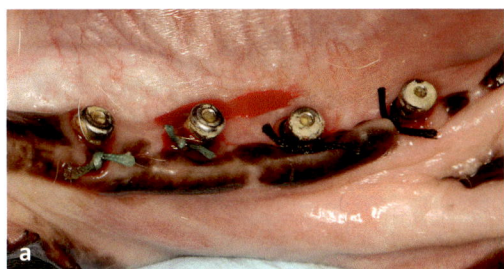

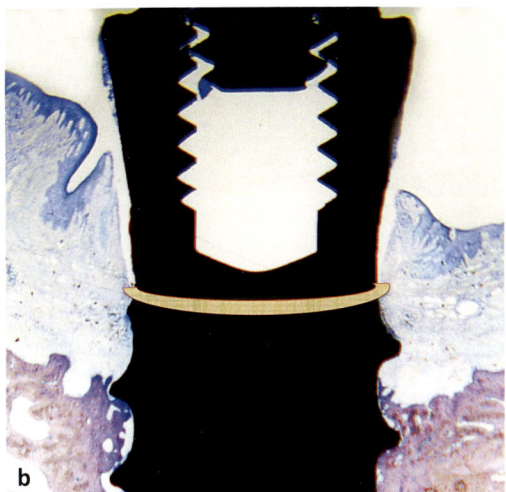
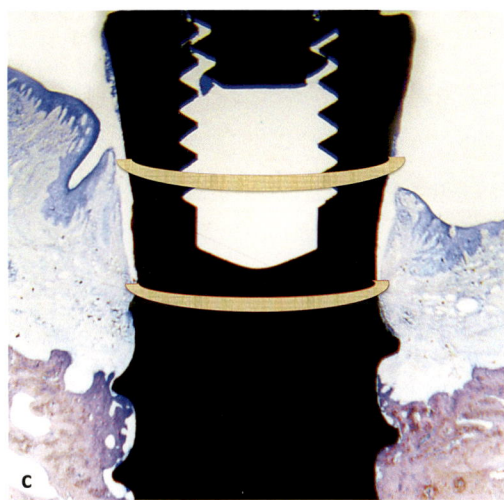

Fig 13-7 Ligature-induced peri-implantitis in canine – layered application. (**a**) Braided cotton ligatures of two different sizes (3-0 and 4-0) are layered at each experimental implant site. (**b**) Step 1: submucosal aspect. Application, knotting (three times) and gentle placement of a 4-0 cotton ligature in a submucosal position employing a surgical elevator. Rationale: The unavoidable swelling of the cotton ligature subsequent to its application *in vivo* will increase the risk for a premature ligature, loss when sizes >4-0 are used. Note: Conical abutment designs/transmucosal implant parts will support the ligature, preserving its original position and potentially prevent coronal sliding. Step 2: Perimucosal aspect. Application and knotting (three times) of a 3-0 cotton ligature in a paramucosal position employing a surgical elevator. Rationale: The paramucosal application of a 3-0 ligature size will accelerate marginal plaque biofilm formation.

Currently, it is impossible to estimate to what extent these data derived from experimental studies performed in dogs may be transferred to other species (i.e., nonhuman primates, minipig).

Ligatures and Modes of Application
Cotton and silk ligatures (4-0) are most commonly used to establish a peri-implant pocket during the active breakdown period. However, the specific mode of ligature application has been reported only in a few studies. This rudimentary information ranges from a "supramucosal" to a "submucosal" application in either a mono- or layered mode (Fig 13-7 and Fig 13-8). A distinct heterogeneity was also observed with respect to ligature replacement. While most authors preferred a single application, a minority of the available publications reported ligature replacement at individual time points, or just renewal in case of loss of a ligature (Tables 13-2 to 13-4).

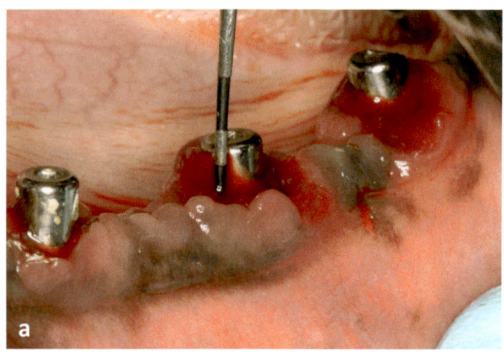
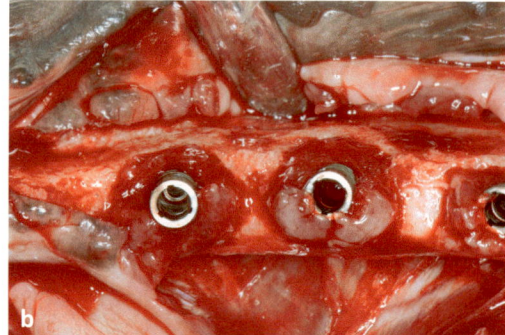
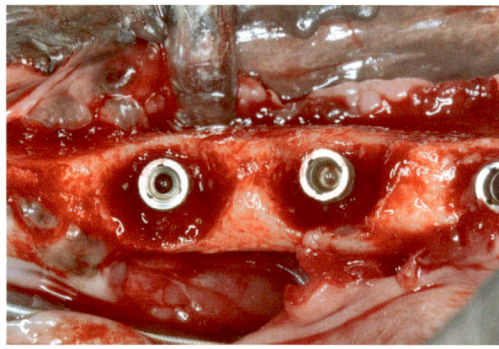
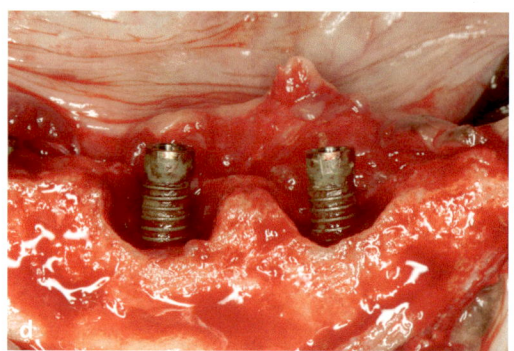

Fig 13-8 Ligature-induced peri-implantitis in the canine – baseline positioning in therapeutic studies. (**a**) Clinical situation at the end of the progression period indicating manifest inflammatory reactions at the experimental implant sites. Note: this situation must be defined as baseline in any studies aimed at investigating nonsurgical therapy of peri-implantitis. (**b**) Elevation of a mucoperiosteal flap clearly reveals the peri-implant bone resorption. Note the typical circumferential arrangement of loose granulation tissue around the screw-type titanium implants. (**c**) Subsequent to removal of all granulation tissue, the typical circumferential-type (i.e., Class Ie [see Box 13-1]) defect configuration is apparent. Note: This situation must be defined as baseline in any studies aimed at investigating surgical therapy of peri-implantitis. (**d**) Lateral view indicating a supracrestal exposure of the titanium implants (i.e., Class II).

For ligature application, renewal and replacement, intramuscular sedation/short-acting anesthesia is mandatory (i.e., acepromazine + medetomidine). Figure 13-7 illustrates the clinical procedure for layered ligature application, as routinely employed.

Factors Potentially Accelerating Disease Progression
Canine
Basically, spontaneous progression of ligature-induced peri-implantitis occurred around implants with different geometry and surface characteristics (Albouy *et al.*, 2008, 2009). However, limited evidence suggests that progression of untreated lesions may be more pronounced around moderately rough titanium implant surfaces compared with polished surfaces (Berglundh *et al.*, 2007b) (Fig 13-9).

In studies aimed at investigating the pathogenesis of peri-implantitis in the canine, the mean active breakdown and progression period (mean ligature application/replacement 3.8 ± 1.8) was 12.2 ± 5.2 weeks and 21.1 ± 19.9 weeks, respectively. This resulted in a calculated mean bone loss of approximately 40%

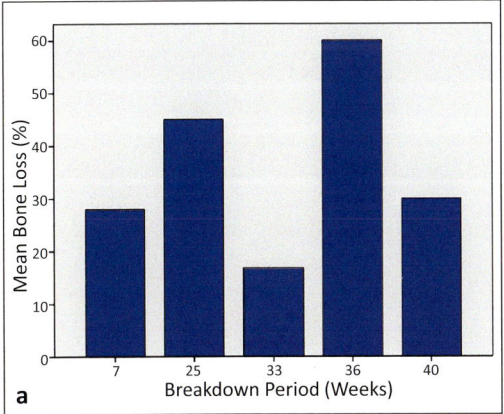
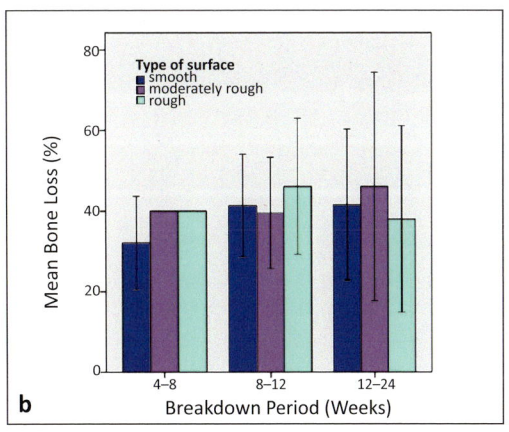
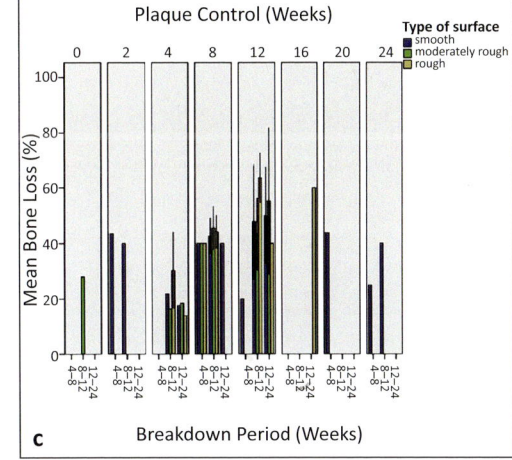

Fig 13-9 Ligature-induced peri-implantitis in canine – bone loss. (a) Mean bone loss as reported for various types of implant surfaces was most pronounced after an active breakdown period of 36 weeks. (b) Evaluation of the available literature seems to point to an accelerated disease progression at moderately rough and rough titanium implant surfaces. (c) Highest mean bone loss is observed for moderately rough and rough titanium implant surfaces after an active breakdown period of 8 to 24 weeks, which was followed by a plaque-controlled progression period of 12 weeks.

relative to the original implant length. The mean active breakdown period in therapeutic studies was 14.3 ± 6.4 weeks (mean ligature application/replacement 2.3 ± 2.2), which was followed by a mean progression period of 5.5 ± 10.4 weeks. This resulted in a calculated mean bone loss of 40.0 ± 14.0% relative to the original implant length (Table 13-2).

Nonhuman Primate
One group of authors inoculated monkeys with pathogenic *Porphyromonas gingivalis* three times weekly for 2 weeks, 1 month after ligature placement (Schou et al., 2003a). The potential influence of this methodological approach to hasten disease progression is currently unknown.

Most of the available studies have investigated the pathogenesis of peri-implantitis. The mean active breakdown (mean ligature application/replacement 2.8 ± 3.3) and progression period was 30.0 ± 13.2 weeks and 0.7 ± 1.5 weeks, respectively. This resulted in a calculated mean bone loss of 27.0 ± 16.3% relative to the original implant length. The mean active breakdown (mean ligature application/replacement 16.0 ± 6.0) period in therapeutic studies was 59.0 ± 19.0 weeks, which was followed by a mean progression period of 3.5 ± 0.5 weeks. This resulted in a calculated mean bone loss of 37.5 ± 12.5% relative to the original implant length (Table 13-3).

Minipig
The available two studies reporting the pathogenesis and therapy of peri-implantitis employed an active breakdown period (singular ligature application) of 45 days and 6 weeks, respectively. Without the implementation of a progression period, the induced inflammatory reactions were associated with a significant breakdown of the implant-supporting tissues (Table 13-4).

For an evaluation of animal studies investigating treatment of peri-implantitis, see the most recent review of the literature (Renvert et al., 2009).

Configuration of Peri-implantitis Defects
Based on preclinical and clinical data, peri-implantitis bone defects can be subdivided in definable classes (Schwarz et al., 2007). In particular, it has been reported that both naturally occurring human and ligature-induced peri-implantitis lesions in animals most commonly featured a combined defect configuration including a supracrestal (Class II) (humans: 79%; dogs: 53.3%) as well as an intrabony aspect. The latter were differentiated into five characteristic defect classes (Ia-e; Box 13-1) (Fig 13-10 and Fig 13-11) (Schwarz et al., 2007). In particular, defects most frequently (humans: 55.3%; dogs: 86.6%) exhibited a circular pattern of bone resorption under the buccal and oral compact bone, whose width was maintained (i.e., Class Ie). This was followed by buccal dehiscence defects with semicircular bone resorption near the middle of the implant body (i.e., Class Ib) (humans: 15.8%; dogs: 0%), and buccal dehiscence defects with circular bone resorption with either maintenance (i.e., Class Ic)

(humans: 13.3%; dogs: 6.7%) or loss (i.e., Class Id) (humans: 10.2%; dogs: 0%) of the lingual compact bone. Conventional buccal dehiscence defects were observed the least frequently (i.e., Class Ia) (humans: 5.4%; dogs: 6.7%) (Schwarz et al., 2007).

> **Box 13-1 Intrabony defect components** (Fig 13-10a) (Schwarz et al., 2007):
> **Class Ia**: vestibular or oral dehiscence defects with the implant body located within or beyond the envelope.
> **Class Ib**: vestibular or oral dehiscence defects with semicircular bone resorption around the middle of the implant body (implant body within or beyond the envelope).
> **Class Ic**: dehiscence defect with circular bone resorption and maintenance of the vestibular or oral compact bone (implant body within or beyond the envelope).
> **Class Id**: circular bone resorption with vestibular and oral loss of the compact layer (implant body within or beyond the envelope).
> **Class Ie**: circular bone resorption with maintenance of the vestibular and oral compact bone.

For clinical documentation of the classes Ia to Ie, as shown in Fig 13-10b, the **intrabony defect components (i)** beginning with the crestal area of the alveolar process to the bottom of the intrabony defect can be measured at four locations (mesial, distal, vestibular and oral). The **circumferential defect components s(c)** determine the linear distance between the mesial, distal, vestibular, and oral bone wall and the implant body. The extension of the dehiscence defect can be assessed from the crestal area of the alveolar process in height s(a) and width s(b). The **supracrestal component** is considered as the distance between the transitions from structured to machined implant portion (bony and transmucosal part, BTB) and the bordering crestal aspect of the implant-supporting alveo-

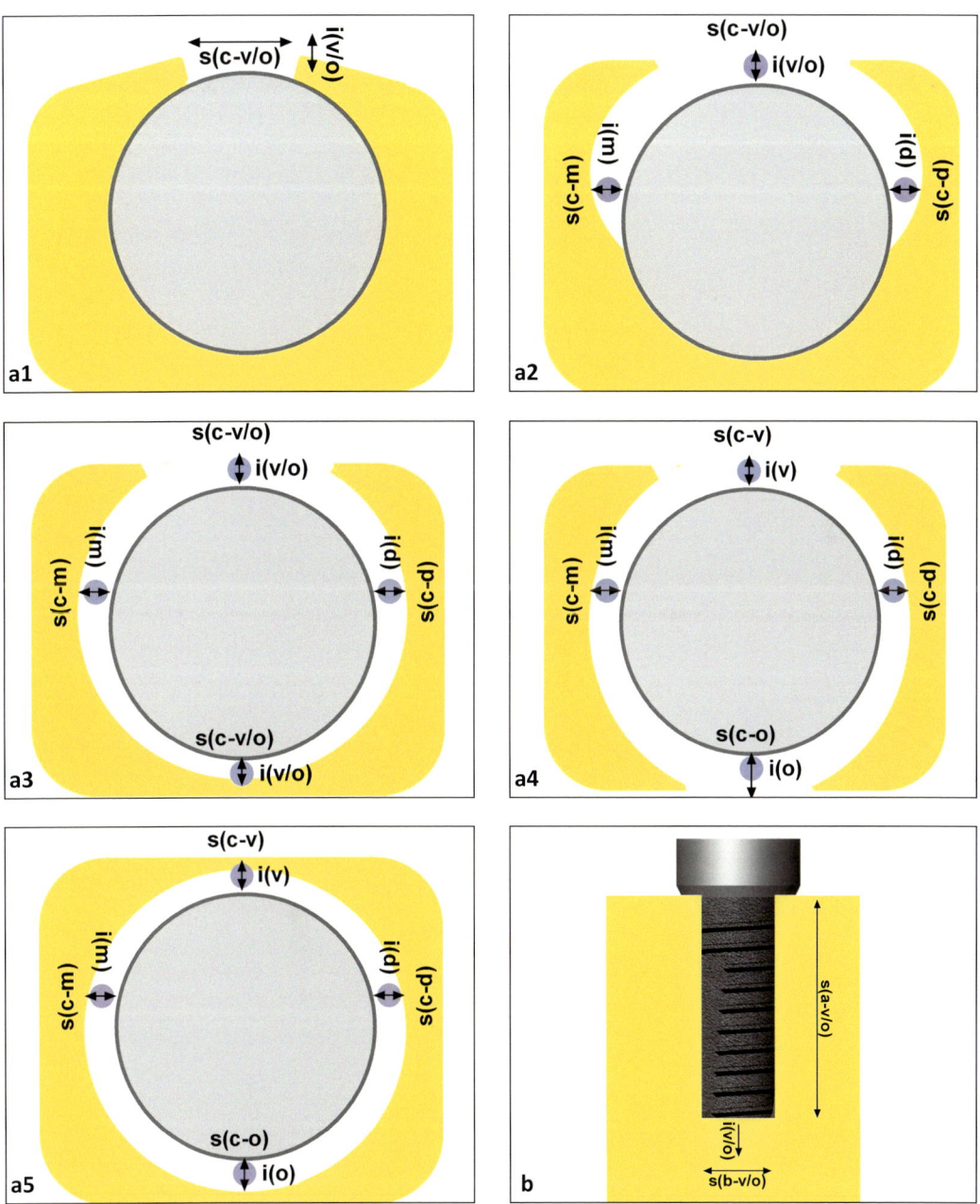

Fig 13-10 (a) Configuration of peri-implantitis bone defects - **intrabony components (i)** – cross-sections. **Circumferential component–s(c)** of the defect, measured as the linear distance from the vestibular–s(c-v), mesial–s(c-m), distal–s(c-d), and oral–s(c-o) bone wall of the defect to the implant surface. **Intrabony component of the defect (i)**, measured as the linear distance from the alveolar bone crest to the bottom of the defect (v, m, d, o). (**b**) **Intrabony component (I)** – extension of the dehiscence defect. s(a): maximum linear mesial or distal distance from the borderline between the bony and transmucosal part (BTB) of the implant to the alveolar bone crest.

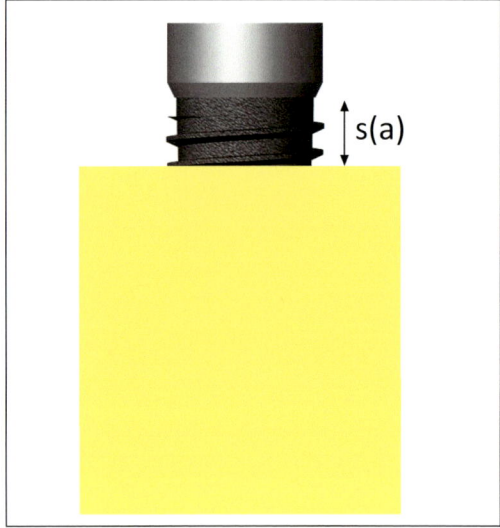

Fig 13-11 Configuration of peri-implantitis bone defects – supracrestal component (II). s(a): maximum linear mesial or distal distance from the borderline between the bony and transmucosal part (BTB) of the implant to the alveolar bone crest.

lar bone. It describes the extent of the supracrestally exposed structured parts of the implant (Fig 13-11). Generally, a combination of Class I and Class II defects is commonly observed around one implant.

End of the Experiment
Animal Sacrifice and Retrieval of Specimens
After the scheduled healing period, the animals are routinely sacrificed by induction of deep anesthesia followed by an overdose of a barbiturate (e.g., sodium pentobarbital 3%; 200 mg/kg intravenously). Even though formaldehyde penetrates tissues quickly (small molecules), this process may be delayed by the cortical bone, which is particularly pronounced in the dog mandible. Accordingly, animal perfusion with a fixative is widely used in the available literature employing either canine (Persson et al., 1996) or nonhuman primates (Schou et al., 2003c) and may stop or greatly reduce autolysis. However, it is to be noted that intravital perfusion with the fixative is not acceptable under animal welfare regulations and should not be done. Basically, the available studies reporting on animal perfusion most commonly employed a fixative consisting of a mixture of 5% glutaraldehyde and 4% formaldehyde buffered to a pH of 7.2 (Karnowsky, 1965). The combination of formaldehyde with glutaraldehyde as a standard fixative for electron microscopy takes advantage of the rapid penetration of small HCHO molecules, which initiate the structural stabilization of the tissue. Basically, mixtures containing formaldehyde and glutaraldehyde may not be required for conventional histologic processing of the specimens. Postmortem fixation is usually prepared after intravenous injection of 50,000 IU of heparin, which basically is given during euthanasia. Afterwards (i.e., postmortem), the carotid arteries are bilaterally prepared and catheterized. In order to facilitate the management of toxic waste and accelerate the perfusion of the corpse, decapitation may be performed and the head of the animal can be fixed intra-arterially with 1000 mL of 4% buffered formalin solution. Finally, the jaws are dissected and cut into single blocks for each experimental implant site. Afterwards, all specimens must be fixed in 10% neutral buffered formalin solution for 4 to 7 days.

Histologic Processing
The specimens are usually dehydrated using ascending grades of alcohol and xylene, infiltrated, and embedded in methylmethacrylate for nondecalcified sectioning. During this procedure, any negative influence of polymerization heat must be avoided by means of controlled polymerization in a cold atmosphere (–4 °C). After 20 hours the specimens are usually completely polymerized.

Each implant site must be cut along the long axis of the implant using a diamond band saw (Exakt®, Apparatebau, Norderstedt, Germany) in either the buccal-oral, mesiodistal, or a combination of both directions (Fig 13-12). Serial sections are usually prepared from the central

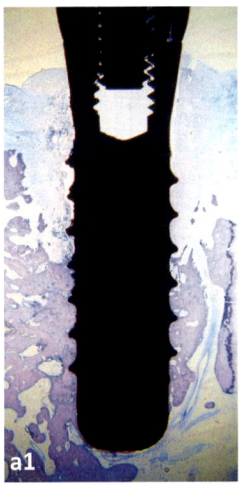 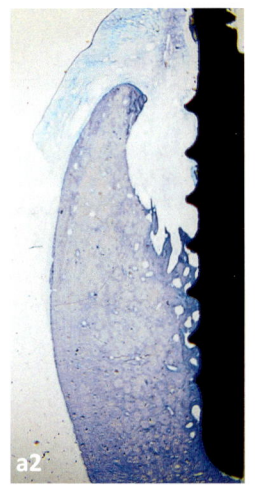 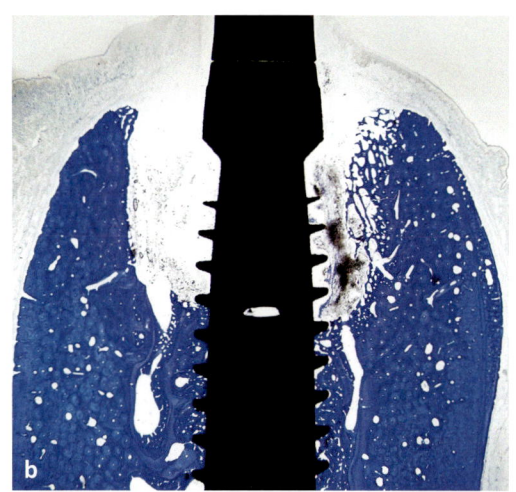 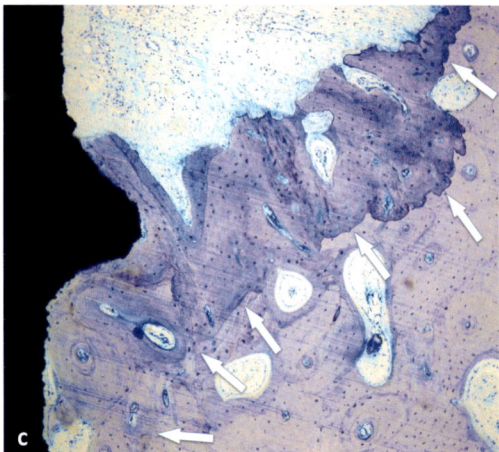

Fig 13-12 (a) Representative histologic views of a ligature-induced peri-implantitis defect in the canine. One-part implant: mesio-distal section (left), buccal aspect (right), toluidine blue stain; original magnification ×12.5. (b) Two-part implant: mesio-distal section; toluidine blue stain; original magnification ×12.5. (c) Demarcation line (arrows) of newly formed bone after 3 months of healing following surgical therapy of peri-implantitis using an Er:YAG laser device (submerged healing). Mesio-distal section; toluidine blue stain; original magnification ×40.

defect area, resulting in about two to four sections of approximately 300 μm in thickness each (Donath, 1985). Subsequently, all specimens are glued with acrylic cement to opaque Plexiglas and ground to a final thickness of approximately 40 μm.

All sections are routinely stained with toluidine blue followed by basic fuchsin to evaluate new bone formation. With this technique, old bone stains light blue, whereas newly formed bone stains dark blue because of its higher protein content (Schenk *et al*. 1984).

13.2.7 Postoperative Care
See the detailed descriptions of the postoperative care in Section 13.2.6.

13.2.8 Endpoint Measurements

Clinical
For the clinical endpoint measurements, see Section 13.2.6 (Implant uncovering + healing period III (optional) – clinical parameters).

Osteology Guidelines for Oral and Maxillofacial Regeneration

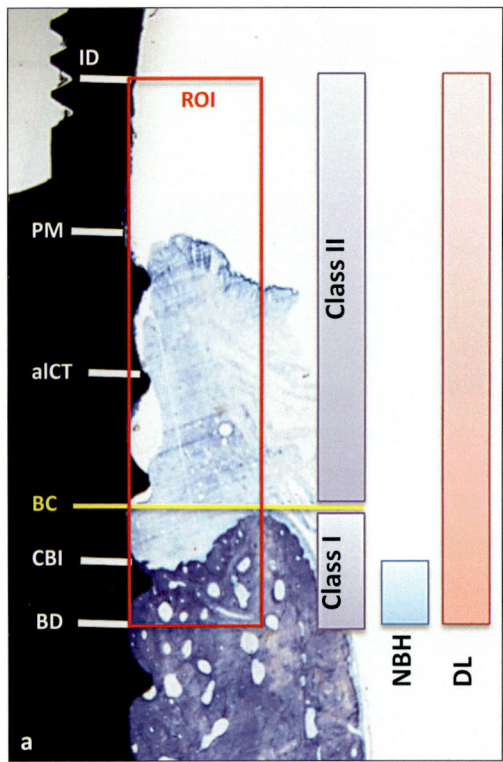
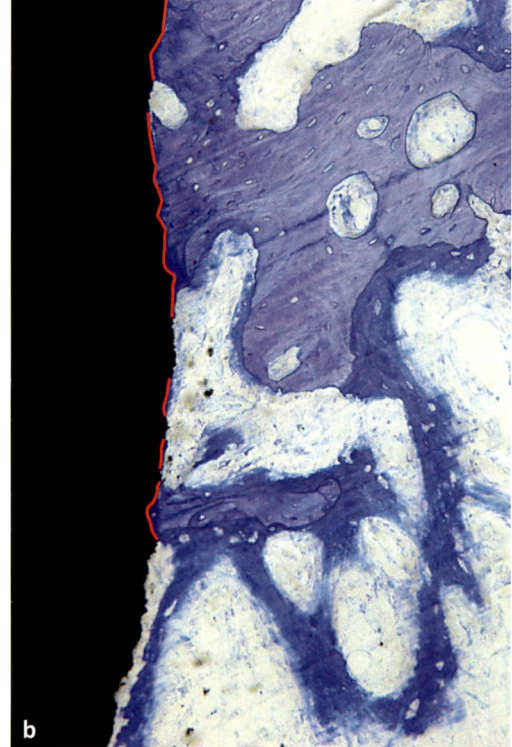

Imaging
For the radiological endpoint measurements, see Section 13.2.6 (Implant uncovering + healing period III (optional) – radiological parameters).

Histomorphometric Analysis
Histomorphometric analyses as well as microscopic observations should be performed by one experienced investigator masked to the specific experimental conditions. For image acquisition a color charge-coupled device (CCD) camera should be mounted on a binocular transmitted light microscope. Digital images (e.g., original magnification ×200) can be evaluated using a variety of commercially available software programs. The landmarks shown in Fig 13-13 are usually identified in the stained sections:

- Borderline between the machined and structured aspects (corresponding to the initial insertion depth) (ID)
- PM: mucosal margin
- The bottom of the former bone defect (BD)
- BC: the level of the alveolar bone crest
- The most coronal level of bone in contact with the implant at respective sites (CBI)
- aICT: the apical extension of the inflammatory cell infiltrate

BC determines the borderline between Class I (i.e., intrabony) and Class II (i.e., supracrestal) defect components. Linear measurements are made by drawing a vertical line, following the long axis of the implant (Fig 13-13a):
- Defect length (DL) is measured from ID to BD (mm)

13.2 Animal Models

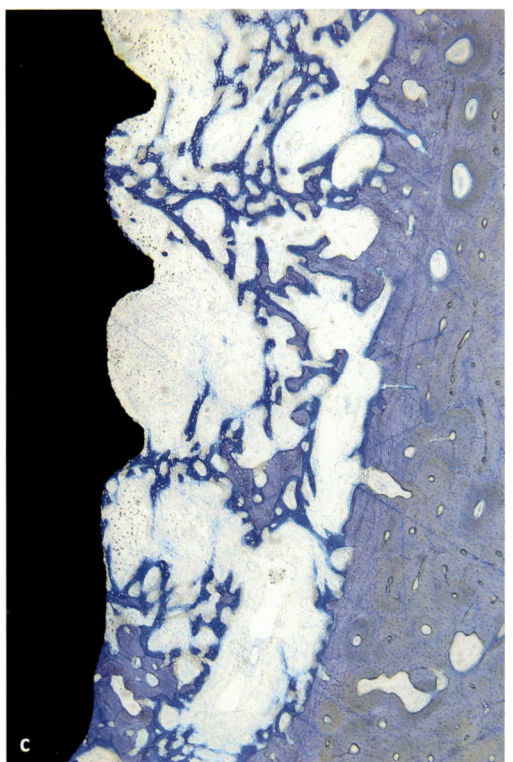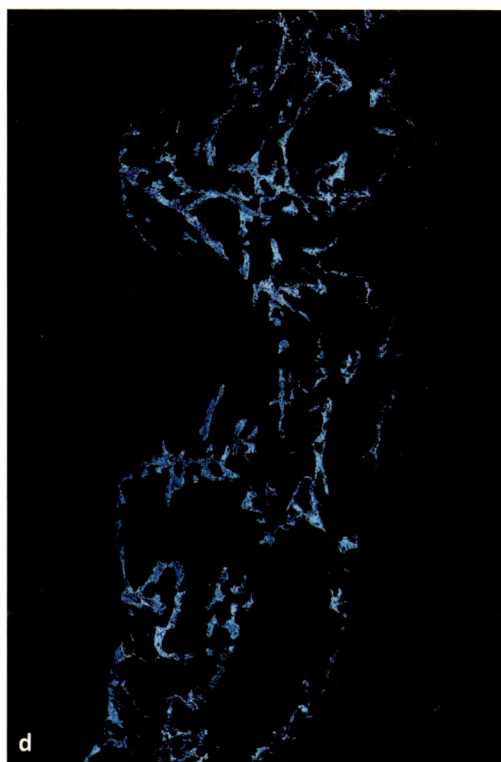

Fig 13-13 Histologic landmarks – ligature-induced peri-implantitis defect in canine. (**a**) One-part implant: buccal aspect, toluidine blue stain; original magnification ×12.5. ID: borderline between the machined and structured aspects; PM: mucosal margin; aICT: the apical extension of the inflammatory cell infiltrate; BC: the level of the alveolar bone crest; BD: the bottom of the former bone defect; CBI: the most coronal level of bone in contact with the implant; ROI: region of interest to assess surface area of bone formation; bone to implant contact (BIC) is measured from BD to ID, serving as 100%; NBH: new bone height; DL: defect length.
Note: BC determines the borderline between Class I (i.e., intrabony) and Class II (i.e., supracrestal) defect components (**b**) Assessment of new BIC excludes any non-mineralized tissue areas, including bone marrow spaces. Toluidine blue stain, original magnification ×40. (**c**) Histologic landmarks – ligature-induced peri-implantitis defect in canine. Histologic view of a new woven bone formation within the Class Ie defect component. Toluidine blue stain, original magnification ×25. (**d**) The image analysis software automatically assesses the surface area (mm²) of newly formed mineralized tissue within any ROI. Note: The vertical dimension of ROI is usually defined from BD to ID. The horizontal dimension of ROI usually correlates with s(c) at the respective site (see Fig 13-10).

- New bone height (NBH) is measured from BD to CBI (mm)
- Percent linear fill (PLF) is defined as NBH divided by DL
- The amount of new bone (mineralized tissue) to implant contact (BIC) in the defect is measured as percentage of the distance from BD to ID, serving as 100% (Fig 13-13b).

The regenerated area (RA), defined as the surface area of mineralized tissue (MT) (mm²) in the region of interest (ROI) can automatically be estimated by the image analysis software (Figs 13-13c and 13-13d). While the vertical dimension of ROI is usually defined from BD to ID, the horizontal dimension correlates with s(c) at the respective site (see Fig 13-10). In case of an augmentative therapy, RA also includes residual bone graft particles.

Prior to the start of the morphometric analysis, a calibration procedure should be conducted for the experienced investigator as well as for the image analysis software.

Fluorescence Microscopy
For these purposes, the microscope needs to be equipped with a fluorescence illuminator. Basically, unstained sections are illuminated with light of a specific wavelength (or wavelengths), which is absorbed by the fluorophores, causing them to emit light of longer wavelengths (i.e., of a different color than the absorbed light). The illumination light is separated from the much weaker emitted fluorescence through the use of a spectral emission filter. Fluorochromes used for bone labeling are calcium-seeking substances that are irreversibly deposited at sites of mineralized tissue formation. This procedure improves the assessment of both direction and topographic localization of new bone formation in studies aimed at assessing therapeutic interventions of peri-implantitis lesions.

Canine
The following fluorochromes (intravenous injection in the jugular vein) and corresponding protocols (e.g., multiple labeling) have been employed in the available literature:
- Xylenol orange (60 mg/kg) at 2 weeks/ oxytetracycline (25 mg/kg) administered at 6 weeks (Persson *et al.*, 1999)
- Oxytetracycline (16 mg/kg) administered at 2 weeks after therapy and repeated after 24 hours (Persson *et al.*, 2001a,b, 2004)
- Oxytetracycline (25 mg/kg) administered at 2 or 19 weeks after therapy (Shibli *et al.*, 2003c, 2006)
- Alizarin red complex (30 mg/kg) at 2 weeks/ tetracycline (15 mg/kg) at 5 weeks/ calcein green (10 mg/kg) at 8 weeks, and xylenol orange (90 mg/kg) at 12 weeks after therapy.

No undesired side effects have been reported in these studies at these dose levels.

Microbiological Analysis
Only three studies have investigated microbiologic changes in dogs subsequent to peri-implantitis therapy employing either antimicrobial photodynamic therapy (Shibli *et al.*, 2003c; Hayek *et al.*, 2005) or Er:YAG laser application (Takasaki *et al.*, 2007) for implant surface decontamination during open flap surgery.

In particular, the original procedure described by Shibli *et al.* (2003c) comprised the removal of one implant from an animal, which was processed for scanning electron microscopy to verify the presence of bacterial cells, thus providing proof of implant surface contamination. Subsequently, microbial samples were obtained before and immediately after treatment by means of sterile paper points and analyzed (quantitatively: colony forming units CFU/ mL; qualitatively: Gram stain, aero tolerance, colony morphology, esculin hydrolysis, nitrate reduction, indole production, α-glucosidase and N-benzoyl-DL-arginine-2-naphthylamide (BANA) hydrolysis, oxidase, and catalase activities) for the presence of *P. gingivalis*, *Prevotella* species, *Fusobacterium* species and group B streptococcus.

Takasaki *et al.* (2007) undertook bacterial detection by polymerase chain reaction (PCR) to identify five major periodontopathogenic bacteria (i.e., *Aggregatibacter actinomycetemcomitans*, *P. gingivalis*, *Prevotella intermedia*, *Treponema forsythia*, and *Treponema denticola*) in submarginal plaque collected by sterile paper points.

Experimental studies aimed at investigating pathogenesis of peri-implantitis employed a wide range of microbiological approaches, including CFU, darkfield microscopy, and PCR (Hickey *et al.*, 1991; Akagawa *et al.*, 1993; Schou *et al.*, 1996; Eke *et al.*, 1998; Nociti *et al.*, 2001a).

13.2.9 Statistical Analysis Plan (see Chapter 4)

Power Analysis
For the power analysis, a standard normal distribution should be assumed. The probability of a type I error is usually set at 0.05. In order to get a study power of 0.80 the probability of a type II error must be set at 0.20. Sigma, which allows for the possibility of different standard deviations in all test and control groups, must be estimated based on the standard deviations observed in previous studies reporting on similar groups. Defining a specific parameter (most commonly BIC) as primary outcome variable, a clinically relevant difference may be set at 10%.

Statistical Analysis
Mean values and standard deviations among animals must be calculated for each variable and group. The data rows should be examined with the Kolmogorov–Smirnov test for normal distribution. According to the data distribution, either nonparametric or parametric tests should be used for the statistical evaluation of the changes within and between groups. The α error is usually set at 0.05.

13.2.10 Materials, Consumables, Equipment

For detailed information on materials, consumables, and equipment see Section 13.2.6.

References

1. Abrahamsson I, Berglundh T, Wennstrom J, Lindhe J (1996). The peri-implant hard and soft tissues at different implant systems. A comparative study in the dog. *Clin Oral Implants Res* 7:212–219.
2. Abrahamsson I, Berglundh T, Glantz PO, Lindhe J (1998). The mucosal attachment at different abutments. An experimental study in dogs. *J Clin Periodontol* 25:721–727.
3. Akagawa Y, Matsumoto T, Kawamura M, Tsuru H (1993). Changes of subgingival microflora around single-crystal sapphire endosseous implants after experimental ligature-induced plaque accumulation in monkeys. *J Prosthet Dent* 69:594–598.
4. Albouy JP, Abrahamsson I, Persson LG, Berglundh T (2008). Spontaneous progression of peri-implantitis at different types of implants. An experimental study in dogs. I: clinical and radiographic observations. *Clin Oral Implants Res* 19:997–1002.
5. Albouy JP, Abrahamsson I, Persson LG, Berglundh T (2009). Spontaneous progression of ligatured induced peri-implantitis at implants with different surface characteristics. An experimental study in dogs II: histological observations. *Clin Oral Implants Res* 20:366–371.
6. Berglundh T, Lindhe J (1996). Dimension of the periimplant mucosa. Biological width revisited. *J Clin Periodontol* 23:971–973.
7. Berglundh T, Lindhe J, Ericsson I, Marinello CP, Liljenberg B, Thomsen P (1991). The soft tissue barrier at implants and teeth. *Clin Oral Implants Res* 2:81–90.
8. Berglundh T, Lindhe J, Marinello C, Ericsson I, Liljenberg B (1992). Soft tissue reaction to de novo plaque formation on implants and teeth. An experimental study in the dog. *Clin Oral Implants Res* 3:1–8.
9. Berglundh T, Abrahamsson I, Welander M, Lang NP, Lindhe J (2007a). Morphogenesis of the peri-implant mucosa: an experimental study in dogs. *Clin Oral Implants Res* 18:1–8.
10. Berglundh T, Gotfredsen K, Zitzmann NU, Lang NP, Lindhe J (2007b). Spontaneous progression of ligature induced peri-implantitis at implants with different surface roughness: an experimental study in dogs. *Clin Oral Implants Res* 18:655–661.
11. Deppe H, Horch HH, Henke J, Donath K (2001). Peri-implant care of ailing implants with the carbon dioxide laser. *Int J Oral Maxillofac Implants* 16:659–667.
12. Deppe H, Greim H, Brill T, Wagenpfeil S (2002). Titanium deposition after peri-implant care with the carbon dioxide laser. *Int J Oral Maxillofac Implants* 17:707–714.
13. Donath K (1985). The diagnostic value of the new method for the study of undecalcified bones and teeth with attached soft tissue (Sage-Schliff (sawing and grinding) technique). *Pathol Res Pract* 179:631–633.
14. Eke PI, Braswell LD, Fritz ME (1998). Microbiota associated with experimental peri-implantitis and periodontitis in adult Macaca mulatta monkeys. *J Periodontol* 69:190–194.
15. Ericsson I, Lindhe J (1993). Probing depth at implants and teeth. An experimental study in the dog. *J Clin Periodontol* 20:623–627.
16. Ericsson I, Lindhe J, Rylander H, Okamoto H (1975). Experimental periodontal breakdown in the dog. *Scand J Dent Res* 83:189–192.
17. Ericsson I, Berglundh T, Marinello C, Liljenberg B, Lindhe J (1992). Long-standing plaque and gingivitis at implants and teeth in the dog. *Clin Oral Implants Res* 3:99–103.
18. Ericsson I, Nilner K, Klinge B, Glantz PO (1996a). Radiographical and histological characteristics of submerged and nonsubmerged titanium implants. An experimental study in the Labrador dog. *Clin Oral Implants Res* 7:20–26.

19. Ericsson I, Persson LG, Berglundh T, Edlund T, Lindhe J (1996b). The effect of antimicrobial therapy on peri-implantitis lesions. An experimental study in the dog. *Clin Oral Implants Res* 7:320–328.
20. Etter TH, Hakanson I, Lang NP, Trejo PM, Caffesse RG (2002). Healing after standardized clinical probing of the perlimplant soft tissue seal: a histomorphometric study in dogs. *Clin Oral Implants Res* 13:571–580.
21. Faggion CM Jr, Schmitter M, Tu YK (2009). Assessment of replication of research evidence from animals to humans in studies on peri-implantitis therapy. *J Dent* 37:737–747.
22. Gotfredsen K, Berglundh T, Lindhe J (2002). Bone reactions at implants subjected to experimental peri-implantitis and static load. A study in the dog. *J Clin Periodontol* 29:144–151.
23. Grunder U, Hurzeler MB, Schupbach P, Strub JR (1993). Treatment of ligature-induced peri-implantitis using guided tissue regeneration: a clinical and histologic study in the beagle dog. *Int J Oral Maxillofac Implants* 8:282–293.
24. Hanisch O, Cortella CA, Boskovic MM, James RA, Slots J, Wikesjo UM (1997a). Experimental peri-implant tissue breakdown around hydroxyapatite-coated implants. *J Periodontol* 68:59–66.
25. Hanisch O, Tatakis DN, Boskovic MM, Rohrer MD, Wikesjo UM (1997b). Bone formation and reosseointegration in peri-implantitis defects following surgical implantation of rhBMP-2. *Int J Oral Maxillofac Implants* 12:604–610.
26. Hayek RR, Araujo NS, Gioso MA, Ferreira J, Baptista-Sobrinho CA, Yamada AM et al. (2005). Comparative study between the effects of photodynamic therapy and conventional therapy on microbial reduction in ligature-induced peri-implantitis in dogs. *J Periodontol* 76:1275–1281.
27. Hickey JS, O'Neal RB, Scheidt MJ, Strong SL, Turgeon D, Van Dyke TE (1991). Microbiologic characterization of ligature-induced peri-implantitis in the microswine model. *J Periodontol* 62:548–553.
28. Huja SS, Beck FM (2008). Bone remodeling in maxilla, mandible, and femur of young dogs. *Anat Rec (Hoboken)* 291:1–5.
29. Hurzeler MB, Quinones CR, Morrison EC, Caffesse RG (1995). Treatment of peri-implantitis using guided bone regeneration and bone grafts, alone or in combination, in beagle dogs. Part 1: Clinical findings and histologic observations. *Int J Oral Maxillofac Implants* 10:474–484.
30. Hurzeler MB, Quinones CR, Schupback P, Morrison EC, Caffesse RG (1997). Treatment of peri-implantitis using guided bone regeneration and bone grafts, alone or in combination, in beagle dogs. Part 2: Histologic findings. *Int J Oral Maxillofac Implants* 12:168–175.
31. Jepsen S, Ruhling A, Jepsen K, Ohlenbusch B, Albers HK (1996). Progressive peri-implantitis. Incidence and prediction of peri-implant attachment loss. *Clin Oral Implants Res* 7:133–142.
32. Joss A, Adler R, Lang NP (1994). Bleeding on probing. A parameter for monitoring periodontal conditions in clinical practice. *J Clin Periodontol* 21:402–408.
33. Jovanovic SA (1993). The management of peri-implant breakdown around functioning osseointegrated dental implants. *J Periodontol* 64(Suppl 11):1176–1183.
34. Jovanovic SA, Kenney EB, Carranza FA, Jr., Donath K (1993). The regenerative potential of plaque-induced peri-implant bone defects treated by a submerged membrane technique: an experimental study. *Int J Oral Maxillofac Implants* 8:13–18.
35. Junker R, Dimakis A, Thoneick M, Jansen JA (2009). Effects of implant surface coatings and composition on bone integration: a systematic review. *Clin Oral Implants Res* 20(Suppl 4):185–206.
36. Karnowsky MJ (1965). A formaldehyde-glutaraldehyde fixative of high osmolality for use in electron microscopy. *J Cell Biol* 27:137A–138A.
37. Kennedy JE, Polson AM (1973). Experimental marginal periodontitis in squirrel monkeys. *J Periodontol* 44:140–144.
38. Lang NP, Adler R, Joss A, Nyman S (1990). Absence of bleeding on probing. An indicator of periodontal stability. *J Clin Periodontol* 17:714–721.
39. Lang NP, Bragger U, Walther D, Beamer B, Kornman KS (1993). Ligature-induced peri-implant infection in cynomolgus monkeys. I. Clinical and radiographic findings. *Clin Oral Implants Res* 4:2–11.
40. Lang NP, Wetzel AC, Stich H, Caffesse RG (1994). Histologic probe penetration in healthy and inflamed peri-implant tissues. *Clin Oral Implants Res* 5:191–201.
41. Lekholm U, Ericsson I, Adell R, Slots J (1986). The condition of the soft tissues at tooth and fixture abutments supporting fixed bridges. A microbiological and histological study. *J Clin Periodontol* 13:558–562.
42. Leonhardt A, Berglundh T, Ericsson I, Dahlen G (1992). Putative periodontal pathogens on titanium implants and teeth in experimental gingivitis and periodontitis in beagle dogs. *Clin Oral Implants Res* 3:112–119.
43. Lindhe J, Hamp SE, Loe H (1975). Plaque induced periodontal disease in beagle dogs. A 4-year clinical, roentgenographical and histometrical study. *J Periodontal Res* 10:243–255.
44. Lindhe J, Berglundh T, Ericsson I, Liljenberg B, Marinello C (1992). Experimental breakdown of peri-implant and periodontal tissues. A study in the beagle dog. *Clin Oral Implants Res* 3:9–16.
45. Löe H, Silness J (1963). Periodontal disease in pregnancy, I. Prevalence and severity. *Acta Odontol Scand* 21:533–551.
46. Machado MA, Stefani CM, Sallum EA, Sallum AW, Tramontina VA, Nociti FH Jr (1999). Treatment of ligature-induced peri-implantitis defects by regenerative procedures: a clinical study in dogs. *J Oral Sci* 41:181–185.
47. Machado MA, Stefani CM, Sallum EA, Sallum AW, Tramontina VA, Nogueira-Filho GR, et al. (2000). Treatment of ligature-induced peri-implantitis defects by regenerative procedures. Part II: A histometric study in dogs. *J Oral Sci* 42:163–168.

References

48. Marinello CP, Berglundh T, Ericsson I, Klinge B, Glantz PO, Lindhe J (1995). Resolution of ligature-induced peri-implantitis lesions in the dog. *J Clin Periodontol* 22:475–479.
49. Martins MC, Abi-Rached RS, Shibli JA, Araujo MW, Marcantonio E Jr (2004). Experimental peri-implant tissue breakdown around different dental implant surfaces: clinical and radiographic evaluation in dogs. *Int J Oral Maxillofac Implants* 19:839–848.
50. Martins MC, Shibli JA, Abi-Rached RS, Marcantonio E Jr (2005). Progression of experimental chronic peri-implantitis in dogs: clinical and radiographic evaluation. *J Periodontol* 76:1367–1373.
51. Mombelli A, van Oosten MA, Schurch E Jr, Land NP (1987). The microbiota associated with successful or failing osseointegrated titanium implants. *Oral Microbiol Immunol* 2:145–151.
52. Mombelli A, Muhle T, Bragger U, Lang NP, Burgin WB (1997). Comparison of periodontal and peri-implant probing by depth-force pattern analysis. *Clin Oral Implants Res* 8:448–454.
53. Nociti FH Jr, Caffesse RG, Sallum EA, Machado MA, Stefani CM, Sallum AW (2000). Evaluation of guided bone regeneration and/or bone grafts in the treatment of ligature-induced peri-implantitis defects: a morphometric study in dogs. *J Oral Implantol* 26:244–249.
54. Nociti FH Jr, Cesco De Toledo R, Machado MA, Stefani CM, Line SR, Goncalves RB (2001a). Clinical and microbiological evaluation of ligature-induced peri-implantitis and periodontitis in dogs. *Clin Oral Implants Res* 12:295–300.
55. Nociti FH Jr, Machado MA, Stefani CM, Sallum EA (2001b). Absorbable versus nonabsorbable membranes and bone grafts in the treatment of ligature-induced peri-implantitis defects in dogs: a histometric investigation. *Int J Oral Maxillofac Implants* 16:646–652.
56. Parlar A, Bosshardt DD, Cetiner D, Schafroth D, Unsal B, Haytac C et al. (2009). Effects of decontamination and implant surface characteristics on re-osseointegration following treatment of peri-implantitis. *Clin Oral Implants Res* 20:391–399.
57. Pearce AI, Richards RG, Milz S, Schneider E, Pearce SG (2007). Animal models for implant biomaterial research in bone: a review. *Eur Cell Mater* 13:1–10.
58. Persson LG, Ericsson I, Berglundh T, Lindhe J (1996). Guided bone regeneration in the treatment of periimplantitis. *Clin Oral Implants Res* 7:366–372.
59. Persson LG, Araujo MG, Berglundh T, Grondahl K, Lindhe J (1999). Resolution of peri-implantitis following treatment. An experimental study in the dog. *Clin Oral Implants Res* 10:195–203.
60. Persson LG, Berglundh T, Lindhe J, Sennerby L (2001a). Re-osseointegration after treatment of peri-implantitis at different implant surfaces. An experimental study in the dog. *Clin Oral Implants Res* 12:595–603.
61. Persson LG, Ericsson I, Berglundh T, Lindhe J (2001b). Osseointegration following treatment of peri-implantitis and replacement of implant components. An experimental study in the dog. *J Clin Periodontol* 28:258–263.
62. Persson LG, Mouhyi J, Berglundh T, Sennerby L, Lindhe J (2004). Carbon dioxide laser and hydrogen peroxide conditioning in the treatment of periimplantitis: an experimental study in the dog. *Clin Implant Dent Relat Res* 6:230–238.
63. Polimeni G, Koo KT, Qahash M, Xiropaidis AV, Albandar JM, Wikesjo UM (2004). Prognostic factors for alveolar regeneration: bone formation at teeth and titanium implants. *J Clin Periodontol* 31:927–932.
64. Renvert S, Polyzois I, Maguire R (2009). Re-osseointegration on previously contaminated surfaces: a systematic review. *Clin Oral Implants Res* 20(Suppl 4):216–227.
65. Rovin S, Costich ER, Gordon HA (1966). The influence of bacteria and irritation in the initiation of periodontal disease in germfree and conventional rats. *J Periodontal Res* 1:193–204.
66. Samuel JL, Woodall PF (1988). Periodontal disease in feral pigs (*Sus scrofa*) from Queensland, Australia. *J Wildl Dis* 24:201–206.
67. Schenk RK, Olah AJ, Herrmann W (1984). Preparation of calcified tissues for light microscopy. In: Methods of calcified tissue preparation. Dickson GR, editor. Amsterdam: Elsevler, pp. 53–71.
68. Schou S, Holmstrup P, Reibel J, Juhl M, Hjorting-Hansen E, Kornman KS (1993a). Ligature-induced marginal inflammation around osseointegrated implants and ankylosed teeth: stereologic and histologic observations in cynomolgus monkeys (Macaca fascicularis). *J Periodontol* 64:529–537.
69. Schou S, Holmstrup P, Stoltze K, Hjorting-Hansen E, Kornman KS (1993b). Ligature-induced marginal inflammation around osseointegrated implants and ankylosed teeth. *Clin Oral Implants Res* 4:12–22.
70. Schou S, Holmstrup P, Keiding N, Fiehn NE (1996). Microbiology of ligature-induced marginal inflammation around osseointegrated implants and ankylosed teeth in cynomolgus monkeys (Macaca fascicularis). *Clin Oral Implants Res* 7:190–200.
71. Schou S, Holmstrup P, Stoltze K, Hjorting-Hansen E, Fiehn NE, Skovgaard LT (2002). Probing around implants and teeth with healthy or inflamed peri-implant mucosa/gingiva. A histologic comparison in cynomolgus monkeys (Macaca fascicularis). *Clin Oral Implants Res* 13:113–126.
72. Schou S, Holmstrup P, Jorgensen T, Skovgaard LT, Stoltze K, Hjorting-Hansen E et al. (2003a). Anorganic porous bovine-derived bone mineral (Bio-Oss) and ePTFE membrane in the treatment of peri-implantitis in cynomolgus monkeys. *Clin Oral Implants Res* 14:535–547.
73. Schou S, Holmstrup P, Jorgensen T, Skovgaard LT, Stoltze K, Hjorting-Hansen E et al. (2003b). Implant surface preparation in the surgical treatment of experimental peri-implantitis with autogenous bone graft and ePTFE membrane in cynomolgus monkeys. *Clin Oral Implants Res* 14:412–422.

74. Schou S, Holmstrup P, Jorgensen T, Stoltze K, Hjorting-Hansen E, Wenzel A (2003c). Autogenous bone graft and ePTFE membrane in the treatment of peri-implantitis. I. Clinical and radiographic observations in cynomolgus monkeys. *Clin Oral Implants Res* 14:391–403.
75. Schwarz F, Jepsen S, Herten M, Sager M, Rothamel D, Becker J (2006). Influence of different treatment approaches on non-submerged and submerged healing of ligature induced peri-implantitis lesions: an experimental study in dogs. *J Clin Periodontol* 33:584–595.
76. Schwarz F, Herten M, Sager M, Bieling K, Sculean A, Becker J (2007). Comparison of naturally occurring and ligature-induced peri-implantitis bone defects in humans and dogs. *Clin Oral Implants Res* 18:161–170.
77. Schwarz F, Mihatovic I, Ferrari D, Wieland M, Becker J (2010). Influence of frequent clinical probing during the healing phase on healthy peri-implant soft tissue formed at different titanium implant surfaces: a histomorphometrical study in dogs. *J Clin Periodontol* 37:551–562.
78. Sennerby L, Persson LG, Berglundh T, Wennerberg A, Lindhe J (2005). Implant stability during initiation and resolution of experimental periimplantitis: an experimental study in the dog. *Clin Implant Dent Relat Res* 7:136–140.
79. Shibli JA, Martins MC, Lotufo RF, Marcantonio E Jr (2003a). Microbiologic and radiographic analysis of ligature-induced peri-implantitis with different dental implant surfaces. *Int J Oral Maxillofac Implants* 18:383–390.
80. Shibli JA, Martins MC, Nociti FH Jr, Garcia VG, Marcantonio E Jr (2003b). Treatment of ligature-induced peri-implantitis by lethal photosensitization and guided bone regeneration: a preliminary histologic study in dogs. *J Periodontol* 74:338–345.
81. Shibli JA, Martins MC, Theodoro LH, Lotufo RF, Garcia VG, Marcantonio EJ (2003c). Lethal photosensitization in microbiological treatment of ligature-induced peri-implantitis: a preliminary study in dogs. *J Oral Sci* 45:17–23.
82. Shibli JA, Martins MC, Ribeiro FS, Garcia VG, Nociti FH Jr, Marcantonio E Jr (2006). Lethal photosensitization and guided bone regeneration in treatment of peri-implantitis: an experimental study in dogs. *Clin Oral Implants Res* 17:273–281.
83. Silness J, Löe H (1964). Periodontal Disease In Pregnancy. Ii. Correlation Between Oral Hygiene And Periodontal Condtion. *Acta Odontol Scand* 22:121–135.
84. Singh G, O'Neal RB, Brennan WA, Strong SL, Horner JA, Van Dyke TE (1993). Surgical treatment of induced peri-implantitis in the micro pig: clinical and histological analysis. *J Periodontol* 64:984–989.
85. Stubinger S, Henke J, Donath K, Deppe H (2005). Bone regeneration after peri-implant care with the CO2 laser: a fluorescence microscopy study. *Int J Oral Maxillofac Implants* 20:203–210.
86. Takasaki AA, Aoki A, Mizutani K, Kikuchi S, Oda S, Ishikawa I (2007). Er:YAG laser therapy for peri-implant infection: a histological study. *Lasers Med Sci* 22:143–157.
87. Tillmanns HW, Hermann JS, Cagna DR, Burgess AV, Meffert RM (1997). Evaluation of three different dental implants in ligature-induced peri-implantitis in the beagle dog. Part I. Clinical evaluation. *Int J Oral Maxillofac Implants* 12:611–620.
88. Tillmanns HW, Hermann JS, Tiffee JC, Burgess AV, Meffert RM (1998). Evaluation of three different dental implants in ligature-induced peri-implantitis in the beagle dog. Part II. Histology and microbiology. *Int J Oral Maxillofac Implants* 13:59–68.
89. Warrer K, Buser D, Lang NP, Karring T (1995). Plaque-induced peri-implantitis in the presence or absence of keratinized mucosa. An experimental study in monkeys. *Clin Oral Implants Res* 6:131–138.
90. Weber HP, Buser D, Donath K, Fiorellini JP, Doppalapudi V, Paquette DW et al. (1996). Comparison of healed tissues adjacent to submerged and non-submerged unloaded titanium dental implants. A histometric study in beagle dogs. *Clin Oral Implants Res* 7:11–19.
91. Weinberg MA, Bral M (1999). Laboratory animal models in periodontology. *J Clin Periodontol* 26:335–340.
92. Wetzel AC, Vlassis J, Caffesse RG, Hammerle CH, Lang NP (1999). Attempts to obtain re-osseointegration following experimental peri-implantitis in dogs. *Clin Oral Implants Res* 10:111–119.
93. You TM, Choi BH, Zhu SJ, Jung JH, Lee SH, Huh JY et al. (2007). Treatment of experimental peri-implantitis using autogenous bone grafts and platelet-enriched fibrin glue in dogs. *Oral Surg Oral Med Oral Pathol Oral Radiol Endod* 103:34–37.
94. Zechner W, Kneissel M, Kim S, Ulm C, Watzek G, Plenk H Jr. (2004). Histomorphometrical and clinical comparison of submerged and nonsubmerged implants subjected to experimental peri-implantitis in dogs. *Clin Oral Implants Res* 15:23–33.
95. Zitzmann NU, Berglundh T, Ericsson I, Lindhe J (2004). Spontaneous progression of experimentally induced periimplantitis. *J Clin Periodontol* 31:845–849.

Compromised Bone Healing: Implantation Model

Reinhard Gruber, Stefan Tangl, and Ulrike Kuchler

14.1 General Overview

The success of implant dentistry strongly depends on the healing capacity of bone (Schenk and Buser, 1998). Osseointegration of dental implants and the consolidation of grafted materials are the consequence of bone regeneration, a highly orchestrated process of cells, growth factors, and the extracellular matrix. Bone regeneration is a sequential process (Ai-Aql et al., 2008; Schindeler et al., 2008). The defect site is filled by a blood clot which is replaced by a blood vessel-rich granulation tissue. This microenvironment is a prerequisite for bone formation to occur. Immature woven bone grows into this microenvironment and provides a first physical anchorage for dental implants. Immature woven bone is replaced by mature lamellar bone as a consequence of bone modeling and remodeling. These sequential events have been observed in a dog model (Berglundh et al., 2003) and human biopsies (Trombelli et al., 2008). Bone remodeling continues for life as functional loading necessitates the repair of fatigue microdamage (Chapurlat and Delmas, 2009). Thus, the success of implant dentistry depends on both bone regeneration and bone remodeling.

Under the physiologic situation, the sequential process of bone regeneration and bone remodeling runs with the robustness of a clockwork. However, while clockworks are based on mechanical movement, bone regeneration and remodeling are biologic processes. Even subtle changes in these biologic processes can influence the regenerative capacity of bone, and may therefore have a negative impact on the early phase of osseointegration. Moreover, systemic diseases and their pharmacologic therapy can cause a shift in bone remodeling, where osteoclast bone resorption exceeds osteoblastic bone formation (Riggs and Parfitt, 2005). The consequence is a net loss of bone mass and bone quality (Seeman and Delmas, 2006). Net loss of bone mass can have a negative impact on the late phase of osseointegration. Thus, changes of the physiologic situations can affect bone regeneration and bone remodeling, which reflect the early and late phases of osseointegration, respectively. Compromised bone regeneration and bone remodeling therefore have a negative impact on the survival rate of implants. Implant research basically focuses on strategies that maximize the survival rate of implants.

Implant research follows a clear strategy. First, characterize the patients that are at risk for implant failures to reveal possible "risk factors". Second, analyze the time point of implant failures to distinguish between early and late implant failures. Third, develop preclinical models that reflect the clinical situation to study the mechanisms of implant failures. Fourth, design therapeutic strategies that specifically take these mechanisms into account. Fifth, use preclinical models to test the new targeted therapeutics to evaluate if they can compensate the mechanisms of implant failures. Implant research following this strategy provides the basis for preclinical studies in higher animals and clinical studies (Muschler *et al.*, 2010). In general, implant research occurs in cycles of clinical studies to test new approaches to find new risk factors. Preclinical studies help to understand the cause of implant failure and to develop strategies to overcome these limitations.

In this chapter, we focus on the rat as a model for preclinical implant research, which is the lowest species in the phylogenetic tree. For higher animal models such as dog, sheep, pig, and nonhuman primates we refer to other chapters and publications (Pearce *et al.*, 2007; Pellegrini *et al.*, 2009). The rat model offers a situation where potential "risk factors" in patients can be produced under standardized conditions. Moreover, the rat model allows generating metric "endpoints" of osseointegration. It is thus possible to study the impact of "risk factors" associated with compromised bone healing, on "endpoints" which are the parameters of osseointegration. However, inflammation and functional loading of implants cannot be easily studied in rats, suggesting that this model is not suitable to investigate the late phase of osseointegration. We therefore focus in this chapter on rat models with compromised bone healing and thus the early phase of osseointegration. We also focus on four parameters of preclinical studies: the "risk factors", the implantation site, the time points, and the "endpoints".

What are the physiologic situations in a patient which can be considered "risk factors" in implant dentistry? Epidemiologic studies revealed that systemic diseases such as osteoporosis and Crohn's disease (Alsaadi *et al.*, 2007) as well as uncontrolled diabetes (Javed and Romanos, 2009) have been associated with a higher risk for implant loss. Also habits such as smoking are considered "risk factors" in implant dentistry (Abt, 2009). Moreover, radiotherapy is associated with a higher risk for implant loss (Carr, 2010). In addition, the incidence of osteonecrosis of the jaw, which occurs as a side effect of high-dose bisphosphonate therapy mainly in tumor patients, is associated with dental procedures (Woo *et al.*, 2006; Ruggiero *et al.*, 2009). Pharmacological therapies including bisphosphonates are therefore "risk factors" in implant dentistry.

Risk factors are differentially associated with early and late implant failures. Early implant failures are mainly caused by compromised bone regeneration, whereas late implant failures are mainly caused by inflammation or overloading. With regard to the clinical relevance of the rat model, it is thus necessary to understand which risk factors are associated with compromised bone healing and therefore early implant loss, prior to abutment connection (Alsaadi *et al.*, 2007). Rat models allow investigating bone regeneration and thus the early phase of osseointegration. Larger models allow studying alveolar inflammation and functional loading and thus the late phase of osseointegration.

What "anatomic location" in the rat is suitable for implant placement? The rat model allows implant placement in the long bones, usually the tibia, which is an ectopic region for this indication. Long bones consist of a cortical envelope for the bone marrow, with negligible amounts of trabecular bone in the diaphyseal region. The advantage of this anatomic situation is that a differential analysis of osseointegration in the cortical and the medullar compartments is possible. The disadvantage of this anatomic situation is that the regeneration in the tibia may follow a different kinetic than alveolar bone. These limitations have to be kept in mind when drawing conclusions that relate to the clinical situation. We thus have to hypothesize that systematic changes affecting bone regeneration in the long bones also have an impact on bone regeneration in the alveolar bone – even though the kinetics might be different. A few reports indicate that implant placement in the alveolar bone of rats is possible, but as we have no experience with this protocol, readers are referred to the original publications (Fujii *et al.*, 1998; Dunn *et al.*, 2005). Therefore, the tibia model is a model to test the proof of principles.

What are the relevant "time points" in the rat model of compromised bone regeneration? The key time points are related to (i) disease induction (induction of the risk factor), (ii) implant insertion, and (iii) termination of the experiments (evaluation of endpoints). For example, implants can be inserted in the tibia before or after disease induction. In the first case, the impact of a risk factor on the already osseointegrated implants can be evaluated, e.g., the effect of catabolic changes caused by ovariectomization. In the latter case, the impact of a risk factor on the early phase of osseointegration can be evaluated. The very early time points after implantation provide insights into the process of granulation tissue formation and woven bone formation while later time points show the presence of lamellar bone. Thus, the selection of time points has to match the research objectives. There is no consensus about one general study design that allows answering the various research questions. However, there are similarities between the studies that can lead to the development of a basic protocol. This basic protocol can be adapted according to the individual research objectives.

What are the relevant "endpoints" in rat models of implant research? The selection of endpoints provides the basis for statistical planning and communication of the results. The endpoints should closely be associated with the clinical success of a therapy, and consequently the survival rate of implants. However, implants will not get lost when osseointegration is studied in the tibia of rats. Thus, implant research with rat models has to be based on surrogate parameters that are associated with implant success. The key metric parameters are provided by bone histomorphometry, for example the amount of bone formed in the peri-implant area ("bone volume per tissue volume"; BA) and the peri-implant surface in intimate contact with bone ("bone-to-implant contact"; BIC) (Kuchler *et al.*, 2011; Mair *et al.*, 2009). Endpoints may also be based on the chemical characterization of the peri-implant mineralized matrix, e.g., the mineral distribution and the cross-linking of collagen (Schupbach *et al.*, 2005; Roschger *et al.*, 2008). Finally, biomechanical testing provides insights into the mechanical performance on an implant, e.g., the resistance to pull-out forces (Li *et al.*, 2010). All these preclinical observations in rat models are "soft" parameters for the "hard" endpoint of implant function. These surrogate endpoints are translated into clinical endpoints based on the relevant studies. However, in preclinical research with rat implantation models, study endpoints have to meet the research objectives and not necessarily the clinical outcome.

In summary, in this chapter we will focus on osseointegration in a rat tibia implantation model of compromised bone regeneration. The chapter has two main parts: (1) The selection of the "risk factors", which is the simulation of a systemic disease and/or a pharmacologic therapy that can cause an impairment of bone regeneration, and thus the early phase of osseointegration, and (2) the surgical technique of implant insertion and the histomorphometric evaluation of surrogate endpoints. This chapter might be helpful for selecting the appropriate protocol when studying implant osseointegration in rats. As research questions differ, a general recommendation for a uniform model cannot be made but the current chapter might serve as a primer during the planning phase of a related project.

14.2 Animal Model

The experimental setup is guided by the research question. The key questions are "What is the impact of a systemic conditions and/or pharmacologic treatment" ("risk factor") on the early phase of osseointegration ("endpoints"). For example, intermittent administration of parathyroid hormone (PTH) is generally accepted as a treatment to improve the process of bone regeneration and, therefore, should also stimulate osseointegration (Skripitz and Aspenberg, 2004; Barnes et al., 2008). However, such effects may not be evident during the compromised physiologic state of diabetes. Therefore, a preclinical study to determine whether the beneficial effects of PTH on osseointegration are also observed under hyperglycemic conditions is feasible. In this case, the study design requires four groups: diabetes, diabetes plus PTH, control, and control plus PTH. Based on this approach, possible association of the factors can be calculated by statistical analysis. Easier questions, that is, if just a systemic condition or pharmacologic therapy is considered a "risk factor", require only two groups.

Selecting the rat tibia implantation model is also based on the research question. The model is appropriate for answering questions related to the impact of a compromised situation on the early phase of osseointegration. Moreover, the rat tibia implantation model allows differential evaluation of osseointegration in the cortical and the medullary compartment using a fast and cheap approach. However, there are concerns with regard to the low species and the ectopic sites that are considered limitations of this model. The chapter provides a primer for the selection of risk factors, time points, the surgical technique, and endpoints.

14.2.1 The Selection of the "Risk Factors"

The basis for the development of a rat model of compromised bone regeneration in our laboratory was our experience (Kuchler et al., 2011; Mair et al., 2009) and a review on rat models simulating osteoporosis or diabetes (Glösel et al., 2010). For other rat models that reflect "risk factors" in implant dentistry such as smoking (Glowacki et al., 2008) and radiation (Renou et al., 2001), readers are referred to the relevant studies. Based on our current studies, we have included rat research models simulating colitis. However, it is not the intention of this chapter to provide a detailed protocol of the induction of osteoporosis, diabetes or colitis, but rather an impression of what situations of compromised bone regeneration are possible in the rat – independent of the surgical procedure.

Postmenopausal osteoporosis is a systemic disease where hypogonadism ultimately leads to bone loss (Riggs and Parfitt, 2005). Bone loss in the axial and the appendicular skeleton proceeds until bone volume and bone quality fall below a critical threshold where the risk of atraumatic fractures increases. Osteoporosis is also a potential risk factor for alveolar bone resorption, tooth loss (Bollen et al., 2004), and

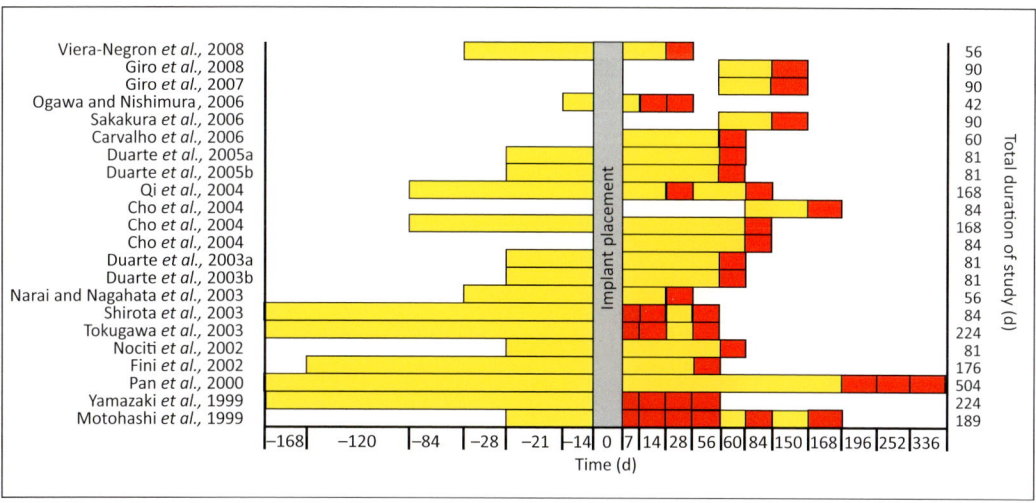

Fig 14-1 Observation periods (I): OVX rats. (Yellow indicates disease induction and red indicates euthanasia). OLETF, Otsuka Long Evans Tokushima Fatty. Adapted with permission from Glösel B, Kuchler U, Watzek G, Gruber R (2010). Review of dental implant rat research models simulating osteoporosis or diabetes. *Int J Oral Maxillofac Implants* 25:516–524. For the full details of the studies cited in this figure, please see the original article.

early implant failures (Alsaadi *et al.*, 2007). In the rat model, hypogonadism can be induced by surgical removal of the ovaries. Ovariectomized (OVX) rat develop a rapid onset bone loss that affects the trabecular and the cortical bone, including the alveolus (Rawlinson *et al.*, 2009). Conflicting data exist that hypogonadism is associated with compromised bone healing, in particular fracture healing. Some studies support this assumption (Meyer *et al.*, 2001; McCann *et al.*, 2008; Beil *et al.*, 2010) while others do not (Cao *et al.*, 2002; Melhus *et al.*, 2007). Thus, even though osseointegration in OVX rats is significantly reduced compared with sham operated control animals (Glösel *et al.*, 2010), this might be the result of a negative turnover rather than impaired bone regeneration. This model is, however, useful to study if pharmacologic therapies that control bone remodeling also have an impact on osseointegration.

According to our recent review on dental implant rat research models simulating osteoporosis (Glösel *et al.*, 2010), the insertion of implants can be performed 3 weeks after OVX (Fig 14-1 and Table 14-1). Implants remain *in situ* for a period ranging between 4 and 8 weeks before analysis. Moreover, if implants are already osseointegrated before OVX, a model situation of patients with implants that undergo postmenopausal osteoporosis is simulated. In this case, implant insertion is performed 8 weeks prior to OVX, and 4 and 8 weeks after OVX, the implants are subjected to analysis.

Diabetes, both type 1 (lack of insulin) and type 2 (insulin resistant), is a systemic disease where hyperglycemia is considered the main pathologic factor that causes serious long-term complications including cardiovascular disease, renal failure, and retinal damage. However, diabetes is also a "risk factor" related to osteoporosis, suggesting that among the long-term complications is negative-balance bone remodeling. Diabetes is also associated with compromised wound healing that typically causes the formation of diabetic ulcers. It is thus not surprising that diabetes is associated with compro-

Table 14-1 Implant locations and characteristics in OVX rats

Study	Location	Implant characteristics	Dimensions
Veira-Negron et al., 2008	Maxilla, nr	Microscrew Ti	3.0 mm long/1.0 mm wide
Giro et al., 2008	Tibia, pm	Microimplant, SAE surface	4.0 mm long/2.2 mm wide
Giro et al., 2007	Tibia, pm	Microimplant Ti, SAE surface	4.0 mm long/2.2 mm wide
Ogawa and Nishimura et al., 2006	Femur, 7.0 mm from d edge	Inner chamber, Ti	3.0:180: 3.0 × 0.8 mm
Sakakura et al., 2006	Tibia, pm	Microimplant, SAE surface	4.0 mm long/2.2 mm wide
Carvalho et al., 2006	Tibia, nr	Screw, Ti	4.0 mm long/2.2 mm wide
Duarte et al., 2005a	Tibia, nr	Screw, Ti	4.0 mm long/2.2 mm wide
Duarte et al., 2005b	Tibia, nr	Screw, Ti	4.0 mm long/2.2 mm wide
Qi et al., 2004	Tibia, pm	Screw, Ti	5.0 mm long/2.0 mm wide
Cho et al., 2004	Tibia, pm	Ti bar, sandblasted	3.0 mm long/1.5 mm wide
Duarte et al., 2003a	Tibia, nr	Screw, Ti	4.0 mm long/2.2 mm wide
Duarte et al., 2003b	Tibia, nr	Screw, Ti	4.0 mm long/2.2 mm wide
Narai and Nagahata, 2003	Femur, dm	Screw, Ti, machined surface	4.0 mm long/2.0 mm wide
Shirota et al., 2003	Tibia, pm	Screw, Ti	5.0 mm long/2.2 mm wide
Tokogawa et al., 2003	Tibia, p, anteromedial	Screw, Ti	5.0 mm long/2.2 mm wide
Nociti et al., 2002	Tibia, nr	Screw, Ti	4.0 mm long/2.2 mm wide
Fini et al., 2002	Femur, d	Cylindric nails, grade 5 Ti-6Al-4V	5.0 mm long/2.0 mm wide
Pan et al., 2000	Tibia, p, anteromedial	Cylindric, Ti, HA surface	3.0 mm long/2.0 mm wide
Yamazaki et al., 1999	Tibia, pm	Screw, Ti	5.0 mm long/2.0 mm wide
Motohashi et al., 1999	Tibia, pm	Cylindric, Ti, HA surface	3.0 mm long/2.0 mm wide

Data source was the original work corresponding to the reference. p, proximal; pm, proximal metaphysis; d, distal; dm, distal metaphysis; Ti, commercially pure titanium; SAE, sandblasted/acid-etched; HA, hydroxyapatite; Ti-6Al-4V, titanium-aluminum-vanadium alloy; nr, not reported. Adapted with permission from Glösel B, Kuchler U, Watzek G, Gruber R (2010). Review of dental implant rat research models simulating osteoporosis or diabetes. *Int J Oral Maxillofac Implants* 25:516–524. For the full details of the studies cited in this table, please see the original article.

mised bone regeneration, typically observed in rat fracture healing models (Kayal et al., 2007). Interestingly, the impact of hyperglycemia in rats on the parameters of osseointegration is not consistent, even causing an increase in osseointegration (Glösel et al., 2010).

Diabetes can be induced by streptozotocin (STZ) or alloxan, which are toxic to β-cells and thus induce a situation of type 1 diabetes. Typically, a single injection of STZ (60 to 100 mg/kg, intraperitoneal) is sufficient to cause hyperglycemia with blood glucose levels exceeding 200 mg/dL. Spontaneous type 1 diabetes models are also available (diabetes-prone BB rat). Research can also be performed with type 2 diabetes models, e.g., the OLETF (Otsuka Long

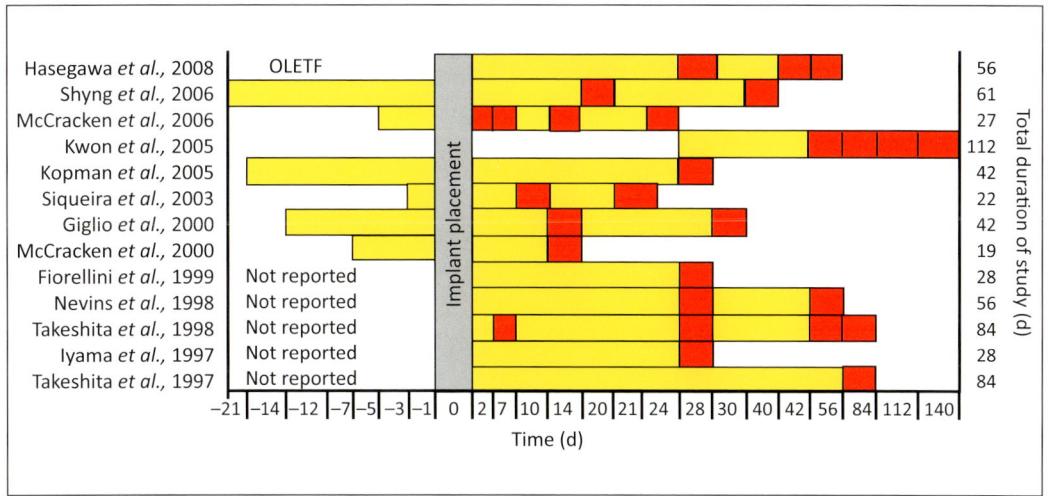

Fig 14-2 Observation periods (II): diabetic rats. (Yellow indicates disease induction and red indicates euthanasia). Adapted with permission from Glösel B, Kuchler U, Watzek G, Gruber R (2010). Review of dental implant rat research models simulating osteoporosis or diabetes. *Int J Oral Maxillofac Implants* 25:516–524. For the full details of the studies cited in this figure, please see the original article.

Evans Tokushima Fatty) obesity-induced diabetes rat model, the obese Zucker fa/fa rat, and the polygenic nonobese Goto-Kakizaki rat. Various reviews are available for rat models of diabetes (Chen and Wang, 2005; Rees and Alcolado, 2005; Chatzigeorgiou et al., 2009). We have used the STZ-induced diabetes model to determine if intermittent PTH can stimulate osseointegration in the hyperglycemic situation (Kuchler et al., 2011). According to recent protocols, depending on the scientific question (e.g., hyperglycemia or compromised bone), diabetes can be induced 7 to 21 days prior to implant insertion. Implants remained *in situ* for 4 and 8 weeks (Fig 14-2 and Table 14-2).

Crohn's disease is a chronic inflammatory process of the gastrointestinal system that has recently been associated with early implant failures (Alsaadi et al., 2007). This inflammatory disease can affects any part of the gastrointestinal tract from oral cavity to anus. Crohn's disease leads to a negative balance of bone remodeling, thereby causing systemic bone loss and thus osteoporosis (Klaus et al., 2002; Hela et al., 2005). Crohn's disease is possibly associated with compromised bone regeneration, which has not yet been shown in rat models. These data are based on preclinical models that closely resemble the clinical picture of colitis (Elson et al., 2005). Widely used protocols of chemically induced intestinal inflammation are based on trinitrobenzene sulfonic acid (TNBS)/ethanol and both acute and chronic dextran sulfate sodium (DSS) colitis (Elson et al., 2005; Wirtz et al., 2007). Ethanol is required to break the mucosal barrier, whereas TNBS is believed to haptenize colonic autologous or microbiota proteins rendering them immunogenic to the host immune system. DSS is directly toxic to gut epithelial cells of the basal crypts and affects the integrity of the mucosal barrier (Elson et al., 2005; Wirtz et al., 2007). The TNBS model of chronic intestinal inflammation is used to model Th1 inflammation in the ileum and colon (Bouma and Strober, 2003), whereas DSS is used to simulate aspects of ulcerative colitis (Okayasu et al., 1990). Rodent models with intestinal inflammation develop severe osteoporotic changes (Lin et al., 1996,

Table 14-2 Implant positions and characteristics in diabetic rats

Study	Location	Implant characteristics	Dimensions
Hasegawa et al., 2008	Femur, 10.0 mm from d edge	Inner chamber, Ti	3.0 × 2.5 × 0.8 mm
Shyng et al., 2006	Maxilla, socket of maxillary molar	Ti	2.0 mm long/0.5 mm wide
McCracken et al., 2006	Tibia, p	Threaded, Ti alloy	8.0 mm long/1.5 mm wide
Kwon et al., 2005	Femur, posterior-lateral aspect	Cylindric, Ti, TPS surface	2.0 mm long/1.0 mm wide
Kopmann et al., 2005	Femur, posterior-lateral aspect	Cylindric, Ti, TPS surface	2.0 mm long/1.0 mm wide
Siqueira et al., 2003	Femur, 10.0 mm d from knee	Cylindric, V-shaped, Ti, SAE surface	3.8 mm long/2.0 mm wide
Giglio et al., 2000	Tibia, nr	Laminar, Ti	6.0 × 1.0 × 0.1 mm
McCracken et al., 2000	Tibia, 8.0 mm p to tibial protuberance	Screws, Ti alloy	8.0 mm long/1.5 mm wide
Fiorellini et al., 1999	Femur, posterior-lateral aspect	Cylindric, Ti, TPS surface	2.0 mm long/1.0 mm wide
Nevins et al., 1998	Femur, posterior-lateral aspect	Cylindric, Ti, TPS surface	2.0 mm long/1.0 mm wide
Takeshita et al., 1998	Femur, 10.0 mm below knee joint	Cylindric, Ti	1.5 mm long/1.0 mm wide
Iyama et al., 1997	Femur, 10.0 mm below knee joint	Cylindric, HA surface	1.5 mm long/1.0 mm wide
Takeshita et al., 1997	Femur, 10.0 mm below knee joint	Cylindric, HA surface	1.5 mm long/1.0 mm wide

Data source was the original work corresponding to the reference.
p, proximal; d, distal; Ti, commercially pure titanium; SAE, sandblasted/acid-etched; HA, hydroxyapatite; TPS, titanium plasma-sprayed; nr, not reported. Adapted with permission from Glösel B, Kuchler U, Watzek G, Gruber R (2010). Review of dental implant rat research models simulating osteoporosis or diabetes. *Int J Oral Maxillofac Implants* 25:516–524. For the full details of the studies cited in this table, please see the original article.

2000; Hamdani et al., 2008). Overall these models indicate that intestinal inflammation can cause a negative balance of bone turnover thereby mimicking the clinical situation of osteoporosis. The question if intestinal inflammation also causes impaired peri-implant bone regeneration still remains an enigma.

According to our protocol, colitis is induced 7 days prior to implant insertion (Kuchler et al., 2011). The implants are removed for analysis after 4 and 8 weeks. For the TNBS colitis model, day 1, TNBS presensitization solution (1% TNBS in acetone/olive oil 4:1 ratio) is applied through the shaved abdominal skin. On day 8, a catheter is inserted into the colon of sedated rats, followed by administration of the TNBS solution (0.5 mL; 50 mg TNBS /mL in 50% ethanol) into the colon lumen. For the DSS-induced colitis, starting on day 1, rats are given 4% DSS (37 to 40 kD) in their drinking water for 7 days. After the first week of disease induction, animals receive drinking water from day 8 until day 21. At day 21, 4% DSS is applied for another 7 days. Body weight, diarrhea, and bloody stool are recorded daily. The severity

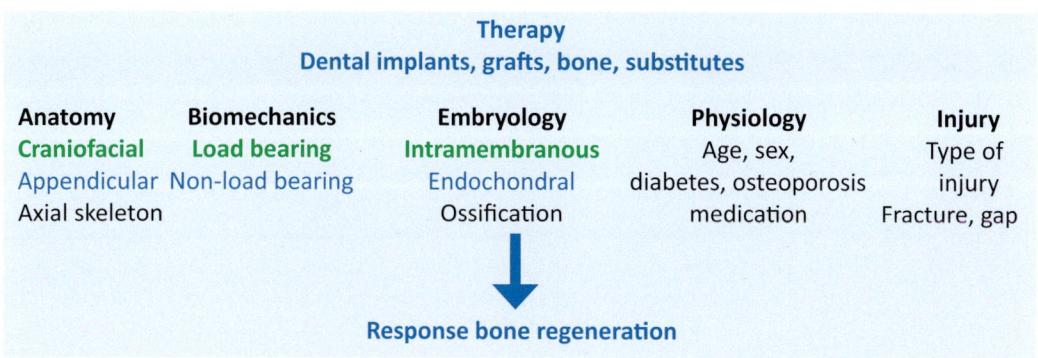

Fig 14-3 Rat models of implant placement have limitations when compared to the clinical situation. In patients, implants are placed in craniofacial bone that develops by intramembranous ossification and are subjected to functional loading. In rats, implants are placed in an appendicular bone of the tibia that develops by endochondral ossification and is not subjected to functional loading. We thus have to assume that the general principles of bone regeneration are similar in different anatomic regions and in bones of different embryologic origin. Moreover, the type of injury does not entirely resemble the clinical situation, considering the different ratio of the cortical and the medullar compartment in the jaw and the soft tissue situation of the implantation site. All these points indicate that the rat implantation model does not fully reflect the anatomic and biomechanical situation in patients. Nevertheless, the model is a valuable tool for simulating the physiologic changes that occur in patients, and thus the impact of these physiologic changes on the early phase of osseointegration. "Response" is a synonym for "endpoint" in our model's histomorphometric parameters. (Green: human clinical situation, blue: rat model situation.)

of colitis is assessed on the basis of clinical parameters indicated above. Detailed protocols on rodent colitis models have recently been published in *Nature Protocols* (Wirtz et al., 2007) and gastroenterology journals (Petersson et al., 2007; Sigalet et al., 2007).

Intravenous application of bisphosphonates (BP) represents an established therapy and prevention strategy of tumor-associated metastasis and severe hypercalcemia. However, patients can develop osteonecrosis of the jaw (ONJ) as a side effect of this therapy. The clinical hallmark is an exposed jawbone with no tendency to heal. Dental treatment such as tooth extraction, and also ill-fitting prostheses, are associated with approximately 80% of the cases, suggesting that suppression of bone turnover at sites requiring modeling and remodeling is the main pathologic factor of this disease (Woo et al., 2006; Ruggiero et al., 2009). Rodent models can help to gain insights into the pathogenesis of ONJ and to test candidate therapies that support bone regeneration under this compromised situation. Rat models are suitable to study regeneration of extraction defects. Defects can be reproduced with high precision and accuracy, also providing a minimum harm to the animal. Rats also tolerate high-dose bisphosphonate therapy. Zoledronic acid, a fourth-generation cyclic amino-bisphosphonate, reduces tumor progression of primary osteosarcoma (Gouin et al., 2006). Rats were treated with 100 µg/kg body weight zoledronic acid twice a week for 8 weeks. No toxic effects were reported. We use the same dosing regimen in our model, being comparable with the common clinical treatment. The life time of a rat can be anticipated with factor 40. Consequently, 3 human years are equivalent to 4 weeks in rat. Patients are usual treated with 4 mg/70kg body weight zoledronic acid, which is equivalent to ~30 µg per day in the rat model. The intended dose of 100 µg/kg subcutaneously zoledronic acid twice a week complies with clinical therapy over 3 years.

We used a protocol where adult Sprague-Dawley rats were treated for 4 weeks before

Table 14-3 Advantages and disadvantages of preclinical rat tibia implantation model under compromised healing situations

Rat model	Advantages	Disadvantages
General aspects of rat models	Cost-effective	Anatomic situation different from clinical situation
	Easy to handle	Different healing kinetic
	Short development and lifecycles	Continuous tooth eruption
	Genetically similar individuals	
	Established tools are available	
	Evaluation of aging	
Tibia implantation model	Easy access	Different skeletal origin of the tibia than the mandible and the maxilla
		Possible different healing response
	Atraumatic and fast	Restricted space for implant placement
	Analysis of medullary and cortical compartment	No simulated inflammation or functional loading
	Low burden for the animals	No Haversian remodeling
Osteoporosis	Established surgical procedure and OVX rat are commercially available	Systemic bone loss might cause a wrong impression of compromised bone healing
	Rapid onset bone loss that affects the trabecular and cortical bone	Control of disease induction requires micro-computed tomography analysis or histology
	Useful model to study impact of pharmacologic therapies	
Type 1 diabetes	Single injection of STZ is sufficient to cause hyperglycemia	Represents type 1 diabetes, not type 2 diabetes
	Rapid onset of hyperglycemia	Major burden for the animals
	Control of disease induction by measuring glucose levels	
Colitis	Many models of disease induction are available, including with DSS and TNBS	Does not represent the autoimmune disease and the complex clinical picture of Crohn's disease
	Easy application of DSS in the drinking water	Control of disease induction requires stool sampling and analysis of the gut
	Widely accepted model in the field of gastroenterology	
Bisphosphonate treatment	Controlled application of bisphosphonates via intravenous injection	Model is not fully representative of the clinical picture of ONJ
	No severe side effects	Control of disease induction only post mortem
		Only limited number of references

surgical intervention, twice a week with subcutaneous 100 µg zoledronic acid/kg body weight or vehicle control (Fügl and Gruber; Osteology Foundation, Grant #06–12). Under anesthesia, the first molars of the mandible are removed. At 1, 2, and 4 weeks after the tooth extraction and continued treatment, histomorphometry and micro-computed tomography (micro-CT) analysis are carried out to quantify bone formation. Histologic specimens can be evaluated for the possible appearance of necrotic bone and wound healing deficits. Readers might also consider similar protocols and evaluation techniques, depending on the underlying research question as indicated for rats (Hokugo et al., 2010) and mice (Bi et al., 2010; Kobayashi et al., 2010).

The basis for the surgical protocol and consequently the writing of this chapter was our experience with the relevant preclinical experiments. We provide detailed information on aspects related to the surgical protocol and implant position. We also include a brief description of our histologic approach to evaluate the relevant histomorphometric endpoints. It is the intention of the chapter to give a detailed protocol on the implantation of titanium screws in the rat tibia – in a situation of compromised bone regeneration.

14.2.2 Advantages/Disadvantages of the Rat Tibia Implantation Model (Table 14-3)

Advantages of the tibia implant model are that inbred animals can be used, which allows a minimum of variation in the animal model and thus the outcome parameters. Short variations and reproducible outcomes lead to a minimum number of animals based on the sample size calculation. Moreover, inbred animals are available worldwide, allowing comparison of results not only within but also between laboratories. Rats can be ordered at different ages. Aged animals can be purchased from certified vendors or can be retired animals from breeding stocks. Moreover, rats have short development and lifecycles keeping the duration of experiments short. Rat models are widely established and numerous tools are available, e.g., antibodies, genetic sequence, immunoassays etc. Moreover, the size of the animal implicates easy handling, simple housing, and low costs. An ideal area to investigate the osseointegration in rats is the tibia. The particular advantage of this rat implantation model is that the access to the tibia bone is atraumatic and fast, keeping the burden for the animals at a minimum. As mentioned in the legend to Fig 14-3, rat models can reflect the physiologic changes that occur in patients and are associated with compromised osseointegration. Thus the impact of these physiologic changes on the process of osseointegration can be studied in rat models.

Disadvantages of the implantation model are that the skeletal origin of the tibia is endochondral whereas the mandible and the maxilla mostly develop by desmal ossification, which might have a different healing response. However, osseointegration in the rat tibia is strictly desmal with no cartilage intermediates, indicating that the developmental situation is of minor relevance for the model. The diaphyseal part of the tibia is composed of a cortical layer that surrounds the bone marrow, which – at least partially – resembles the situation in the alveolar bone. Another determining factor is the restricted space for implant placement in the tibia (Table 14-1 and Table 14-2). Once implants are inserted, the early phase of osseointegration, which is bone regeneration, can be measured. The late phase of osseointegration, which is formed by the response of bone to inflammation and functional loading, cannot be measured. In addition, bone remodeling in rats does not involve the formation of Haversian canals, which is a hallmark of bone remodeling in humans. Moreover, rat bones continue to grow throughout their life, as indicated by the open growth plates. Bone regeneration in rats is generally faster than in humans. Based on these limitations, careful selection of the research questions is mandatory when considering implant research in the rat tibia model.

14.2.3 Timing

Starting with the approval by the local ethics committee, the project is introduced to the staff including the personnel in the animal facilities. Important points are the source, the total number, and the number of animals per cage. A critical issue is the availability of space, which dictates the time point of the delivery of animals to the institution. Once the animals have arrived, they are allowed to adapt for 2 weeks in their new environment before any further steps in the protocol are taken. Time management is particularly relevant when animals are subjected to disease induction, e.g., OVX and diabetes. It takes time until the "disease" becomes manifest and implants are inserted. For example, OVX and the sham-operation can be performed 8 weeks prior to implantation (Fig 14-1). For induction of diabetes, STZ injections are applied usually 1 to 4 weeks prior to implantation (Fig 14-2). The surgical procedure has to be organized including booking the operation theatre, surgical equipment, anesthesia, veterinarian team, staff assistance, and documentation. After surgery, implants remain *in situ* for usually 4 to 8 weeks; also longer time points can be used. Thus the overall time requirements in the animal facilities can range from 10 to 20 weeks.

While biomechanical testing should be done immediately after necropsy, histology and chemical characterization of the peri-implant surface requires processing of the specimens. Our histologic approach follows cutting and grinding (Donath, 1992). The preparation of histologic specimens requires approximately 4 to 8 weeks, including fixation, dehydration, and plastic embedding. The morphometric analysis is particularly challenging because the automatic scanning has to be controlled by light microscopy. In our experience, preparation and histomorphometric analysis of one specimen takes approximately 10 hours. If we assume that an average project has 30 specimens, one person has to work for about 60 days (12 weeks) on this task. Thus, the overall time necessary for conducting the whole project is between 20 and 40 weeks.

14.2.4 Surgical Procedures, Preparation, and Detailed Methodology

Anesthesia should be performed in a familiar surrounding for the animals to avoid stress and therefore to keep the drug administration at a minimum. Animals usually receive ketamine (100 mg/kg) and xylazine hydrochloride (5 mg/kg) by intramuscular injection. Anesthesia is effective once there is no reaction in the rat's whiskers when the toes are pinched. Note that rats with a severely impaired metabolic situation, as observed in the diabetes rats, can barely tolerate high doses of anesthesia. In this case, inhalational anesthesia is recommended. Inhalational starts with the supply of 100% oxygen close to the snout for 1 minute to avoid hypoxia and laryngospasm during the endotracheal procedure. A cannula (G14, orange, diameter 2 mm) fixed with a suture is an appropriate instrument for endotracheal intubation. The inhalation of isoflurane starts with 2% to 3% isoflurane and is continued with 0.6% to 1.0% isoflurane in air and O_2 mixture with 30% O_2. Note: the cannula can only be use for a limited time as it has no cuff.

Surgery requires aseptic conditions. The (left) leg is shaved by the nonsterile staff. Eyes are covered with ointment to avoid desiccation. Disinfection is performed by dipping the claws up to the ankle in a bowl filled with povidone-iodine in 10% alcohol (Betadine) for roughly 20 seconds. The nonsterile staff member places the animal on its back and fixes the front legs with adhesive tape on the operation table. Skin disinfection is repeated by swabbing the leg with betadine twice. Sterile towels are placed around the leg and fixed with clamps.

Hint: When exploring the anterior margin of the tibia, after betadine disinfection, a white line becomes visible that marks the area of incision (Fig 14-4a).

Spontaneous breathing is checked prior to surgery. When heavy breathing the animal is

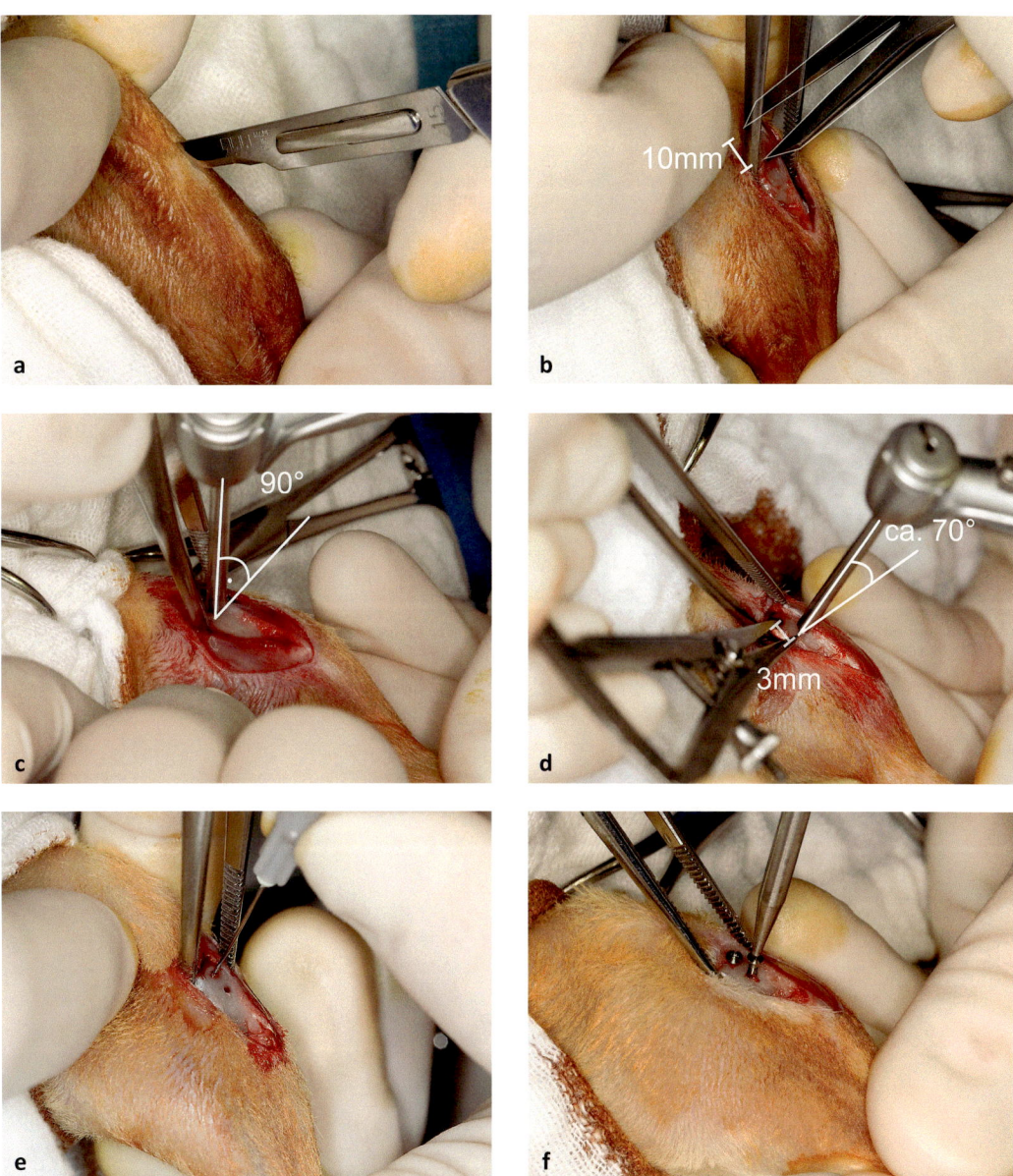

Fig 14-4 (a) After skin disinfection and palpating the anterior crest a bright line can be seen that marks the incision line. The incision starts at the protuberance along the tibia crest (2 cm) with blade number #15. (b) After the incision the tissue is reflected to expose the medial surface of the tibia and retracted by the assistant with forceps. The joint space is palpated and the end of the caliper/circle is placed on the tibia plateau (10 mm). It is not necessary to open the intra-articular space. (c) The first osteotomy is made at a distance of 10 mm from the tibia plateau. The osteotomy is placed in the middle of medial surface's diameter at a 90° angle to it. The osteotomy is 1 mm in diameter and 3 mm deep. Saline irrigation is continued during the drilling procedure. To prevent "drill dust" in the specimens, edgeless drills should be avoided. (d) The second osteotomy on the medial surface of the tibia is 3 mm lateral to the first osteotomy. The angle between the surface and the anterior crest is about 70°. (e) The implant sites are checked with a syringe to ensure the integrity of the walls. (f) The "study implants" are inserted and the wound closed.

turned into a lateral position (left side) and subjected to inhalational anesthesia. The assistant is sitting opposite and holds the ankle and the knee joint. The incision (#15 blade) starts at the protuberance of the tibia along the anterior crest (2 cm). The soft tissue is reflected to expose the medial flat surface of the tibia. The joint capsule of the knee remains intact. The assistant retracts the soft tissue in, holding the tibia with forceps. The joint space can be palpated and marked with a caliper/compass. A first osteotomy is drilled 10 mm distal of the joint under irrigation with sterile physiologic saline (Fig 14-4b). The first osteotomy is placed in the middle of the tibia at a right angle to the medial surface (Fig 14-4c). A second osteotomy is drilled 13 mm distal of the joint. The second osteotomy is positioned slightly toward the anterior crest of the medial surface at an angle of approximately 70° to the surface (Fig 14-4d). The integrity of the drilling channel can be estimated by probing with a needle (Fig 14-4e). If a perforation is noticed, another osteotomy can be drilled 1 mm distal to the perforated site. The bone surface is rinsed with sterile saline prior to implant placement. Titanium screws with a diameter of 1 mm and a length of 3 mm can be inserted (Fig 14-4f). The surgical site is closed with cutaneous resorbable sutures (e.g., Vicryl 4-0).

Hint: Make sure that the drills are sharp to keep the "drilling debris" in the channel at a minimum as this complicates histomorphometry.

14.2.5 Postoperative Care

Wound management is performed with merbromin 2% after surgery. When animals undergo inhalational anesthesia the amount of isoflurane is cut back to 0% in the last minutes of the surgery. The anaesthetic machine is disconnected and the rat observed until unassisted breathing starts. After 60 seconds of no breathing the machine has to be connected again to support breathing (oxygen should not be above 21%). This procedure has to be repeated until unassisted breathing starts. Animals have to be placed on their flank and kept in a warm place (infrared lamp) to avoid hypothermia. Attention has to be given to provide an area that is not too warm as the animals might dehydrate. For postoperative pain relief the following drugs can be administered by subcutaneous injection: butorphanol (1 to 2 mg/kg), or buprenorphine (0.05 to 0.1 mg/kg), or ketoprofen (5 mg/kg). Continuing analgesia per os, buprenorphine 0.01 to 0.02 mg/mL in drinking water, is recommended for 2 days.

Animals are sacrificed by an overdose of a barbiturate (thiopental 150 mg/kg) or carbon dioxide. An incision is made on the anterior margin of the tibia. The tibia is cut off at both ends with a saw at a distance of 5 to 10 mm from the implant. Opening of the medullary space allows the fixative to penetrate the bone marrow and the peri-implant bone tissue. Sawing has to be done carefully, because the tibia might crack especially in compromised bone. The muscles and the fibula have to be removed without damaging the soft tissue immediately above the implants. The tibia is exarticulated by cutting the ligaments with a scalpel or scissors. Each biopsy specimen is placed in a container (200 mL) with neutral-buffered formalin.

Hint: The "ID" of the biopsy specimen is written with a pencil on the container and on paper which is placed in the container.

14.2.6 Endpoint Measurements

Our main focus is related to bone histomorphometry, and its most commonly used parameters "bone volume per tissue volume" (which is the amount of bone tissue in a defined region of interest) and bone-to-implant contact (BIC) (the percentage of the implant surface in contact with bone) (Mair et al., 2009; Kuchler et al., 2011). Other metric endpoints, which are not described here, are related to chemical characterization of the peri-implant mineralized matrix (Schupbach et al., 2005; Roschger et al., 2008) and biomechanical testing (Li et al.,

2010). Neither of the methods to determine endpoint data will be described in detail as this is beyond the scope of this chapter. Imaging techniques based on X-rays, such as live animal CT or micro-CT are not as reliable in implant research because the interface between the implant and the bone cannot be evaluated at high resolution due to artifacts caused by interface scattering and beam hardening. Synchrotron-radiation-based micro-CT systems can overcome these problems, but the method requires massive equipment and cannot be used for routine measurements (Bernhardt et al., 2004).

Bone histomorphometry can be carried out on thin-ground sections of undecalcified plastic embedded tissue blocks. To avoid demineralization, buffered formalin is recommended for fixation. Diffusion of the fixative is facilitated when the proximal and distal parts of the tibia are removed. Tissue samples are dehydrated in ascending grades of alcohol and embedded in light-curing resin (Technovit 7200 VLC + BPO; Kulzer, Wehrheim, Germany). A number of comparable, equally reliable products with different modes of polymerization are commercially available (methyl methacrylate; Epon, Fluka Chemie, Buchs, Switzerland). Plastified blocks are processed with cutting and grinding equipment, for example Exakt (Exakt Apparatebau, Norderstedt, Germany) or Buehler (Lake Bluff, Il, USA). The thin-ground sections (Donath, 1992) should be precisely oriented in the longitudinal axis of the implants. It is highly advisable to plan the direction of the slice using radiographic images of the plastic blocks. It is safer to grind down the block until the midplane is reached instead of trying to cut the implant in half. The thickness of the thin-ground sections should not exceed 30 μm which is equivalent to one or two cell layers, because the interface is difficult to analyze and depict in thicker sections. Applied staining methods should allow to reproducibly distinguish between old and newly formed bone (i.e., Levai-Laczko, toluidine blue, Giemsa).

For histomorphometric analyses, high-resolution overview images are a prerequisite for reliable results. Motorized stages (Märzhäuser Wetzlar, Wetzlar-Steindorf, Germany), high-resolution digital cameras (Nikon DXM 1200, Nikon, Tokyo, Japan) and specialized "stitching" software produce microscopic images depicting the entire implant at resolution of at least 1 pixel equal to ~2 μm. In a next step, images are manually divided into a medullar and a cortical compartment using Adobe Photoshop, (Adobe, San Jose, CA, USA). This is necessary because osseointegration is different in these two regions. Before the amount of bone tissue or the length of the contact between bone and implant surface can be measured, these structures have to be reliably determined or classified. Manual retracing of bone and implant areas is an old-fashioned but reliable method for this, although time consuming. Advanced histomorphometry software can help to automate the process to a high degree. For the segmentation and classification of implant and bone, a rule set for this software is devised. This algorithm considers the color and shape of the objects, as well as their relations to neighboring objects. This automatic classification should be confirmed and improved by visually assigning the few falsely classified areas to the correct tissue class.

The percentage of the implant surface in contact with mineralized bone, referred to as BIC, is a standard parameter for the quantification of histological osseointegration. BV/TV, also termed "bone area", is determined in the immediate neighborhood of the implant. Measurements within a distance of 200 μm around the implant contour, in our experience, yield reasonable results. BIC and BV/TV are determined separately for the medullar and the cortical compartment. For the medullar portion, those parts of the implants that partially penetrated the cortical bone of the dorsal side of the tibia are not included into the analysis. If one flank of the screw is in close proximity to cortical bone, only the other side

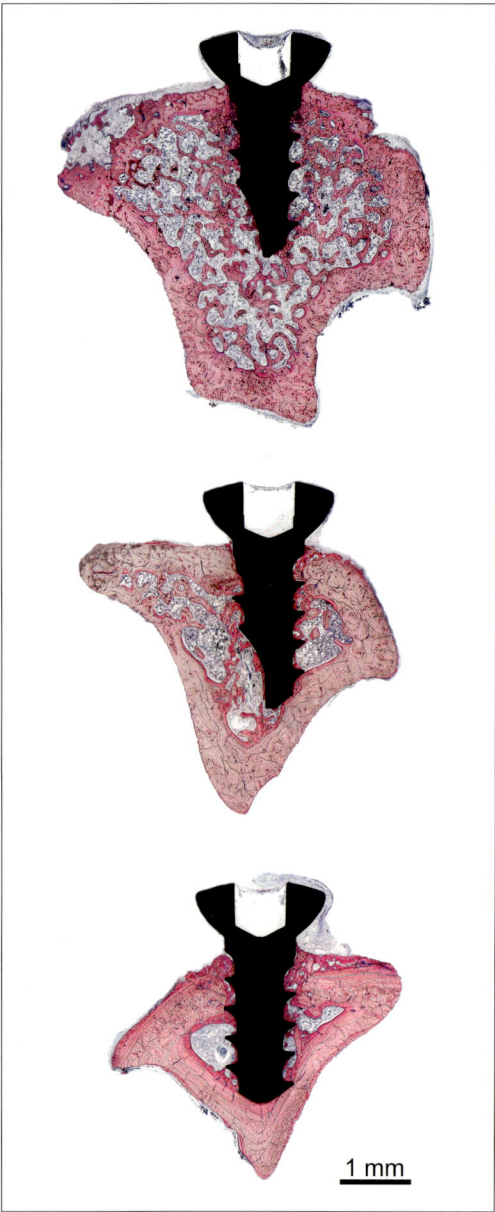

Fig 14-5 The proximal part of the tibia is wide and contains large amounts of cancellous bone whereas the distal regions have a smaller cross-section and consist almost exclusively of cortical bone. The correct implant position is therefore a critical parameter to keep the variability at a minimum. Preliminary experiments with cadavers may help to find the appropriate implant positions.

facing the marrow cavity is evaluated. This is necessary because bone regeneration usually originates from old bone. Parts of the implant surface in closer proximity to pristine bone therefore have a better chance of osseointegration. Histology also reveals variations of bone quality and composition dependent on the distance of the implant from the joint. While the proximal part is wide and contains large amounts of cancellous bone, the distal regions have a smaller cross-section and consist almost exclusively of cortical bone (Fig 14-5).

14.2.7 Statistical Analysis Plan (see Chapter 4)

Pre-data analysis in experimental statistics is called power analysis. A power analysis in the planning phase of a study is used to anticipate the likelihood that the study will yield a significant effect. It is required to answer the following question: How many subjects per group are needed in order to have a desired power for detecting a meaningful difference? The calculation is based on the same factors as the post-data analysis. In order to indicate the sample size using the power analysis, we need to specify the following: significance level (typically 5%), a desired power (e.g., 80% or 90%), a meaningful difference (comparing the treatment with the control group), and the standard deviation. There are various online tools that allow sample size calculation. Moreover, when planning preclinical studies, we have to consider losing animals, e.g., during surgery, the pre- and postsurgical period, and that not all animals can be included in the analysis, for example, because of unexpected inflammation. Also histology might reveal that implants are not positioned adequately for histomorphometry analysis. Thus, the calculated sample size is usually an underestimation for the number of animals to be included in the study. As a rule of thumb, the calculated sample size can be increased by 20%. Overall, variables in the protocol (e.g., observation periods, treatments) should be kept at a minimum to answer the research question with sufficient power. Details on sample size calculation can also be included in a publication (Charles et al., 2009).

Pre-data analysis depends on whether or not the data are normally distributed. Basically, two groups of ordinal and metric measures can be compared with *t* test (if normally distributed) or Mann-Whitney U or Wilcoxon signed-rank test (if not normally distributed). Three or more groups of ordinal and metric measures can be compared with analysis of variance (ANOVA; if normally distributed) or Kruskal-Wallis one-way ANOVA by ranks (if not normally distributed). Multiple comparisons require alpha adjustment, which are considered in the *post-hoc* tests. Two-way ANOVA may be used to examine the effects of two categorical variables, e.g., aging and PTH pharmacologic therapy (Mair et al., 2009), both individually and together, on an experimental response (change in BA, BIC). Two-way ANOVA, in combination with *post-hoc* testing, can answer the following questions: Is there an effect of aging on osseointegration? Is there an effect of PTH therapy on osseointegration? Is there interaction between the factors? It is always advisable to consult a statistician in the planning phase of a study.

14.2.8 Materials, Consumables, Equipment
- Scalpel with #15 blade
- Caliper
- Adson forceps
- Dressing forceps straight (16 cm)
- Freer elevator
- Drill, 1.0 diameter, 3 mm length
- Titanium screws, 1.0 diameter, 3.0 length,
- Screwdriver
- 5 mL, 10 mL syringes
- 22G needles
- Needle holder
- 4-0 Vicryl sutures
- Physiologic saline
- Scissors
- Anesthetics: ketamine (100 mg/kg) + xylazine hydrochloride (5 mg/kg)
- Analgesics post operative:
  – Buprenorphine (0.05 to 0.1 mg/kg) subcutaneous, buprenorphine 0.01 to 0.02 mg/mL in drinking water
  – Alternatively: butorphanol tartrate (1 to 2 mg/kg) (Torbugesic), subcutaneous ketoprofen (Toradol) (5 mg/kg)
- Towel clamps
- Sterile towels (1 piece per animal)
- Rescue: inhalational anesthetic
- Cannula (14G; orange, diameter 2 mm) for endotracheal tube
- Anesthetic machine with application mode for isoflurane in air and O_2.

14.3 Acknowledgments

First, thank you to the co-authors for their contributions (Stefan Tangl, 13.9, Figs 12-15; Ulrike Kuchler, 14.2.4–14.2.8, Fig 2-11) Also, the authors wish to thank Jeffrey O Hollinger, Hans Plenk Jr., William V. Giannobile, and Georg Watzek for being our teachers, colleagues, and mentors.

References

1. Abt E (2009). Smoking increases dental implant failures and complications. *Evid Based Dent* 10:79–80.
2. Ai-Aql ZS, Alagl AS, Graves DT, Gerstenfeld LC, Einhorn TA (2008). Molecular mechanisms controlling bone formation during fracture healing and distraction osteogenesis. *J Dent Res* 87:107–118.
3. Alsaadi G, Quirynen M, Komarek A, van Steenberghe D (2007). Impact of local and systemic factors on the incidence of oral implant failures, up to abutment connection. *J Clin Periodontol* 34:610–617.
4. Barnes GL, Kakar S, Vora S, Morgan EF, Gerstenfeld LC, Einhorn TA (2008). Stimulation of fracture-healing with systemic intermittent parathyroid hormone treatment. *J Bone Joint Surg Am* 90(Suppl 1):120–127.
5. Beil FT, Barvencik F, Gebauer M, Seitz S, Rueger JM, Ignatius A et al. (2010). Effects of estrogen on fracture healing in mice. *J Trauma* Jul 20 [Epub ahead of print].
6. Berglundh T, Abrahamsson I, Lang NP, Lindhe J (2003). De novo alveolar bone formation adjacent to endosseous implants. *Clin Oral Implants Res* 14: 251–262.

7. Bernhardt R, Scharnweber D, Muller B, Thurner P, Schliephake H, Wyss P et al. (2004). Comparison of microfocus- and synchrotron X-ray tomography for the analysis of osteointegration around Ti6Al4V implants. Eur Cell Mater 7:42–51; discussion 51.
8. Bi Y, Gao Y, Ehirchiou D, Cao C, Kikuiri T, Le A et al. (2010). Bisphosphonates cause osteonecrosis of the jaw-like disease in mice. Am J Pathol 177:280–290.
9. Bollen AM, Taguchi A, Hujoel PP, Hollender LG (2004). Number of teeth and residual alveolar ridge height in subjects with a history of self-reported osteoporotic fractures. Osteoporos Int 15:970–974.
10. Bouma G, Strober W (2003). The immunological and genetic basis of inflammatory bowel disease. Nat Rev 3:521–533.
11. Cao Y, Mori S, Mashiba T, Westmore MS, Ma L, Sato M et al. (2002). Raloxifene, estrogen, and alendronate affect the processes of fracture repair differently in ovariectomized rats. J Bone Miner Res 17:2237–2246.
12. Carr AB (2010). Implant location and radiotherapy are the only factors linked to 2-year implant failure. J Evid Based Dent Pract 10:49–51.
13. Carvalho MD, Benatti BB, Cesar-Neto JB et al (2006). Effect of cigarette smoke inhalation and estrogen deficiency on bone healing around titanium implants: A histometric study in rats. J Periodontol 77:599–605.
14. Chapurlat RD, Delmas PD (2009). Bone microdamage: a clinical perspective. Osteoporos Int 20:1299–1308.
15. Charles P, Giraudeau B, Dechartres A, Baron G, Ravaud P (2009). Reporting of sample size calculation in randomised controlled trials: review. Br Med J 338:b1732.
16. Chatzigeorgiou A, Halapas A, Kalafatakis K, Kamper E (2009). The use of animal models in the study of diabetes mellitus. In Vivo 23:245–258.
17. Chen D, Wang MW (2005). Development and application of rodent models for type 2 diabetes. Diabetes Obes Metab 7:307–317.
18. Cho P, Schneider GB, Krizan K, Keller JC (2004). Examination of the bone-implant interface in experimentally induced osteoporotic bone. Implant Dent 13:79–87.
19. Donath K (1992). Die Trenn-Dünnschliff-Technik zur Herstellung histologischer Präparate von nicht schneidbaren Geweben und Materialien. Der Präparator 34:197–206.
20. Duarte PM, Goncalves PF, Casati MZ, Sallum EA, Nociti FH Jr (2005a). Age-related and surgically induced estrogen deficiencies may differently affect bone around titanium implants in rats. J Periodontol 76:1496–1501.
21. Duarte PM, de Vasconcelos Gurgel BC, Sallum AW, Filho GR, Sallum EA, Nociti FH Jr (2005b). Alendronate therapy may be effective in the prevention of bone loss around titanium implants inserted in estrogen-deficient rats. J Periodontol 76:107–114.
22. Duarte PM, Cesar Neto JB, Goncalves PF, Sallum EA, Nociti FH (2003a). Estrogen deficiency affects bone healing around titanium implants: A histometric study in rats. Implant Dent 12: 340–346
23. Duarte PM, Cesar-Neto JB, Sallum AW, Sallum EA, Nociti FH Jr (2003b). Effect of estrogen and calcitonin therapies on bone density in a lateral area adjacent to implants placed in the tibiae of ovariectomized rats. J Periodontol 74:1618–1624
24. Dunn CA, Jin Q, Taba M Jr, Franceschi RT, Bruce Rutherford R, Giannobile WV (2005). BMP gene delivery for alveolar bone engineering at dental implant defects. Mol Ther 11:294–299.
25. Elson CO, Cong Y, McCracken VJ, Dimmitt RA, Lorenz RG, Weaver CT (2005). Experimental models of inflammatory bowel disease reveal innate, adaptive, and regulatory mechanisms of host dialogue with the microbiota. Immunol Rev 206:260–276.
26. Fini M, Giavaresi G, Rimondini L, Giardino R (2002). Titanium alloy osseointegration in cancellous and cortical bone of ovariectomized animals: Histomorphometric and bone hardness measurements. Int J Oral Maxillofac Implants 17:28–37.
27. Fiorellini JP, Nevins ML, Norkin A, Weber HP, Karimbux NY (1999). The effect of insulin therapy on osseointegration in a diabetic rat model. Clin Oral Implants Res 10:362–368.
28. Fujii N, Kusakari H, Maeda T (1998). A histological study on tissue responses to titanium implantation in rat maxilla: the process of epithelial regeneration and bone reaction. J Periodontol 69:485–495.
29. Giglio MJ, Giannunzio G, Olmedo D, Guglielmotti MB (2000). Histomorphometric study of bone healing around laminar implants in experimental diabetes. Implant Dent 9:143–149
30. Giro G, Goncalves D, Sakakura CE, Pereira RM, Marcantonio E Jr, Orrico SR (2008). Influence of estrogen deficiency and its treatment with alendronate and estrogen on bone density around osseointegrated implants: Radiographic study in female rats. Oral Surg Oral Med Oral Pathol Oral Radiol Endod 105:162–167.
31. Giro G, Sakakura CE, Goncalves D, Pereira RM, Marcantonio E Jr, Orrico SR (2007). Effect of 17beta-estradiol and alendronate on the removal torque of osseointegrated titanium implants in ovariectomized rats. J Periodontol 78:1316–1321.
32. Glösel B, Kuchler U, Watzek G, Gruber R (2010). Review of dental implant rat research models simulating osteoporosis or diabetes. Int J Oral Maxillofac Implants. 25(3):516–524.
33. Glowacki J, Schulten AJ, Perrott D, Kaban LB (2008). Nicotine impairs distraction osteogenesis in the rat mandible. Int J Oral Maxillofac Surg 37(2):156–161.
34. Gouin F, Ory B, Redini F, Heymann D (2006). Zoledronic acid slows down rat primary chondrosarcoma development, recurrent tumor progression after intralesional curretage and increases overall survival. Int J Cancer 119:980–984.
35. Hamdani G, Gabet Y, Rachmilewitz D, Karmeli F, Bab I, Dresner-Pollak R (2008). Dextran sodium sulfate-induced colitis causes rapid bone loss in mice. Bone 43:945–950.

References

36. Hasegawa H, Ozawa S, Hashimoto K, Takeichi T, Ogawa T (2008). Type 2 diabetes impairs implant osseointegration capacity in rats. *Int J Oral Maxillofac Implants* 23:237–246.
37. Hela S, Nihel M, Faten L, Monia F, Jalel B, Azza F et al. (2005). Osteoporosis and Crohn's disease. *Joint Bone Spine* 72:403–407.
38. Hokugo A, Christensen R, Chung EM, Sung EC, Felsenfeld AL, Sayre JW et al. (2010). Increased prevalence of bisphosphonate-related osteonecrosis of the jaw with vitamin D deficiency in rats. *J Bone Miner Res* 25:1337–1349.
39. Iyama S, Takeshita F, Ayukawa Y, Kido MA, Suetsugu T, Tanaka T (1997). A study of the regional distribution of bone formed around hydroxyapatite implants in the tibiae of streptozotocin-induced diabetic rats using multiple fluorescent labeling and confocal laser scanning microscopy. *J Periodontol* 68:1169–1175.
40. Javed F, Romanos GE (2009). Impact of diabetes mellitus and glycemic control on the osseointegration of dental implants: a systematic literature review. *J Periodontol* 80:1719–1730.
41. Kayal RA, Tsatsas D, Bauer MA, Allen B, Al-Sebaei MO, Kakar S et al. (2007). Diminished bone formation during diabetic fracture healing is related to the premature resorption of cartilage associated with increased osteoclast activity. *J Bone Miner Res* 22:560–568.
42. Klaus J, Armbrecht G, Steinkamp M, Bruckel J, Rieber A, Adler G et al. (2002). High prevalence of osteoporotic vertebral fractures in patients with Crohn's disease. *Gut* 51:654–658.
43. Kobayashi Y, Hiraga T, Ueda A, Wang L, Matsumoto-Nakano M, Hata K et al. (2010). Zoledronic acid delays wound healing of the tooth extraction socket, inhibits oral epithelial cell migration, and promotes proliferation and adhesion to hydroxyapatite of oral bacteria, without causing osteonecrosis of the jaw, in mice. *J Bone Miner Metab* 28:165–175.
44. Kopman JA, Kim DM, Rahman SS, Arandia JA, Karimbux NY, Fiorellini JP (2005). Modulating the effects of diabetes on osseointegration with aminoguanidine and doxycycline. *J Periodontol* 76:614–620.
45. Kuchler U, Spilka T, Baron K, Tangl S, Watzek G, Gruber R (2011). Intermittent PTH fails to stimulate osseointegration in diabetic rats. *Clin Oral Implants Res Jan 20* [Epub ahead of print].
46. Kwon PT, Rahman SS, Kim DM, Kopman JA, Karimbux NY, Fiorellini JP (2005). Maintenance of osseointegration utilizing insulin therapy in a diabetic rat model. *J Periodontol* 76:621–626.
47. Li Y, Zou S, Wang D, Feng G, Bao C, Hu J (2010). The effect of hydrofluoric acid treatment on titanium implant osseointegration in ovariectomized rats. *Biomaterials* 31:3266–3273.
48. Lin CL, Moniz C, Chambers TJ, Chow JW (1996). Colitis causes bone loss in rats through suppression of bone formation. *Gastroenterology* 111:1263–1271.
49. Lin CL, Moniz C, Chow JW (2000). Treatment with fluoride or bisphosphonates prevents bone loss associated with colitis in the rat. *Calcified Tissue Int* 67:373–377.
50. Mair B, Tangl S, Feierfeil J, Skiba D, Watzek G, Gruber R (2009). Age-related efficacy of parathyroid hormone on osseointegration in the rat. *Clin Oral Implants Res* 20:400–405.
51. McCann RM, Colleary G, Geddis C, Clarke SA, Jordan GR, Dickson GR et al. (2008). Effect of osteoporosis on bone mineral density and fracture repair in a rat femoral fracture model. *J Orthop Res* 26:384–393.
52. McCracken MS, Aponte-Wesson R, Chavali R, Lemons JE (2006). Bone associated with implants in diabetic and insulin-treated rats. *Clin Oral Implants Res* 17:495–500
53. McCracken M, Lemons JE, Rahemtulla F, Prince CW, Feldman D (2000). Bone response to titanium alloy implants placed in diabetic rats. *Int J Oral Maxillofac Implants* 15:345–354.
54. Melhus G, Solberg LB, Dimmen S, Madsen JE, Nordsletten L, Reinholt FP (2007). Experimental osteoporosis induced by ovariectomy and vitamin D deficiency does not markedly affect fracture healing in rats. *Acta Orthop* 78:393–403.
55. Meyer RA Jr, Tsahakis PJ, Martin DF, Banks DM, Harrow ME, Kiebzak GM (2001). Age and ovariectomy impair both the normalization of mechanical properties and the accretion of mineral by the fracture callus in rats. *J Orthop Res* 19:428–435.
56. Motohashi M, Shirota T, Tokugawa Y, Ohno K, Michi K, Yamaguchi A (1999). Bone reactions around hydroxyapatite-coated implants in ovariectomized rats. *Oral Surg Oral Med Oral Pathol Oral Radiol Endod* 87:145–152
57. Muschler GF, Raut VP, Patterson TE, Wenke JC, Hollinger JO (2010). The design and use of animal models for translational research in bone tissue engineering and regenerative medicine. *Tissue Eng Part B Rev* 16:123–145.
58. Narai S, Nagahata S (2003). Effects of alendronate on the removal torque of implants in rats with induced osteoporosis. *Int J Oral Maxillofac Implants* 18:218–223.
59. Nevins ML, Karimbux NY, Weber HP, Giannobile WV, Fiorellini JP (1998). Wound healing around endosseous implants in experimental diabetes. *Int J Oral Maxillofac Implants* 13:620–629.
60. Nociti FH Jr, Sallum AW, Sallum EA, Duarte PM (2002). Effect of estrogen replacement and calcitonin therapies on bone around titanium implants placed in ovariectomized rats: A histometric study. *Int J Oral Maxillofac Implants* 17:786–792.
61. Ogawa T, Nishimura I (2006). Genes differentially expressed in titanium implant healing. *J Dent Res* 85:566–570.
62. Okayasu I, Hatakeyama S, Yamada M, Ohkusa T, Inagaki Y, Nakaya R (1990). A novel method in the induction of reliable experimental acute and chronic ulcerative colitis in mice. *Gastroenterology* 98:694–702.
63. Pan J, Shirota T, Ohno K, Michi K (2000). Effect of ovariectomy on bone remodeling adjacent to hydroxyapatite-coated implants in the tibia of mature rats. *J Oral Maxillofac Surg* 58:877–882.
64. Pearce AI, Richards RG, Milz S, Schneider E, Pearce SG (2007). Animal models for implant biomaterial research in bone: a review. *Eur Cell Mater* 13:1–10.

65. Pellegrini G, Seol YJ, Gruber R, Giannobile WV (2009). Pre-clinical models for oral and periodontal reconstructive therapies. *J Dent Res* 88:1065–1076.
66. Petersson J, Schreiber O, Steege A, Patzak A, Hellsten A, Phillipson M et al. (2007). eNOS involved in colitis-induced mucosal blood flow increase. *Am J Physiol* 293:G1281–1287.
67. Qi MC, Zhou XQ, Hu J et al (2004). Oestrogen replacement therapy promotes bone healing around dental implants in osteoporotic rats. *Int J Oral Maxillofac Surg* 33:279–285.
68. Rawlinson SC, Boyde A, Davis GR, Howell PG, Hughes FJ, Kingsmill VJ (2009). Ovariectomy vs. hypofunction: their effects on rat mandibular bone. *J Dent Res* 88:615–620.
69. Rees DA, Alcolado JC (2005). Animal models of diabetes mellitus. *Diabet Med* 22:359–370.
70. Renou SJ, Guglielmotti MB, de la Torre A, Cabrini RL (2001). Effect of total body irradiation on peri-implant tissue reaction: an experimental study. *Clin Oral Implants Res* 12:468–472.
71. Riggs BL, Parfitt AM (2005). Drugs used to treat osteoporosis: the critical need for a uniform nomenclature based on their action on bone remodeling. *J Bone Miner Res* 20:177–184.
72. Roschger P, Paschalis EP, Fratzl P, Klaushofer K (2008). Bone mineralization density distribution in health and disease. *Bone* 42:456–466.
73. Ruggiero SL, Dodson TB, Assael LA, Landesberg R, Marx RE, Mehrotra B (2009). American Association of Oral and Maxillofacial Surgeons position paper on bisphosphonate-related osteonecrosis of the jaws–2009 update. *J Oral Maxillofac Surg* 67(Suppl5):2–12.
74. Schenk RK, Buser D (1998). Osseointegration: a reality. *Periodontol 2000* 17:22–35.
75. Schindeler A, McDonald MM, Bokko P, Little DG (2008). Bone remodeling during fracture repair: The cellular picture. *Semin Cell Dev Biol* 19:459–466.
76. Schupbach P, Glauser R, Rocci A, Martignoni M, Sennerby L, Lundgren A et al. (2005). The human bone-oxidized titanium implant interface: A light microscopic, scanning electron microscopic, back-scatter scanning electron microscopic, and energy-dispersive x-ray study of clinically retrieved dental implants. *Clin Implant Dent Relat Res* 7(Suppl 1):S36–43.
77. Seeman E, Delmas PD (2006). Bone quality – the material and structural basis of bone strength and fragility. *N Engl J Med* 354):2250–2261.
78. Shirota T, Tashiro M, Ohno K, Yamaguchi A (2003). Effect of intermittent parathyroid hormone (1-34) treatment on the bone response after placement of titanium implants into the tibia of ovariectomized rats. *J Oral Maxillofac Surg* 61:471–480.
79. Shyng YC, Devlin H, Ou KL (2006). Bone formation around immediately placed oral implants in diabetic rats. *Int J Prosthodont* 19:513–514.
80. Sigalet DL, Wallace LE, Holst JJ, Martin GR, Kaji T, Tanaka H et al. (2007). Enteric neural pathways mediate the anti-inflammatory actions of glucagon-like peptide 2. *Am J Physiol* 293:G211–221.
81. Siqueira JT, Cavalher-Machado SC, Arana-Chavez VE, Sannomiya P (2003). Bone formation around titanium implants in the rat tibia: Role of insulin. *Implant Dent* 12:242–251.
82. Skripitz R, Aspenberg P (2004). Parathyroid hormone – a drug for orthopedic surgery? *Acta Orthop Scand* 75:654–662.
83. Takeshita F, Murai K, Iyama S, Ayukawa Y, Suetsugu T (1998). Uncontrolled diabetes hinders bone formation around titanium implants in rat tibiae. A light and fluorescence microscopy, and image processing study. *J Periodontol* 69:314–320.
84. Takeshita F, Iyama S, Ayukawa Y, Kido MA, Murai K, Suetsugu T (1997). The effects of diabetes on the interface between hydroxyapatite implants and bone in rat tibia. *J Periodontol* 68:180–185.
85. Tokugawa Y, Shirota T, Ohno K, Yamaguchi A (2003). Effects of bisphosphonate on bone reaction after placement of titanium implants in tibiae of ovariectomized rats. *Int J Oral Maxillofac Implants* 18:66–74.
86. Trombelli L, Farina R, Marzola A, Bozzi L, Liljenberg B, Lindhe J (2008). Modeling and remodeling of human extraction sockets. *J Clin Periodontol* 35:630–639.
87. Viera-Negron YE, Ruan WH, Winger JN, Hou X, Sharawy MM, Borke JL (2008). Effect of ovariectomy and alendronate on implant osseointegration in rat maxillary bone. *J Oral Implantol* 34:76–82
88. Wirtz S, Neufert C, Weigmann B, Neurath MF (2007). Chemically induced mouse models of intestinal inflammation. *Nat Protoc* 2:541–546.
89. Woo SB, Hellstein JW, Kalmar JR (2006). Narrative [corrected] review: bisphosphonates and osteonecrosis of the jaws. *Ann Intern Med* 144:753–761.
90. Yamazaki M, Shirota T, Tokugawa Y et al (1999). Bone reactions to titanium screw implants in ovariectomized animals. *Oral Surg Oral Med Oral Pathol Oral Radiol Endod* 87:411–418.

Index

A
acellular dermal matrix 58
American Dental Association 53
American Society for Testing and Materials (ASTM) 55
Animal Rights Movement 12
animal welfare 7
archivists 28

B
back-scattered electron microscopy 168–169
biocompatibility 45
biologics 5–6, 86, 90, 95, 97
biomaterials
 biocompatibility 45
 for bone repair 4
 evaluation methodologies 6–7, 111–120
 tissue response 47
 see also osseoIntegration
biomechanical tests 118–120
biostatistics 31
 replication 37–38
 sample size 35–37
 split-mouth design 38–39
 see also statistical analysis
bisphosphonates 226, 233
bone healing 46, 225–244
bone implant models 48–50
bone regeneration 225–227
 canine model 144, 161–167
 ectopic 161
 screening models 45–47
 see also guided bone regeneration
bone remodeling 225

C
calvarium standardized defect model 49
canine models 6
 dentition 123
 horizontal ridge augmentation 144–156
 osseointegration 108–110
 peri-implantitis defects 199
 periodontal defects 90–94
 periodontal lesions 85–89
 ridge preservation 124–126, 126–138
 sinus floor augmentation 183, 184
 soft tissue volume 65–74
 vertical ridge augmentation 163–171
circumscribed defect model 48–59
clinical trials 5
collagen, graft 58
combination products 6
computed tomography 189
 see also micro-computed tomography
contractualism 14

D
defect reconstruction 1–8
devices, definition 5
diabetes 229–231
documentation 29

E
ectopic bone models 50–54
ethical considerations 9–21
 ethical theories 16
 moral status 10
 weighing up interests 15–17

F
F test 40
false positive/negative rates 35
fluorescence microscopy 220

G
goat models, sinus floor augmentation 178, 185, 186
good laboratory practice 23–30
 archivist 28–29
 compliance 24
 documentation 29
 framework 24–26
 IT personnel 29
 multisite studies 30
 study director 27–28
grafting 57
guided bone regeneration (GBR) 19, 142–144, 153, 159, 190, 191
guided tissue regeneration (GTR) 97, 163
guidelines
 animal welfare 7
 OECD test guidelines 24

H
histomorphologic analysis 190
histomorphometry 114, 115, 152–155, 169, 190, 191, 218

horizontal ridge augmentation 141–158, 159
 canine model 144–156
 model selection 142–144
 hypotheses 34

I
immunohistochemical analysis 153, 190, 191
implants 48–56
 biomechanical tests 118–120
 bone-to-implant contact 114–115
 osseointegration 103–121, 225–241
 osseous response 48
 tibia model 227–240
 research strategy 226
 risk factors 226, 228–235
 screening protocols 46–56
 selection 109
 testing 46
 tissue response 47
International Standards Organization (ISO) 55
intrabony defects 214–216
intrabony regeneration model 90–94

K
Kantianism 11
keratinized tissues
 animal models 58–59
 porcine model 60–65

L
laboratories, good practice 23–30
large animal models 85

M
magnetic resonance imaging 190
mandibular symphyseal defect model 49
maxillary sinus 175
 see also sinus floor augmentation
medical devices 5
micro-computed tomography 117, 168, 189, 190
microradiography 155, 189
minipig models 138
 peri-implantitis defects 198–201
 sinus floor augmentation 179, 186, 187
model selection 2, 161
moral status 10

Index

N

new medical formulations 1, 3
nonhuman primate models 6
    peri-implantitis defects 199
    periodontal defects 94–97
    periodontal regeneration 85
    sinus floor augmentation 192, 193

O

Office of Combination Products (OCP) 6
osseointegration 103
    bone quality 114–118
    canine models 108–110
    evaluation methods 110–120
    of implants 103–120
    rabbit model 106–108
    rat models 104–106, 228–241
    osteoporosis 228

P

parathyroid hormone 228
peri-implantitis defect models 197–221, 199–201, 206–208
    canine 199, 203–208
    detailed methodology 203–219
    nonhuman primate model 199, 206–208
periodontal defects 90–97
    nonhuman primate models 94–97
periodontal lesions
    canine model 86–89
    nonhuman primate models 97–99
periodontal regeneration 77–102
    fenestration model 79
    large animal models 85–89
    small animal models 78–85
periodontium 77, 78
pig models, keratinized tissue 60–65
preclinical studies, purpose 5–6
primate models *see* nonhuman primate models

Q

quality assurance 26–27, 28
quality systems, good laboratory practice 23–30

R

rabbit models, osseointegration 106–108
radiographic analysis 189
ramus trephine defect model 49
rat models
    implant research 228–241
    osseointegration 104–106

rat models
    periodontal regeneration 6, 79–85
    ridge preservation 138
reconstructive therapies 1–8
    surgical models 7
replication (biostatistics) 37
research design 31–43
    hypotheses 34
    sample size 35
ridge augmentation *see* horizontal ridge augmentation; vertical ridge augmentation
ridge preservation 123–139
    canine models 126–138
    minipig model 138

S

sample size 35
screening
    models 45–56
    recommended practices 50–55
sheep models
    sinus floor augmentation 177, 178, 179–182
sinus floor augmentation 175–196
    canine model 176, 177
    goat model 178, 185, 186
    minipig model 186–188
    model selection 175–179
    pig model 178, 179
    primate model 192, 193
    sheep model 177, 178, 179–182
soft tissues
    graft models 58–60
    grafting 57
    implant models 48–50, 50
    regeneration 57–75
    volume augmentation 57, 65–74
    see also keratinized tissues
speciesism 10
split-mouth studies, design 38–39
statistical analysis 39–43, 137
    ANOVA 40
    chi-squared test 41–42
    error 35
    F test 40
    Fisher's exact test 42
    hypotheses 34
    non-independent data 43
    rank tests 40–41
    t test 39–40
    useful methods 42
statistical significance 155, 191
strong egalitarianism 12
study design *see* research design
study director 27–28

surgical procedures
    canine horizontal ridge augmentation model 146–150
    canine osseointegration model 109
    canine periodontal defects model 90–94
    canine periodontal lesions model 87–88
    canine ridge preservation model 128–132
    canine sinus floor augmentation model 183
    canine soft tissue augmentation model 66–70
    minipig sinus floor augmentation model 187, 188
    nonhuman primate periodontal defects 95–96
    nonhuman primate periodontal lesions 97
    peri-implantitis defect models 203–207
    porcine keratinized tissue model 60–62, 63
    primate sinus floor augmentation model 192
    rabbit osseointegration model 108
    rat osseointegration model 105
    rat periodontal regeneration model 80–83
    rat tibia implantation model 236–238
    sheep sinus floor augmentation model 181, 182
    vertical ridge augmentation 165–167

T

t test 39–40
test facilities, management 26
tissue engineering, screening models 45–56
tissue grafts see soft tissues
tissue regeneration 57–75
    models 3
    see also soft tissues
translational continuum 2
type I/II errors 35

U

US Pharmacopeia 53
utilitarianism 13

V

vertical ridge augmentation 159–173
    canine model 161–171
    model selection 161, 162
    research protocol 160